Psycholo   s
and Gyn

Jayne Cockburn and Michael E. Pawson (Eds)

Psychological Challenges in Obstetrics and Gynecology

The Clinical Management

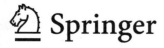 Springer

Jayne Cockburn, MD, FRCOG
Frimley Park Foundation
Trust Hospital
Portsmouth Road
Frimley Surrey GU16 7UK
UK

Michael E. Pawson, FRCOG
Consulting Obstetrician
  and Gynaecologist (Retired)
Chelsea and Westminster Hospital
London SW10 9NH
UK

British Library Cataloguing in Publication Data
Psychological challenges in obstetrics and gynecology : the clinical management
  1. Gynecology – Psychological aspects 2. Gynecology – Psychosomatic aspects 3. Obstetrics –
  Psychological aspects 4. Obstetrics – Psychosomatic aspects 5. Physician and patient
  I. Cockburn, Jayne II. Pawson, Michael E. 618 .019

ISBN-13: 978-1-84628-807-4   e-ISBN-13: 978-1-84628-808-1

Library of Congress Control Number: 2007921197

Printed on acid-free paper

9 8 7 6 5 4 3 2 1

Springer Science+Business Media
springer.com

Foreword

This book goes a long way to remind us that the patient is both mind and body, and that the best medical practice recognises this and is learned in this context. It is therefore a great pleasure for me to have been asked to introduce and recommend this book, which represents a very considerable volume of work, enhanced by the contributions of so many distinguished practitioners and specialists. Whether for learning and knowledge, or used as a reference, this book will meet a need that is now both recognised and better understood. Many of the chapters are a real pleasure in themselves, and the book is packed with sound evidence, factual material and new information.

Don't delay being acquainted with its contents. It has been my pleasure and privilege to have been asked to review the book and to write this foreword.

ALLAN TEMPLETON
Regius Professor of Obstetrics
and Gynaecology
University of Aberdeen
Aberdeen, Scotland

Foreword

I am delighted to write a foreword for this innovative and thought-provoking book, which gives an excellent overview of the field.

Psychological challenges in obstetrics vary from the expected adjustments that every new mother faces through to high-risk pregnancies in which infant or maternal death is a possibility. It is crucial to know that suicide is the leading cause of maternal death in the United Kingdom and to realise that prevention of suicide needs psychological and psychiatric problems to be recognized early in pregnancy by everyone involved in maternity care.

A woman's mental state will also affect other aspects of her health and her ability to access both obstetric and gynecologic services. At the Royal College of Psychiatrists, we assert that there is no health without mental health. This book supports our assertion, and I hope readers have a better understanding of their own role in helping women to achieve health outcomes through recognising this.

PROFESSOR SHEILA HOLLINS
President
Royal College of Psychiatrists
London, UK

Preface

We have set out to make this a practical book to help all those working in Obstetrics and Gynecology to incorporate psychological aspects of care into their everyday work. By listening to our patients and colleagues, it has become increasingly clear to us that integration of mind and body is essential to the future of our specialty. When highly trained doctors find that their technical expertise is of no benefit to their patients, or indeed on occasion harmful, they are left feeling lost and inadequate. Their patients are also lost when the emotional aspects of their symptoms are neither recognised nor acknowledged. The patients tend to wander from doctor to doctor, using up resources and losing faith in the health system.

There is accumulating scientific evidence that mind and body are connected. The discipline of science has been evolved to look at that which is measurable, relegating the feelings and emotions that make us human and disconnecting them from the organic processes of the body. This narrow scientific approach has its limitations; it is not a reason to dismiss what we refer to as psycho somatic medicine. The scientific community is beginning to recognise research which shows that emotions and physiology are indeed connected. We in medicine must move forward and embrace this integrated approach. Psycho-somatic is a maligned and misunderstood word, but it is only incorporating the mind and the body, which is the ideal way to practise all medicine.

But where to start? We wanted to write this book to collect together our current knowledge of the role of the psyche in obstetrics and gynecology, and also to be practical in showing how this can be used in the clinical situation. There is much we can do and learn, recognising at the same time that there is much we do not know or understand. We need to learn to modify our approach, to use both the medical models, but be able to incorporate psychological thinking as well. This book provides an introduction to some of the more common issues in obstetrics and gynecology. The chapters are easily read, are short enough to read in an evening, and also have useful references and websites to help the reader find out more. This book is unique in that the experts have covered both an up to date theory base and also given useful tools for immediate application to the clinical situation. It can be read as a stand-alone handbook or used as a reader after an interesting clinic or case when you want to think and explore more about a single issue or feeling that has come up. It covers topics not covered in other textbooks.

Part One covers basic issues, from improving "listening" in the clinic – important for all training and medical practice – and covers some basic issues that are changing in this advanced technological age. Obstetrics and gynecology is the specialty of life, love, sex and death, all the big things that underpin our lives as human beings. Our experience of these has been changing as society changes. We have also included some basic ideas as to how psychosomatic medicine should be incorporated in training. Continental Europe is more advanced in this respect than the UK.

Part Two gathers together both techniques to help the normal obstetrician understand how the patient is coping and how that manifests itself physically, giving some structure to our thoughts. We then cover some of the commonly seen topics in obstetrics.

Part Three is conventionally gynecology. Fifty per cent of the patients in a gynecology clinic have significant distress as well as the physical problem they present with. The topics covered are again the more common topics that challenge us everyday.

After reading this we expect you to feel more in control and more understanding of the issues and their complexity. You will have the tools to actually recognise if the patient is not coping, rather than just having "a gut feeling". We hope you will have a structure for your intuitive thoughts, as well as some practical ideas on easily helping the majority of women, at least by recognition and validating and getting the problems out in the open so that they can be thought about. This will also give you the confidence to make good and appropriate referrals to the limited-support psychological services that are so pitiful in today's health system.

We particularly wanted to write this book for those who are training in obstetrics and gynecology. Too often the technical solutions seem inadequate. Despite trying your best, the consultation feels unsatisfactory. Complex patients are demanding and difficult, and there is no training for these situations. Too often trainers hide behind dismissive attitudes and blame the patient, or just delegate the difficult patients, or if it doesn't respond to surgery discharge them to the GP.

This book can also provide information and help to GPs who already have some training in the social and psychological aspects of ill health, to work more closely with patients in the community setting. Sadly, being a hospital doctor these days seems to mean that you leave the community behind. We regret this and feel that it dilutes the quality of care.

Midwives, nurses, physiotherapists and all health workers in related fields will find plenty that is relevant to them, particularly as often the patient will speak to you, rather than the doctor. Whilst training in these areas may include more community aspects, we hope to provide a useful grounding in what is known in psychology and psychotherapeutic practice, that is useful to add to the repertoire.

We hope that medical students will read this book and gain inspiration. Many medical students are reported to feel that their humanity and caring are removed during their training. We believe this is because the feelings and psychological aspects are removed both for the patient and for the doctor, leaving the new enthusiast feeling sterile and removed from the patients. This book is easy to understand, and we hope it will inspire you to stay with your enthusiasm for healing. Technology has a very important place, accept that, but be prepared to look out for the practitioners who are able to be with their patients in understanding the problems in the context of the patients' lives, not just a set of algorithms.

We also have enjoyed reading all the contributions and have learned a lot, and clarified our thinking. Thus, we hope that many more senior clinicians will enjoy and learn from this book. Many of us have had to learn the hard way, seeking out information that was scrappy and not integrated. We also hope it will help all trainers by providing a basic text and starting point.

This book is not to make us psychologists – that has its own training – but should help make us more aware, help provide an integrated psychological, social and biological approach for our patients, thus helping many more than we do. Giving us confidence to work in this area, providing better service for our patients, and helping us feel more satisfied with our work and less scared of the complex problems for which we were previously ignorant and untrained.

JAYNE COCKBURN
MICHAEL E. PAWSON

Contents

List of Contributors

Ian Ainsworth-Smith
St Georges Healthcare NHS Trust
Canon Emeritus – Southwark Cathedral
London, UK

Susan Ayers, PhD, BSc, CPsychol
Psychology Department
University of Sussex
Brighton, UK

Bronwyn B. Bell, MBChB, MRCOG
Department of Obstetrics and Gynecology
Poole NHS Trust
Poole, UK

Johannes Bitzer, MD
University Hospital of Basel
CH 4031
Switzerland

Audrey H. Brown, MBChB, MRCOG, DFFP
Sandyford Initiative
Glasgow, UK

Jayne Cockburn, MD, FRCOG
Consultant Obstetrician and Gynecologist
Frimley Park Hospital NHS Trust
Frimley, UK

Catherine Coulson, MBCHB, DRCOG
Reproductive Medicine Clinic
St Michael's Hospital
Bristol, UK

John Cox, BM BCh, DM(oxon), MA, DPM, FRCpsych, FRCP(Edin), FRCP(Lon)
Academic Psychiatry Unit
Keele University
Keele, UK

Ken Daniels, MA
University of Canterbury, School of Social Work Services
Christchurch, New Zealand

Michael Dooley, MBBS, FFFP, FRCOG
The Poundbury Clinic
Dorset County Hospital
Dorchester, UK

Dimitrios Doumplis, MD
West London Gynecological Centre
Hammersmith Hospital Trust
London, UK

Gillian Gill, BA (Hons)
Department of Medical Social Work
St Michaels Hospital
Bristol, UK

Sandra Goldbeck-Wood, MB ChB, MA Psycho
Obstetrician and Gynecologist
92 Gilbert Road
Cambridge, UK

Josephine M. Green, PhD
Mother and Infant Research Unit
Department of Health Sciences
University of York
York, UK

Carol Henshaw, MD, FRCPsych
Academic Psychiatry
Keele University School of Medicine
Harplands Hospital
Stoke on Trent, UK

Kristina Hofberg, MRCPsych
South Staffordshire Healthcare NHS Trust
St George's Hospital
Stafford, UK

Patricia Hughes, MD, FRCPsych
Division of Mental Health
St George's, University of London,
London, UK

Myra S. Hunter, PhD CPsychol, AFBPS
Department of Psychology
Adamson Centre
St Thomas' Hospital
London, UK

L. Jane Knowles, MBBS, FRCPsych
The Group Analytic Practice
London, UK

Pittu Laungani† Honorary Research Fellow, PhD
Manchester University
Manchester, UK

Kirstie N. McKenzie-McHarg, BBSc (Hons), DClinPsy, C.Psychol
National Perinatal Epidemiology Unit
University of Oxford
Oxford, UK

Michael E. Pawson, FRCOG
Chelsea Westminster Hospital
London, UK

Mary Pillai, MB ChB, DCH, MRCP (UK), MRCPCH, FRCOG, MD MSc
Department of Obstetrics and Gynecology
Gloucestershire Hospitals NHS Trust
Cheltenham General Hospital
Cheltenham, UK

Nigel Sage, BA, MSc, C.Psychol, AFBPS
The Beacon Community Centre for Cancer and Palliative Care
Guildford, UK

W.C.M. Weijmar Schultz, MD, PhD
Department of Obstetrics and Gynecology
University of Groningen Medical Centre
Groningen, The Netherlands

Tom Shakespeare, BA, PhD
University of Newcastle, Bioscience Centre
Newcastle, UK

J. Richard Smith, MB, MD, FRCOG
The Lister Hospital
London, UK

Michelle Sowden, BSc, MSc, PSYCHD, C.Psychol
Department of Psychological Medicine
Frimley Park Hospital, NHS Trust
Frimley, UK

Helen E. Statham, BSc
Centre for Family Research
University of Cambridge
Cambridge, UK

R. William Stones, MD, FRCOG
Princess Anne Hospital
Southampton, UK

H.B.M. van de Wiel, PhD
Department of Health Sciences
University Medical Centre
Medical Faculty
University of Groningen
Groningen, The Netherlands

Mark Ward
South Staffordshire Healthcare NHS Trust
St George's Hospital
Stafford, UK

Catherine White, MB ChB
St Mary's Sexual Assault Referral Centre
St Mary's Hospital
Manchester, UK

Kevan R. Wylie, MB, ChB MMedSc MD DSM
Department of Andrology (Urology)
Royal Hallamshire Hospital
Sheffield, UK

Part One
Background for the Study of Psychosomatic Obstetrics and Gyneocology

1
Teaching Psychosomatic Obstetrics and Gynecology

Johannes Bitzer

1.1. The Essentials of Psychosomatic OB/GYN

Residents in gynecology as well as specialists have been trained for many years in accordance with the concepts of biomedical thinking and practice. This basic way of understanding patients' health problems can be described as follows:

Symptoms are caused by objectively measurable (biological) factors, which constitute disease entities independent of individuals. These diseases are defined in the biomedical code and structured into subunits like etiology, pathophysiology, diagnostic procedures and therapeutic interventions. This code is international, is continuously adapted and the "truth" of the code is evaluated by using scientific evidence, which is the basis of standardized practice.

This approach is very useful and successful in a large number of clinical situations. Daily practical experience shows, however, that in a considerable part of the working time gynecologists and obstetricians are confronted with problems which do not fit into the biomedical model:

- The same disease entity evokes completely different responses in different individuals like a miscarriage, a cancer, a bleeding disorder, and so on. Where do these differences come from and how should the doctor understand them?
- The presented symptoms do not fit into any known disease entity like feeling bad, feeling exhausted and tired, feeling nauseated, feeling pain in different body regions without a detectable cause. Where do these symptoms come from and how should the doctor handle it?
- Patients and gynecologists are confronted with situations in which there is no one single evidence-based solution but patients have to make personal choices. How should gynecologists help in shared decision-making?
- A therapeutic intervention is well founded on scientific evidence but the patient does not comply. The health risks of some behaviors are very well proven but still the patient maintains her risk-prone behavior. What type of disease is this and how should the doctor diagnose and treat it?

- Patients present personal problems like sexual difficulties, partner and family conflicts, stressful life events in the context of adolescence, pregnancy, postpartum, perimenopause, and postmenopause and seek help from their gynecologists. How can the doctor respond to these demands and problems?
- Patients are experienced as difficult and demanding, and the gynecologist feels exhausted and burned out. Is there any disease category relating to the doctor–patient relationship and how should these disorders be treated?

All these situations point to the necessity of a complementary working model. This model can be called the biopsychosocial model of health and disease (1,2).

This model is characterized by the following features:

Symptoms as the manifestation of individual suffering are the result of an interaction of biological, psychological, and social factors, specific to the patient. This means that the basic unit of observation is the interaction of the disease process and the individual person in her life situation.

Diagnostic procedures have therefore to add to the detection of measurable biological abnormalities an understanding of the patient's life situation and patterns of thoughts, feelings, and behavior relevant to the illness state.

Therapeutic plans take into account the characteristics of the motivation, the objectives, the decisions, and the behavior of the patient.

Enabling gynecologists to integrate this model into their daily working routine is the aim of teaching psychosomatic obstetrics and gynecology.

1.2. Teaching Basic Communicative Skills

1.2.1. Contents

As shown above, the principal component of psychosomatic thinking and practice lies in shifting the focus of attention from an isolated disease perspective to a balanced disease–person interaction view. To integrate more of the person into the consultation, physicians need a type of communication style which differs from disease-centered techniques (3,4):

Disease-centered communication: In disease-centered communication, the physician quickly takes the lead and determines the agenda. He/she uses the classical history taking with a catalogue of preformed questions, which usually should be answered as yes or no. These questions are based on disease entities and serve the purpose of reaching a diagnosis quickly. The patient is a passive recipient of a therapeutic prescription.

Patient-centered communication: In patient-centered communication, the patient gets space and time to tell her story (narrative). The questioning is much more of a Socratic dialogue with reference to the patient's expression and feedback. There is respect for and response to emotions. The patient defines the agenda. The patient is an active partner in therapeutic decisions and interventions.

The basic elements of patient-centered communication are as follows (5,6):
Active listening: The gynecologist learns to listen in a way that encourages the patient to tell her story by

- *Waiting*: Giving the patient time to think and express herself. This means that the physician has to learn "not to talk" but use silence and pause as a means of encouragement.
- *Echoing*: Repeating a specific word or expression of the patient to signal attentive listening and that the physician follows the patient's story.
- *Mirroring*: Reflecting body language or a whole verbal sequence in the words of the patient.

Checking back and summarizing: The physician summarizes in his/her words what he/she has understood from the patient's story. This is the basis of mutual understanding by assuring that the physician and the patient have found a common language of exchange of information and the patient's needs and her agenda have been understood.

Response to emotions: This is a difficult task which needs considerable exercise. The different steps are as follows:

- The physician first needs to become aware of his/her own emotions (e.g., feeling irritated, sad, worried, helpless).
- Then the physician has to try to perceive the emotions expressed by the patient (How does she feel?).
- Next the physician should try in his/her mind to verbalize the emotions expressed by the patient (she feels sad, worried, angry, frustrated, overwhelmed, etc.).
- The emotions perceived by the physician can then be reflected to the patient in a respectful way using sometimes the form of a question: "I can see that you are frustrated and angry. This situation must evoke a lot of anger and frustration, mustn't it?"

Information exchange: A large part of a medical consultation deals with information giving. Physicians inform patients about risks and frequency of diseases, diagnostic measures and the diagnosis found, the prognosis of a disease, therapeutic options with success rates and side effects. This educational part needs didactic skills and some basic knowledge about how to transmit information.

Information giving is not a one-way process. It is always an information exchange process (7):

- In the first step the physician has to elicit the patient's needs for information, her expectations, and her preexisting knowledge about the subject she would like to talk about.
- In the second step the physician gives a defined quantity of information. It is important that the information is given in small units and well structured, important parts are announced, and the patient is encouraged to interrupt this phase by direct questioning.
- The third step is equally important. The physician should elicit the patient's understanding and interpretation of the information. This can be done by asking about the quantity, the speed, the clarity, and the understandability of the information given. In some situations (see later), it is equally important to ask the patient about the emotional meaning she gives to the information: "What does this information mean to you? Is it reassuring or worrying? Are there new questions coming up?"

In case of new questions the exchange process described above can restart.

1.2.2. Educational Methods

The above-mentioned techniques and their flexible use can be taught by means of

- *Critical incident reporting*: The resident in training gets the basic format of critical incident reporting. This means that in clinical situations in which the trainee feels that something went wrong she/he will try to recall the sequence of events commenting about the type of difficulty encountered. Then the supervisor can brainstorm together with the trainee about alternative options of communication and so on.
- *Video clips*: Videotaping of consultations including educational videos (videos with real patients and simulated patients).
- *Role play*: This is a useful instrument in which the trainees change roles. The roles are patient, physician, and observer. This helps them to experience the patient's position and feelings.

1.3. Teaching Communicative Skills in Special Clinical Situations

1.3.1. Contents

There are special clinical situations which need specialized skills, based on the above-described techniques. These skills integrate elements of counseling and psychotherapy.

Breaking bad news: The situation of breaking bad news occurs frequently in oncology and infertility, less frequently in pregnancy care. The basic elements are as follows (8,9):

- Preparation for the encounter (Quiet setting, enough time, is all the information needed available? Does the patient come alone or accompanied by a family member or friend? What is the emotional situation of the physician?).
- Introduction (Joining with the patient by using a more personal issue, a brief summary of the previous events, and the objective of the consultation).
- Announcement ("Unfortunately I have to give you bad news").
- Statement (Give the diagnosis in simple words).
- Waiting for the individual reaction of the patient (Stunned, paralyzed, confused, shocked, desperate, crying, stoic, denying, etc.).
- Response to the reaction (Emotion handling, reflecting, summarizing).
- Encouraging questions and giving further information in small pieces.
- Give hope (There is always something that can be done).
- Structure the near future (What is the patient going to do next – define the next steps to be taken and give appointments).

Risk and decision-making counseling: These situations occur in menopause, oncology, and so on. The physician needs some basic knowledge about risks and shared decision-making.

Basic principles of risk counseling are as follows (10,11):

- Clarify the needs, values, and objectives of the patient related to the specific issues of risks and decisions to be made.
- Elicit the need for information and the preexisting knowledge.
- Give a framework of risks relating to everyday experiences.
- Give absolute risk numbers; don't use relative risks and conditional probabilities.
- Visualize risk numbers showing the relationship between risk and chances.
- Point to the other side of the risk, namely the chances.
- Encourage the patient to reflect about her values and the individual importance which she attributes to the benefits and risks shown.

1.3.2. Educational Methods

The techniques can be trained by the following:

- *Video clips*: Videotaping of consultations including educational videos (videos with real patients and simulated patients).
- *Role play*: This is a useful instrument in which the trainees change roles. The roles are patient, physician, and observer. This exposes them to new experiences.

1.4. Teaching the Application of the Biopsychosocial Model in Obstetrics and Gynecology

1.4.1. The Psychosomatic Diagnostic Process

1.4.1.1. Contents

The gynecologist in training and the practicing specialist will meet complicated cases in which a gynecological and/or obstetrical diagnostic entity cannot be established and the standardized somatic interventions cannot be used or are inefficient. The typical clinical situations are as follows:

- The patient with physical symptoms that cannot be explained by organic pathology (the "psychosomatic or somatoform" patient).
- The patient in whom the response to a disease leads to severe psychological symptoms (the "somatopsychic" patient).
- The patient with mental and behavioral problems interacting with gynecological and obstetrical diseases (the "comorbid" patient).
- The patient with sexual and relational problems (the "sexual dysfunction" patient).

For all these patients the psychosomatic diagnostic approach demands the integration of psychosocial information into the working hypothesis of a clinical problem. This means that we need some knowledge and concepts concerning psychosocial pathogenetic factors.

From clinical experience and the literature, we have developed the following mnemonic (12,13):

A = Affect: This means that the physician should be aware of a predominant affective state like depression, anxiety, and so on. This also includes some basic knowledge about the prevalence and the diagnostic possibilities to detect affective disorders.

B = Behavior: Frequently, risk-taking or health-damaging behavior plays an important part in the pathogenesis or complication of clinical disorders in OB/GYN. This is especially true in obstetrics, where behavioral problems have an important impact on the health of the mother and the child.

C = Conflict: Conflicts can be either external or internal and can be subdivided into attraction versus attraction, avoidance versus avoidance, and attraction versus avoidance types of conflicts. Chronic unresolved conflicts lead to chronic stress, reduced motivation, depressive and anxious mood, and social difficulties, which may all together impair health.

D = Distress: Distress describes a condition in which a person is confronted with external or internal stressors, which overwhelm the person's coping capacity. This includes transitional periods in the course of one's life. Distress leads to psychoendocrine, psychovegetative, and psychomotor responses which may be hazardous to the patient's health.

$E = Early\ life\ experiences$: This refers to previous life events, which may date back to childhood and adolescence. Traumatic experiences may have an impact on neurobiological pathways which may increase the patient's vulnerability to later stressful life events and may induce repetitive health-damaging behavior. Also, emotional deprivation and neglect may have long-term consequences regarding the emotional development and interpersonal competence of patients.

$F = False\ beliefs$: False beliefs relate to general patterns of thinking which are likely to increase the vulnerability to life stressors: low self-esteem, pessimism, generalization, self-reference, and so on.

$G = Generalized\ frustration$: Life situations in which essential needs are unmet. These situations may lead to depression, anxiety, loss of self-esteem, and somatization.

In the biopsychosocial diagnostic workup these factors are combined with biological findings in what we call the nine-field diagnosis.

In this nine-field diagnosis there are three types of factors (biological, psychological, and social) which on a timeline are subdivided into predisposing, precipitating, and maintaining factors (Table 1.1). This information is obtained by the use of different techniques and instruments

The final step in the diagnostic workup is the elucidation of the patient's concept about her disease as well as her previous coping style and resources.

1.4.1.2. Educational Methods

In two educational sessions of 2–3 h duration the basic elements of psychosocial pathogenetic factors and the nine-field diagnosis are presented.

In group case discussions and group supervision the trainee will learn to use this diagnostic framework by means of cases the trainee presents either as report or audiotaped or videotaped. Another tool is that the supervisor presents a case which is then discussed in a group of six trainees. The trainees

TABLE 1.1. Nine field diagnosis

	Biological	Psychological	Social
Predisposing	Family risks, pregnancy and birth-related risks	Early trauma, abuse, neglect	Broken family, early separation, migration
Precipitating	Disease, drugs, biological transition	Loss, life transition, separation	Migration, cultural norms, social changes
Maintaining	Side effects of drugs, and so on.	Anxiety, false beliefs, stress responses	Secondary reinforcement in the environment

TABLE 1.2. Techniques and instruments

Biological	Psychological	Social	
Predisposing	Medical history	Biographic history	Social and migration history
Precipitating	Medical history and examination	Psychosocial history, personality characteristics	Communication style, family diagnosis
Maintaining	Medical history and examination	Transference and countertransference	Communication style, family dynamics

should learn to establish a comprehensive biopsychosocial diagnosis in all the patient groups mentioned earlier (Table 1.3).

1.4.2. *Psychosomatic Therapeutic Interventions*

1.4.2.1. **Contents**

For the psychosomatic management of the above-mentioned patient groups the trainee needs to learn to establish a helpful patient–doctor relationship with the help of the three elementary attitudes of empathy, respect, and congruence. Based on this he/she should learn some basic therapeutic techniques which can be summarized under the notion of "supportive and/or coping counseling/psychotherapy." By this we mean an integrative approach which contains different elements directed at the above-described pathogenetic factors. The therapeutic elements can be summarized under CCCISH (14,15):

Catharsis: The gynecologist encourages the patient to express her emotions and talk about her feelings (affects). He/she shares these emotions by nonverbal and verbal reflection, summarizing, and checking back.

Example: A 36-year-old primagravida comes for an ultrasound scan at 20 weeks' gestation. The scan shows a missed abortion with fetal structures without heart activity. The patient is desperate. The physician invites her into a separate room and encourages her to talk about her emotions and the questions she might have. She reveals that at the beginning of the pregnancy she did not want this child and she was thinking about abortion. Now she is convinced that the intrauterine death is god's punishment and that "it is all her fault." The

TABLE 1.3. Comprehensive biopsychosocial diagnosis

Symptoms and problems as descriptive summary

Conditioned
By predisposing, precipitating, and maintaining biological, psychological, and social factors
And
Patient's concepts and resources

physician is just listening and holding the hand of the patient. She keeps on talking about her feelings of guilt and her sadness. After a while the physician responds,

> *Physician:* I can imagine the overwhelming pain you feel about the loss of the child which is even aggravated because you put the blame on yourself. Let me tell you that many women have mixed feelings at the beginning of a pregnancy and that this ambivalence is a normal feeling. I am very sure that you are not responsible for this death. You should give yourself permission to mourn and to be supported in this mourning process.

Clarifying of conflicts and conflict resolution:
The general principles of conflict clarification and resolution are as follows:

- Clarifying the individuals' views of the problem and the related causes.
- Increasing the understanding of biographical factors influencing these views.
- Delineating and verbalizing the elements of the conflict.
- Brainstorming about possible options of conflict resolution.
- Help in conscious and transparent decision-making.

Example: A 35-year-old female suffers from complete loss of libido, which creates a profound conflict with her partner, who feels a deep-rooted sexual desire toward her. During the session with the couple it becomes evident to the male partner that previous traumatizing sexual experiences have conditioned her aversive reactions to his expression of intense desire which is experienced as threatening and aggressive. After encouraging her to verbalize her sexual wishes and needs which are much more directed toward nonpenetrative sex, both can start to negotiate about new ways of sexual expression and encounters.

Cognitive reframing: By reframing the cognitive attributions given by the patient to her disease or her symptoms the physician may attenuate the emotional distress caused by catastrophic and pessimistic explanatory styles of patients.

Example: A 22-year-old para 0 suffers from chronic pain, which could not be explained by laparoscopic findings. After the operation the physician explains the results. The patient is silent and withdrawn.

> *Physician:* This must be somehow disappointing for you, that we could not find a single cause for your pain, which bothers you so much. I can imagine that you might have the impression that we do not understand your suffering.
>
> *Patient:* Yes, this is so frustrating. Do you think that the pain is just in my head...pure fantasy...
>
> *Physician:* Not at all. We know that this pain is real, but that the conditioning factors are complex as we have discussed before. We were talking about the chronic pain as the result of a disturbed processing of signals coming from certain body regions...

Insight and understanding: Increasing insight and understanding of one's symptoms and problems can be obtained either by information and education provided by the physician or through the help the physicians can offer in a dialogue about the patient's self-image, view of the world, way of coping, and so on. Through this dialogue the patient may be enabled to correct destructive and distorted patterns of thinking and behavior.

Example: A 52-year-old patient had undergone treatment for mammary carcinoma with lumpectomy, radiation and adjuvant antihormonal treatment. She feels abandoned by her husband and her family and responds with a depressive mood. The physician tries to clarify with her the expectations she has toward her family. By verbalizing her wishes it becomes clear that she had never expressed her anger and frustration about her disease and the deep feeling of the injustice imposed on her by fate or god. She gains some insight into the influence of her own behavior on the withdrawal of the family and she is able to adapt her expectations to the possibilities of her family.

Stress reduction techniques: Distress is experienced if the challenge (threat, change, etc.) imposed on a person cannot be confronted and coped with. The distress reaction on a cognitive level is the lack of a solution, on an emotional level the experience of anxiety and helplessness, and on a physiological level the activation of the sympathetic system and the endocrine response of the ACTH–Cortisol axis. Stress reduction techniques are based on the following elements:

- *Cognitive level:* Reframing, reducing catastrophic thinking, search for solutions.
- *Emotional level:* Creating awareness of the sequence between event-thoughts and emotions to be able to modify affective responses.
- *Physiological level:* Breathing techniques, progressive muscle relaxation.

Example: A 36-year-old patient and her partner undergo assisted reproduction with ovarian stimulation, ovum-pickup, and embryo transfer. After two failed treatment cycles the female patient exhibits a strong vegetative reaction during the ultrasound evaluation of the ovarian response; she starts crying and reports heart palpitations and headache. The physician teaches her some basic breathing techniques. In a separate consultation her way of coping with the treatment is analyzed, showing the enormous pressure she puts on herself and the anticipatory anxiety she develops. In a counseling session with the couple, different ways of coping are discussed: modifying the "fixed" objective of success by all means, defining a plan B, building up compensatory activities, and initiating the learning of a relaxation technique.

Helping in behavioral change (15): The trainee learns how to practice motivational interviewing. The main elements are the assessment of the patient's readiness for change, which is determined by the importance attributed to changing behavior and the confidence of the patient in her capacity for change. Depending on the degree of readiness the physician can either negotiate issues of importance and confidence or elaborate a detailed plan for change.

Example: A 30-year-old primagravida of 8 weeks' gestation smokes 30 cigarettes a day. In the first consultation she tries to deny a negative impact on her child. It becomes evident that problems with her partner are much more important for her at the moment. After having clarified this the physician can actively re-enter the issue of smoking. She rates the importance to stop at 8 out of 10 points, but her self-confidence in achieving this change is rated by her rather low (4 out of 10). The physician focuses her talk very much on the support of her self-confidence and her ability to learn from previous failures and define an individual strategy. In her case she decided for a compensatory strategy which consisted in active distraction through the Internet.

1.4.2.2.   Educational Methods

In two teaching sessions of 4 h duration, the basic elements of counseling are taught. After this, educational videos are used to show the different interventions in clinical settings. The trainees will then practice these techniques in 4–5 videotaped sessions with simulated patients.

1.5.   Summary

The gynecologist is confronted with many tasks for which he/she needs a biopsychosocial competence: patient education and health promotion, counseling and management of psychosocial problems in various phases of a woman's life cycle, care for patients with unexplained physical symptoms and patients with chronic incurable diseases. To obtain this competence a curriculum is needed which comprises elements of psychology, psychosocial medicine, and psychiatry adapted to the specific needs of gynecologists in their everyday work. A basic part of the curriculum consists of teaching knowledge and skills derived from communication theory and practice including physician- and patient-centered communication with active listening, responding to emotions, and information exchange as well as breaking bad news, risk counseling, and shared decision-making. Building on these skills, trainees are introduced to the biopsychosocial process of diagnosis, establishing a nine-field comprehensive workup using the ABCDEFG guideline (Affect, Behavior, Conflict, Distress, Early life experiences, False beliefs, Generalized frustration). The therapeutic interventions are based on a working alliance between the physician and the patient and are taught as basic elements, which have to be combined according to the individual patient and situation. The overall technique for gynecologists can be summarized as supportive counseling/psychotherapy (CCCISH) including elements like catharsis, clarifying conflicts and conflict resolution, cognitive reframing, insight and understanding, stress reduction techniques, and helping in behavioral change.

References

1. Engel GL. The need for a new medical model: a challenge for biomedical science. *Science.* 1977;196:129.
2. Uexküll ThV. Was heisst Psychosomatik. *Schweiz Med Wochenschr.* 1984;114:1806–1809.
3. Bitzer J. Die Arzt-Aerztin-Patientin Kommunikation in der Konsultation—Grundlagen, Techniken, Schwierigkeiten und Lösungsmöglichkeiten. In: Bodden-Heidrich R, Rechenberger I, Bender HG, eds. *Psychosomatische Gynäkologie und Geburtshilfe.* Giessen: Psychosozial Verlag; 2000.
4. Mead N, Bower P. Patient centeredness: a conceptual framework and review of the empirical literature. *Soc Sci Med.* 2000;51:1087.
5. Stewart M, Stewart M, Belle Brown J, et al. *Patient-Centered Medicine. Transforming the Clinical Method.* Thousand Oaks: Sage; 1995.
6. Bitzer J, Tschudin S, Schwendke A, Alder J. Psychosoziale und psychosomatische Basiskompetenz des Frauenarztes—von der inneren Ueberzeugung zum lernbaren Curriculum. 1. Kommunikation. *Gynakol Geburtshilfliche Rundsch.* 2001;41:158–165.
7. Rollnick S, Mason P, Butler C, eds. *Health Behaviour Change.* Edinburgh, London: Churchill Livingstone; 1999.
8. Fallowfield L. Giving sad and bad news. *Lancet.* 1993;341:476–478.
9. Langewitz W. Arzt-Patient-Kommunikation. Mitteilen schlechter Nachrichten. In: Brähler S, Strauss B, eds. *Lehrbuch der Medizinischen Psychologie und Soziologie.* Göttingen: Hofgrefe; 1998.
10. Gigerenzer G. *Calculated Risks—How to Know When Numbers Deceive You.* New York: Simon and Schuster; 2002.
11. Epstein RM, Alper BS, Quill TE. Communication evidence for participatory decision making. *JAMA.* 2000;291(19):2359.
12. Ustün BT. WHO Collaborative Study: an epidemiological survey of psychological problems in general health care in 15 centers worldwide. *Int J Psychiatry.* 1994;6:357–363.
13. Bitzer J, Tschudin S, Schwendke A, Alder J. Psychosoziale und psychosomatische Basiskompetenz des Frauenarztes von der inneren Ueberzeugung zum lernbaren Curriculum. 2. Biopsychosoziales Modell. *Gynakol Geburtshilfliche Rundsch.* 2001;42:136.
14. Egan G. *The Skills Helper: A Problem Management Approach to Helping.* Pacific Grove, CA: Brooks/Cole; 1994.
15. Rollnick S, Mason P, Butler C, eds. *Health Behaviour Change.* Edinburgh, London: Churchill Livingstone; 1999.

2
The Vaginal Examination

Catherine Coulson

2.1. Introduction

The vaginal examination becomes such a commonplace examination to gynecologists that they may forget its importance to their patients. As doctors, we are privileged not only to hear our patients' anxieties, fears, and fantasies but also to examine their bodies. Many other people will touch bodies as part of their work—masseurs, physiotherapists, hairdressers, and beauticians to mention but a few. However, most people only expose that private part of their body to have their nappy changed as a small child or to be intimate with a lover as an adult. There are strict societal rules and clear boundaries to make the experience safer. However, there is the potential for complaint, misunderstandings, and harm, as well as for helping the patient.

Many misunderstandings can be avoided by being aware of the process and tuning in to the patient. This chapter assumes basic competence in gynecological skills such as locating the cervix, but aims to explore some of the other processes that are going on at a conscious or unconscious level during the practical examination.

2.2. Communication

An examination rarely occurs in the absence of a preceding consultation. Good consultation skills can be taken into the examination. Misunderstandings are usually the result of failure of communication:

- Be alert to clues. The words used by the patient, the *way they are said*, and the *body language* of the patient help you to understand the patient's fears.
- Good communication depends on listening in an active way and then feeding back to the patient to make sure you have understood correctly. The patient can give you the history in her own words and you can clarify it with open-ended questions.
- We cannot reassure the patient until we know what she is concerned about.

- Many people choose medicine as career because they like to put things right. If we can tolerate not knowing what to do for a while, we might help the patient to find her own solutions.

2.3. The Role of a Chaperon

GMC Guidance, December 2001

The GMC regularly receives complaints from patients who feel that doctors have behaved inappropriately during an intimate examination. Intimate examinations, that is examinations of the breasts, genitalia, or rectum, can be stressful and embarrassing for patients. When conducting intimate examinations you should

- Explain to the patient why an examination is necessary and give the patient an opportunity to ask questions.
- Explain what the examination will involve, in a way the patient can understand, so that the patient has a clear idea of what to expect, including any potential pain or discomfort (paragraph 13 of our booklet *Seeking patients' consent* gives further guidance on presenting information to patients).
- Obtain the patient's permission before the examination and be prepared to discontinue the examination if the patient asks you to. You should record that permission has been obtained.
- Keep discussion relevant and avoid unnecessary personal comments.
- Offer a chaperon or invite the patient (in advance if possible) to have a relative or friend present. If the patient does not want a chaperon, you should record that the offer was made and declined. If a chaperon is present, you should record that fact and make a note of the chaperon's identity. If for justifiable practical reasons you cannot offer a chaperon, you should explain that to the patient and, if possible, offer to delay the examination to a later date. You should record the discussion and its outcome.
- Give the patient privacy to undress and dress and use drapes to maintain the patient's dignity. Do not assist the patient in removing clothing unless you have clarified with them that your assistance is required.

Anaesthetised patients
You must obtain consent prior to anaesthetisation, usually in writing, for the intimate examination of anaesthetised patients. If you are supervising students you should ensure that valid consent has been obtained before they carry out any intimate examination under anaesthesia.

The GMC guidelines on intimate examination, 2001, make it perfectly clear that a chaperon should be offered to all patients undergoing intimate examinations. The role of the chaperon is twofold: to protect the patient from abuse by the doctor and to protect the doctor from allegations of abuse by the patient. However, the presence of a third party in the room may make the patient feel doubly exposed. The mere suggestion that a chaperon may be necessary may make the patient feel as if she needs protection!

If the patient says she does not want a chaperon, it should be appropriately documented in the notes and the doctor should ask himself/herself whether he/she feels comfortable to go ahead. If there is any sense of discomfort, it is worth further consideration. Perhaps another doctor could do it, or perhaps a nurse could be called in to help with a practical part of the examination. Where is this unease coming from? Is it the patient's unease projected onto the doctor or a sense of risk from some sexualization of the doctor/patient relationship?

The presence of a third party in the room will impact on the consultation. A patient may often say something important during the examination. She may express a fear, which only surfaces as she removes her clothes. A chaperon may talk to the patient and distract her, or hold her hand as though the examination is going to be painful, or make a noise and clatter with instruments. These potentially negative impacts can be minimized by careful preparation of the chaperon.

An appropriate chaperon might be a member of the clinical team who should be introduced by name and position. A receptionist, unless properly trained, is not considered acceptable. Friends and family of the patient are not suitable, since there could be breaches of confidentiality and embarrassment to the patient and it might prove difficult for the doctor to defend himself/herself, especially against malicious allegations.

2.4. Consent

Verbal consent is usually enough. You should explain what you would like to do and ask the patient if that is acceptable. At each stage, check with the patient that she is happy to continue and it is worth giving her a few moments to consider. If there is any hesitation or body language such as a tightening of the thighs or looking away, which might signify ambivalence or overt distress, then give her chance to say how she feels. If you are still not sure, you could use an open-ended comment such as "Perhaps this is difficult for you."

2.5. Competence to Give Consent

Most of our patients are competent to give consent but in the case of a young girl or a woman with learning difficulties, extra care is needed to avoid unwitting abuse of the patient. A doctor can make an assessment during history taking and usually decide whether the patient is competent (Gillick competence—see Fraser guidelines (1)), or a carer or parent could also be asked to give consent.

Basic Requirements for Examination

Environment:

- Warm room.
- Private area for undressing and putting clothes.
- Minimum bodily exposure, for example use of wraps.
- Interruption-free zone, for example use of "Engaged" sign on door.

Information giving and opportunities for questions:

- Why examination is appropriate?
- What is going to be done stage by stage?
- Verbal consent and checking with patient.
- Ask the chaperon to stand quietly and to respond to requests from the patient instead of assuming a comforting role.

Vaginal Examination

Consider the following:

- Respect
- Explanation

    Information—why/what/when?
    Permission/informed consent
    Gillick competent—see Fraser guidelines (1)

- Chaperon

    Protection/support
    Offered/discussed/documented

- Privacy

    Minimum bodily exposure
    Avoid personal comments

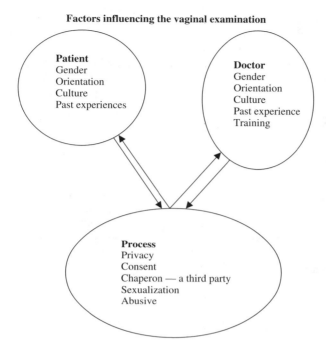

Factors influencing the vaginal examination

Patient
Gender
Orientation
Culture
Past experiences

Doctor
Gender
Orientation
Culture
Past experience
Training

Process
Privacy
Consent
Chaperon — a third party
Sexualization
Abusive

FIGURE 2.1. Factors influencing the vaginal examination.

Sometimes it is helpful to see the examination as a process (Figure 2.1) to which the doctor, patient, and chaperon bring their life experiences, culture, prejudices, and themselves. All these factors can impact on the experience of the examination. If doctors are aware of this process, then misunderstandings are less likely.

For example, we bring our assumptions, which stem from experience, culture, and our gender and orientation. Remember that not all women have male partners, most women remain sexual throughout their lives but some are never sexual, and that religious taboos are interpreted differently by different people. For example, we might *assume* that a nun is not presently sexual but that does not mean to say she has *never* been sexual.

2.6.   Warning

2.6.1.   *How Do You Feel, Doctor?*

As mentioned earlier, social taboos exist and vaginal examination is a strange thing to do. Training helps us here but sometimes it seems more difficult than others. Some patients seem to make it more difficult. Supposing the patient reminds you of your mother or grandmother, supposing it is a colleague who presents to you, supposing it is a patient who is particularly attractive to you, what do you do with these feelings? You could ignore them or you could retreat behind an efficient doctor façade. It may be worth considering these feelings before you act. Perhaps they are warning you of the peril ahead. If you have noticed an attraction, perhaps the patient has noticed it too so you may wish to take particular care over a chaperon. If the patient feels very powerful to you, that could be a sign of the patient finding it very difficult to submit to medical care, or it could be that the patient wishes to see your consultant!

2.6.2.   How Is the Patient Behaving, Doctor?

Clinical findings are not restricted to observations of size, shape, and appearance of genitals. The way the patient conducts herself can be very revealing and may throw light on the presenting symptom. How did she agree to being examined—reluctant and unwilling, keen to be examined?

How does she react to getting up onto the couch? How does she behave? Does she seem to be relaxed and comfortable with her body? Is she tense and anxious? Is she emotionally distanced? Does she make a fuss that is incomprehensible to you?

Example: Mrs A was referred to the infertility clinic. The GP's letter had mentioned a long and irregular cycle and the possibility of polycystic ovarian syndrome. It was the first appointment and I suggested a vaginal scan. She looked doubtful, so I said her husband could wait outside and went to the couch. I explained that most women found it much more comfortable than a smear and asked her to get undressed and get up on the couch and showed her the blanket with which to cover herself. She took ages to get ready. As I approached her, I realized she was still wearing her knickers. Her initial reluctance, sending her husband away, and taking so long to get ready, taken together with her knickers suggested that she was finding it difficult. I said, "Oh dear, this is difficult for you. Do you want to continue?" She was then able to explain that she was worried about the cysts she thought I might see on the scan.

2.6.3.   How Are You Behaving, Doctor?

Clinical findings are also found in the doctor. When patients have powerful feelings, they can be projected onto the doctor. So what sort of a doctor are you being to this patient on this occasion? Are you being very gentle, concerned you may hurt this patient? Are you tempted to laugh and joke—perhaps both patient and doctor running away from a painful subject? Are you confused by mixed messages from the patient: "It's alright, doctor, do what you have to and don't mind if I scream!"

Clinical Findings

Observation of patient physically
Observation of patient psychologically
Behavior of patient
Behavior of doctor
Feelings of patient
Feelings of doctor

Things to Think About

Referral
History
Attitude of patient
Atmosphere in the room
Interaction
Body language
Feelings expressed by the patient
Feelings felt by the doctor

Example: Ms B's GP telephoned to expedite her outpatient appointment. She had intermenstrual bleeding and could not allow a speculum examination— it had been too painful. We made an early appointment, which the patient rearranged, and subsequently did not attend. The GP rang again and this time the patient arrived. She was dowdy looking and hiding behind lank long hair. She gave a short factual account of her bleeding, saying that speculum examinations had always been difficult but last time the nurse had not been able to remove the speculum and had to fetch the GP to remove it. It sounded awful although she spoke without emotion. She got up onto the couch. It was difficult to make eye contact with her. The doctor commented that it seemed as if she did not want to be there. The patient agreed but did not expand on it. The doctor asked again about the previous examination and the patient gave another actual account. "You are telling me about a horrible experience but I do not hear about how awful it was for you." The patient said there was no point in making a fuss and perhaps the doctor could get on with the smear and ignore her if she cried. The doctor said she did not want to hurt the patient and would she like to insert the speculum herself? She was not sure but then put it in easily and the swabs and smear were taken without difficulty. The referral and the patient's behavior showed ambivalence. The body language showed she did not care for herself (appearance) and also emotional distance. She gave little emotionally and although the doctor commented on her lack of feelings, none were revealed. She appeared a retiring woman who, nonetheless, was powerful enough to get and rearrange an appointment. Perhaps she needed to be in control and when she had regained control was able to control the examination.

2.7.   Vulnerability

Generally speaking, people feel vulnerable when they are without their clothes. If a woman is also worried about whether she has a significant disease affecting her sexual organs, which might have an impact on her very womanhood, she will be in a state of heightened arousal, of fear. Thus even innocent comments can be misunderstood and so it is important to think about the language used and indeed to avoid comments of a personal nature during intimate examinations. See quotes below.

Quotes

(*Things that have been said to women with subsequent sexual problems*)

- Looks like a bomb's gone off in here.
- What a lot of discharge!
- You have an erosion of your cervix.
- Looks like a large nabothian follicle.
- Can I have the extra large speculum?
- Your vagina is very long.
- I don't like the look of that.
- Put your legs like a frog.

2.8.   Potential for Abuse

It is a sad fact that some women are traumatized by their experience of vaginal examination and indeed will present with sexual problems years later as a result of a smear test or colposcopy that was traumatic for them (Figure 2.2). They may fail to attend further routine screening tests and avoid medical attention when necessary. This can be avoided with good communication, an empathetic doctor, and appropriate training.

Some such women have had previous experience which has sensitized them to further abuse. For example, a previous bullying relationship where she had little autonomy and was unable to say "no" might make it difficult for a woman to assert herself with a heath-care professional. Previous sexual abuse will have a similar impact. The patient has not had any control over previous access to her genitals by the abuser and so finds it difficult to say "No."

If we follow the guidelines in this chapter we may be able to avoid damaging our patients. However, women do undergo repeated examinations in the

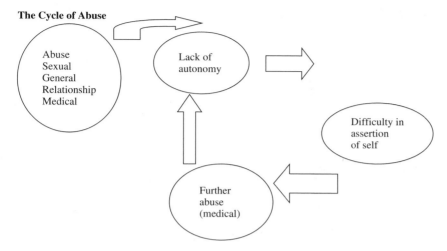

FIGURE 2.2. The cycle of abuse.

colposcopy and GUM clinics, during treatment for cancer and infertility, and it may not be possible to protect them fully. Sometimes it is enough to acknowledge how difficult such examinations are; a statement of the obvious like "It must seem as if everyone has had a look at that part of you" may give her an opportunity to express her distress. This is best said before the examination so that the doctor and the patient can agree whether the examination is necessary. You could also ask if there is anything you could do which would make this examination easier. Some doctors fear inviting patients to say how they feel, anxious that the floodgates may not be stemmed, and the doctor may be overwhelmed with too much distress. Although that is a possibility, in practice it is rare.

2.9.   Is This Examination Really of Benefit to the Patient?

It is always worth considering the *value of this examination to the patient* and to avoid unnecessary intrusions.

2.10.   Avoided Examination

A vaginal examination is part of an outpatient appointment, and patients often expect to be examined. Failure to do an examination in this environment may be more apparent to both patient and doctor. However, in different settings it is easier to avoid, and the reasons are not always obvious.

If your normal practice is to examine then it is worth considering *why not on this occasion*?

- Is it because you have too much to do and are feeling lazy or harassed?
- Is it because there is no chaperon ready for you?
- Is it because you decided not to examine and is that reason a good one?
- Is it because you are picking up on the reluctance from the patient and, if so, what to do about it?

You could ask how she feels about being examined and whether it might be possible. Such enquiries often release the patient to talk about specific anxieties.

2.11.   Refusal for Examination

Informed consent must be obtained and so we must respect a refusal. Such a refusal can be frustrating for the doctor when an opinion is being sought and it is not possible to do the job effectively. If we can receive a refusal with a spirit of interest, then a gentle exploration of what is behind the refusal is better than a long explanation to the patient as to why she should submit to being examined.

2.12.   Some Specific Clinical Problems

2.12.1.   Vaginismus

Some women may come straight to the point and say that they cannot be examined or cannot have intercourse or cannot use tampons. Others will give no warning until the moment of examination. As clinicians, we need to make a specific positive diagnosis of vaginismus, not an assumption that that is the problem. We should rule out anatomical abnormalities, painful vulval and vaginal conditions such as infections or vulvo-vestibulitis first.

An American gynecologist, James Marion Sims, when addressing the Obstetrical Society of London in 1862, first coined the term "vaginismus" when describing one of his patients:

But the most remarkable thing in her history was the fact she had remained a virgin notwithstanding a married state of a quarter of a century...Among other investigations of her case, I attempted to make a vaginal examination but failed completely. The slightest touch at the mouth of the vagina produced the most intense suffering. Her nervous system was thrown into great commotion; there was a general muscular agitation; her whole frame was shivering as if with the rigors of an intermittent fever. She shrieked aloud, her eyes glaring wildly, while tears rolled down her cheeks and she presented the most pitiable appearance of terror and agony. Notwithstanding all these outward involuntary evidences of physical suffering, she had the moral fortitude to hold herself on the couch, and implore me not to desist from any efforts if there was the least hope of finding anything out about her condition. After pressing with all my strength for some minutes, I succeeded in introducing the index finger into the vagina up to the second joint, but not further. The resistance to its passage was so great, and the vaginal contraction so firm, as to deaden the sensation of the finger, and thus the examination revealed only insuperable spasm of the sphincter Vaginae.

2.12.1.1.   How Do You Examine a Woman to Diagnose Vaginismus?

Fortunately, not all women with vaginismus react in the dramatic way described by James Sims. Doctors will develop their own methods. It is essential that the woman feels she is in control:

- Explain she is in control. Explain that you will stop at any stage and not move until she is comfortable. Say also that she can tell you to take it out whenever she likes and you will do so carefully.
- Then ask her to part the labia so you can look.
- Then with her continuing consent, place a fingertip at the vulva and wait for her to settle and then very slowly introduce the tip of your finger into the vagina, watching her face all the time. Some women like to guide your finger with their hand.
- When she expresses discomfort, stop and ask her to let you know when to resume.
- If vaginal tension is detected, ask her to squeeze the finger with her pelvic muscles as tight as she can and then relax the muscles. She may be able to control the pelvic musculature but she may have little control. Typically she relaxes the muscles a little and then unconsciously tightens them up again without knowing about it. You can then draw her attention to what is actually happening. In this way it may be possible to introduce a finger into the vagina.
- Plan to stop when she says she has had enough.
- If the problem is severe, little progress will have been made. You might suggest she practice at home by herself and, depending on the circumstances, see her again or plan to refer her on.

Vaginismus: Definition

The persistent or recurrent difficulties of the woman to allow vaginal entry of a penis or a finger or an object, despite the woman's expressed wish to do so. There is often a phobic avoidance, involuntary pelvic muscle contraction and anticipation/fear/experience of pain. Structural or other physical abnormalities must be ruled out/addressed (1,2).

2.12.2. Vaginal Pain

Vaginal pain may be expressed as a burning sensation or, more dramat-ically, "like a knife going up," "tearing," "searing," or sometimes a more specific area or a deep pain. Pain may be due to a physical cause, vaginismus, or sometimes vaginismus left after a physical problem has resolved. As the patient shows the doctor where it is painful, she may give clues about its origins.

2.12.3. Exploration of Patient's Fantasies

The concerns of the patient may be expressed in the story or may come to light during the examination.

Example: Mrs C presented to the infertility clinic with 5 years' primary infer-tility. It transpired that they were unable to consummate their marriage. They were not sure why, but she said it was painful when they tried and he said, "It just won't go in." His erections were normal and on further questioning were very firm—firm enough to hang a towel on! She got onto the couch to be examined. As the doctor approached the vagina with a gloved finger the patient asked if there might be a blockage in the vagina.

2.13. How Do You Feel Now, Doctor?

Medical training has to partially desensitize young doctors to misery and pain or we might not be able to cope. However, it is possible to learn skills grounded in psychotherapy. These skills allow us to feel something of what the patient brings to us, hold it, process it, and feed it back to the patient in a way that might be helpful. Therefore, if we can be aware of *our* feelings during a consultation or examination we may begin to understand the problem from the perspective of the patient.

Example: Mrs D presented with loss of libido since the birth of her son 18 months ago. Before the pregnancy, sex had been good. The baby had been planned, the pregnancy uneventful, and there were no problems during delivery. She had gone back to work and her husband was a househusband. The arrangement worked very well. She said she felt dead in the genital region. As the doctor examined the patient, the doctor was aware of a sense of loneliness in the room. Unsure of the origins of these feelings, the doctor suggested that perhaps the husband was feeling shut out. The patient cried and said, "No, it is me that is left out. They have all day together and he saw her first steps and I feel so lonely." Further exploration of these feelings after the exami-nation allowed the patient to make some connections and she said she was feeling better at the next appointment although she needed some help with spontaneity!

2.14. Further Training

- The Institute of Psychosexual Medicine (3) offers training in these skills with particular reference to sexual problems, especially about the vaginal examination.
- The Nixon club also offers psychotherapy-type training to obstetricians and gynecologists.
- Balint-based groups for doctors.

2.15. Skills of Psychosexual Medicine

- Active listening
- The use of the genital examination
- Formulation of hypotheses as the consultation progresses
- The use of shared understanding of the facts *and feelings* to help discover the truth.

References

1. Fraser guidelines, http://www.gpnotebook.co.uk.
2. Crowley T, Richardson D, Goldmeier D. Recommendations for the management of vaginismus: BASHH Special Interest Group for Sexual Dysfunction. *Int J STD AIDS*. 2006;17:14–18.
3. Institute of Psychosexual Medicine, http://www.ipm.org.uk.

Suggested Reading

1. Skrine R. *Blocks and Freedoms in Sexual Life—A Handbook of Psychosexual Medicine*. Oxford: Radcliffe Medical Press; 1997.
2. Skrine R, Montford H. *An Introduction to Psychosexual Medicine*. London: Hodder Arnold; 2001.

3
Communication Skills, What You Can Do in 15 Minutes

L. Jane Knowles

We have divided this chapter into two parts. "Communication skills" looks at what is possible in a 15 minutes interview when your prime consideration is gathering facts and making treatment plans. Psychological awareness should improve the consultation for both the patient and yourself. "Breaking bad news" takes your communication skills and psychological understanding several steps further but good communication is never more important than when what we have to communicate is sensitive and difficult for the patient and for ourselves.

3.1. Communication Skills

Good communication takes place in an environment that is perceived as psychologically safe by all participants. This sense of safety is difficult to achieve in a busy OP department. Clear contracts about boundaries help.

A clear statement such as "We have 15 minutes to explore the problems you are experiencing and the ways I may be able to help" makes several statements, some overt, some more covert. It gives a clear message about time boundaries. It helps if there is a clock in the room, so the patient and you maintain a similar sense of that time during the appointment. It says, "I want to hear about your problems" and offers hope that there are ways that you may be able to help. At a more covert level, it says that you are interested and wish to be helpful. By sharing the time boundary at the beginning, you are also helping to equalize the power imbalance that would be within the treatment relationship if the patient did not know when you planned to end.

In such a brief appointment, you need the patients to "open up" rapidly about what is really worrying them. This is difficult to achieve when the woman is anxious, wants to talk about something very personal and possibly shameful to her, and may have previous experience of appointments that have not proved helpful, indeed may have increased her anxieties.

It is also difficult to achieve if there are "blocks" in your own view of the situation. If the referral letter has already given you the impression of a long-standing difficult-to-help problem, for instance, you are likely to approach the appointment with a certain amount of "heartsink." If the woman who walks through the door is obese, your heart may sink further with the thoughts of a difficult examination ahead.

Have a brief internal dialogue about what your assumptions are about the patient at the beginning and review this as the appointment proceeds. This provides a personalized type of self-supervision with every patient. This is particularly important with those patients who seem, superficially at the least, most like the doctor or like many patients the doctor has met before. Let wisdom temper these assumptions. The context of every patient's life is different. Because at the moment of consultation one is a doctor and one a patient, their context is quite different, even if the patient is also a doctor.

It is hard to be honestly interested in each and every patient. Every doctor has bad days, parts of the day when energy is low, times when overworked and tired. But the patient may have put off coming for help for months; they may have been on a waiting list and then spent some time in your waiting room. The potential for disappointment in this meeting is considerable. When emotions are intense and anxiety high, the capacity for disappointment to escalate to a sense of betrayal is high. These are the patients most likely to complain and feel badly treated, however good the subsequent treatment is.

However, what of the patient who seems to bring about a sense of doom and hopelessness even when you started the appointment in good spirits.

The process of "transference" (T) of feelings is complex, but if we have expectations of disappointment and failure in emotional relationships, because of personality or life events, past relationships and "failures," we can make the failure reoccur by our behavior and words. The doctor may be left feeling anxious, depressed, frustrated, or angry by these feelings that feel inappropriate for the present setting. This depends on the doctor's past experience and is called "countertransference" (CT).

One of the problems within T/CT relationships in assessments is that they are at least partially unconscious. We know what we feel but we do not know why. Indeed the feelings may be completely inappropriate to the meeting. However, if you wish to end the appointment on a note of hope you need to be able to "step outside" the T/CT relationship. Sometimes taking a minute or two to write a few notes allows you breathing time to take account of how the interview has left you feeling. This may give you some clues about the patient's basic assumptions. Experience allows you to differentiate between the feelings you brought to the interview and the feelings you are left with and find out who has influenced any change.

Many patients invite us to enter what Karpman (1) originally described as "The drama triangle" (Figure 3.1). The model illustrates the different positions (rescuer, persecutor, or victim) that we may take up in our encounters with others and the relationship between power and responsibility. Each patient comes to us with preconceived ideas about what to expect from the doctor

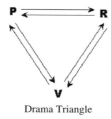

Drama Triangle

FIGURE 3.1. Drama triangle.

and many may act or feel like a helpless victims. It is important to avoid denying the patient the right to be self-determining in our efforts to say or do the "right thing."

In our work, we may favor the rescuer and the persecutor positions in order to avoid experiencing ourselves as victims of our patients or our own anxiety.

This is always a no-win option as none of the three positions allow you to adopt a sensible clinical, nonidealistic summing up or "sewing up clearly" of the appointment. You need a clear head at the end and if you can put forward the options and plans for the patient in that form, it helps them to be more rooted too.

We all know that patients remember very little of the end of interviews. They are psychologically preparing to leave much as you are preparing to finish. Have paper and pen on your desk if they wish to make brief notes and/or put your precis and plans into writing to them as soon as possible.

3.2. Breaking Bad News

Whatever the bad news is, you need to feel calm as you deliver it to the patient and/or relatives. This is sometimes hard, but you can "center" yourself by containing your own anxieties, for instance your anxieties about how the patient might react. Many patients will take their lead from you. If you are calm and contained in how you deliver the news, it is easier for them to listen and hear you. This should become less difficult with experience but will never be easy. Remember, though, that it is always harder for the patient, so you should try to rehearse your parts of the dialogue in order not to sound clumsy or unfeeling. Never rush with lots of words in order to hide your own anxiety about the task. It is helpful to think about the occasions when someone has broken bad news to you. What was good and what was bad about that experience? Most patients, perhaps as many as 90%, will have some idea that bad news is a possibility: they will want to feel that you are being honest with them and this includes saying, "I don't know" if and when that is the case. What may seem obvious to a doctor is not necessarily so for the patient. It is a great skill to be explicit in how you deliver information without being blunt or frightening.

The bad news you deliver will almost certainly make the patient anxious. When we are anxious, we have difficulty in listening, hearing, and remembering; so expect to have the conversation again.

It is useful to consider what sort of social support systems the patient has, both physical and psychological. Who, if anyone, is with the patient? Who can they talk to tonight as your information "sinks in"? Do they need help, support, or advice in telling their family? Do they need to telephone someone straight away? How are they going to get home? Even asking these questions allows the patient to begin to think about what support is available.

Do you have written information to give to the patient? Is there a contact number for a clinic nurse or a counselor? Is it possible for the patient or next of kin to speak to you tomorrow or this week?

Remember, people have many "layers" of vulnerability, but we are all vulnerable, however well we might seem to be coping. Some patients, especially those with whom we can identify, will "haunt" your memories more than others. When the patient has left the room, be aware of how you are feeling. For many people, there is a tightness in the chest where they have held their tension: take a few deep breaths and deliberately let go of that tension.

You need to develop the capacity to "turn off" and give yourself permission to do it or you will suffer from the cumulative effects of the hard parts of your career.

Most patients still invest a great deal of trust in their doctors: you are their partner in both joy and sorrow, life and death. Sometimes we are remarkably helpless practically in that partnership, but we can always be reflective and aware: patients remember what is said and how it is said just as much as what is done to them. Words are the "bridge" between you. Speak kindly and listen intently.

Reference

1. Karpman S. Fairy tales and script drama analysis. *Trans Anal Bull.* 1968;7(26): 39–43.

4
Psychoanalysis for Emergencies: A Toolkit for Trainees

Sandra Goldbeck-Wood

Creative intellectual space is a scarce luxury in obstetric and gynecological specialist training. You are awash with medical and surgical knowledge and skills; you work long hours, manage high levels of clinical risk, negotiate an obstacle course of exams and assessments, and if you are lucky, may even manage a social or family life. Whatever could psychoanalysis possibly offer you? Little, in straightforward consultations in which both doctor and patient are rational, friendly, and working together toward a shared clinical goal. Alas, just as not all cesarean sections are straightforward elective procedures on slim primigravidae, not all doctor–patient interactions are rational, constructive conversations between relaxed adults. When the going gets psychologically tough—and there are few places it gets as tough as a specialty dealing in birth, death, and sex on a daily basis—the following toolkit of common psychotherapeutic ideas may help make your toughest encounters less exhausting and more interesting.

4.1. Transference

The must-have of your psychoanalytic toolkit is the idea of transference. Transference is the phenomenon whereby we are apt to "transfer" experience gained in one situation to other analogous situations (1). This includes a tendency to interpret current relationships, according to rules or patterns learned in early relationships, and to behave accordingly. So my boss may remind me of my indulgent father or my strict mother, and I may respond like a spoilt, or rebellious, child; my junior colleague might remind me of my pesky little sister, eliciting in me the behavior of the bossy older sibling. Transference forms a kind of personal "relationship theory," whose patterns we fall back on unconsciously in unfamiliar situations. It does not imply psychopathology. But like all theories, it may serve us well or badly, depending on how applicable the old data are to the current situation.

4.1.1. How to Manage Negative Transference

Transference can become a kind of "unreasonableness machine" insisting blindly and unhelpfully that a current relationship resembles one from childhood and inducing in me the behaviors which echo or express the child I once was, rather than the adult I now am.

BOX 1 Managing Negative Transference

Do not

- Blindly allow yourself to be transformed into demon or hero.
- Forget your own risk of falling into the child's position.
- Rule out fair criticism.

Do

- Keep thinking.
- Use your awareness to transform destructive, unconscious transference into a useful source of data.
- Look for an appropriate response to the "child" in your patient.

More than any other client–professional relationship, the doctor–patient relationship contains elements especially liable to remind us of powerless, childhood states, and therefore induce transference responses (2). There is always a degree of power imbalance, however sensitively handled, in that treatments can be offered or withheld, care can be given kindly or unkindly, pain can be inflicted or alleviated, and the doctor is ultimately in a position of greater knowledge. In gynecology, the transference stakes are raised still higher by our specific powers to question people about the most private of bodily functions, place patients in potentially humiliating physical positions, and touch parts of the body which are otherwise only ever touched dispassionately by a parent, in infancy. Small wonder that infantile feelings can be brought back.

This takes us away from our usual experience as adults with the resources to meet our own needs. If we are hungry, we buy or cook food; if we are bored, we reach for a chosen entertainment—we need not be overly troubled by feelings of powerlessness or dependency on others. But becoming a patient, with a powerful immediate need such as relief from pain, can remind us powerfully of what it is like to be small, needy, and dependent.

Nor is our professional role a complete protection from such feelings. On a good day, you may be well fed, well rested, well supported, and working well within your range of competence, but during a bad night, exhausted or working at the limits of your competence there is nothing to protect you against your own memories of feeling small, overstretched, and at other people's mercy.

Our responses to dependency in the present will be heavily colored by early experiences of dependency. Was it on balance a positive or at least a bearable experience, in which I mostly felt recognized and dealt with compassionately? Or was it a frightening or unbearable seeming thing? If on balance I had sufficient positive experiences in relation to carers and authority figures, I am likely to be relaxed about dependency, straightforward in expressing my needs and wants clearly and without aggression, able to hear the other person's point of view, and accept disappointment without feeling psychologically "broken." This is psychological maturity.

If I am not fortunate enough to have developed this maturity, I will struggle to deal with difficult experiences such as being denied a much-wanted treatment. I have little mental elasticity to protect me from all the anxiety and powerlessness of the small child's early environment. If these feelings become overwhelming, I may begin to *behave* like the threatened, mistrustful infant I feel like. The doctor may merely be offering a rational view of what he/she sees as my best interests, but in my mind, he/she is a cruelly withholding parent, insensitive to my needs. I may develop a child-like vehemence, becoming distressed and aggressive, and try everything in my power to force or manipulate him/her into delivering the outcome I passionately want. Locked into an internal drama, I will deploy all the primitive weapons at my disposal to try and protect myself from what feels like an attack on my fragile coping mechanisms.

4.1.2. What Not to Do

On a bad day, caught painfully between your own needs and pressures and your patient's vehemence, you might find yourself falling into your own transference responses. You may feel overwhelmed, like a child struggling under a barrage of criticism, and be tempted to lock horns with your patient in an unconscious attempt to overpower her with your own weapons of medical knowledge and intellectual argument, just to win back a bit of psychological space of your own. You may win the battle and comfort yourself by dismissing the patient's irrational behavior, while nevertheless feeling secretly humiliated by your own irrationality. And in getting drawn into counterattack, you probably become much like the harsh parent the patient originally feared. She may succeed, unwittingly, in turning you into the dismissive doctor she most feared.

4.1.3. What to Do Instead

The only alternative to unwittingly accept the role of villain in your patient's transference drama is to notice what is happening and keep thinking. If things go well, you may spot the signs of "child-like vehemence" in your patient's responses, remind yourself that this is really about a power struggle with a past parent, and avoid taking her negative reactions personally. Ideally, you may even be able to see the small, powerless, frightened child she feels she is and find a helpful response—a kindly acknowledgment of the difficulty of her situation.

4.1.4. Positive Transference

Not all of a patient's transference responses are negative—she may view you as a benign parent figure who has solved her menorrhagia with your new magical microwave treatment, given her a much-wanted baby with IVF, or even saved her life. You may be her hero or heroine and reap the reward of effusive gratitude. This kind of "positive transference" is less of a problem than a well-earned perk of practicing medicine. But it does no harm to notice where positive responses may be inflated by transference, if only to protect yourself from distorting your clinical judgment in order to preserve your heroic status.

4.1.5. Fair Comment

Nor do all of a patient's responses to a doctor, however negative, arise in transference; there may be either positive or negative feelings born of the real situation. Try and remain open to the possibility that a patient's response *might* be fair comment on your own behavior or consulting style.

4.2. Countertransference and How to Use It

If transference is "what your patient unconsciously makes of you," countertransference is what you make of her. There is controversy within psychoanalysis about the exact nature of countertransference, but what is agreed is that our responses to the patient, such as irritation or protectiveness, can sometimes tell us something about the patient's psychological situation, as well as our own (3).

For example, a woman I saw with vaginismus seemed to me both very organized and "grown up" and very young and "little-girlish," at the same time. In taking her history, I noticed a tendency in myself to tread gently and carefully in a conversation which has the capacity to feel "penetrative." I took a long time to get round to the physical examination and carried it out especially gently and slowly. Commenting on my awareness of this "woman-girl" contradiction led to my patient describing a sense of being a girl trapped in a woman's body and going on to disclose a previously undisclosed history of sexual abuse in childhood.

The point is not that such countertransference responses are good or bad, but that they are informative. In this consultation, mine suggested to me that "this is a woman who needs things not to go too fast, or perhaps a woman who feels too 'small' for sex, in emotional as well as literal ways."

Your countertransference will not deliver a diagnosis, but it may help you ask the patient the right questions which will make it possible for the patient to tell you what the matter is. When it works, it does so both because your observations are careful and accurate and because your patient, sensing your care and accuracy, develops the trust without which she cannot tell you more. She will sense that you are listening carefully to both spoken and unspoken things—her words and her body language (such as vaginismus itself)—in other words, to her as a whole person.

4.3. Somatization and Embodiment

Somatization, or hysteria, as it was originally known, occurs when the mind fails to contain the anxiety or distress we are exposed to, and "the organism begins to think" (4). Our psychological sense of self or of "wholeness" has its earliest origins in bodily experiences of pleasure, pain, care, or neglect. Primitive anxiety first arises when we are hungry and there is no breast to feed us (5), and all subsequent anxieties can remind us of these early psychological dramas. However, developmentally, we learn about our experience to contain our own anxiety with the help of *thinking* (6).

If we are unable to fully achieve this maturity, or if distress is overwhelming, we may go back, or regress, to the condition of the psychologically immature infant and express our distress in bodily symptoms or " somatize" it. Because distress can no more be "disposed of" than matter, it will express itself physically if it cannot be contained and expressed mentally or verbally. The more unthinkable the thought or feeling, the more likely it is to be "encoded" in physical symptoms.

4.3.1. How to Address Somatized Distress

BOX 2

In managing somatization, remember

- What cannot be held in mind may well be held in body.
- Body language and actions can be read, potentially offering insights into the behavior.
- It is likely that everything makes sense, if only it can be understood.
- You will need to switch into an imaginative, intuitive part of your brain.
- Your patient is likely to appreciate your efforts toward understanding, even where understanding remains partial or limited.

What can you hope to do as a gynecologist, faced with a patient presenting with somatic symptoms untraceable to any known pathology? Having taken all appropriate steps to exclude organic pathology, try the following.

First, briefly notice your own feelings. You may feel frustration at what appears an "illegitimate" use of your time, or you may simply feel overwhelmed and "set up"—expected to produce a biological solution to a psychological problem. Your feelings are allowed, and probably inevitable.

Next, resist the temptation to dispose of the problem, mentally, by labeling your patient as "heartsink patient" (7). Acknowledge that although you might prefer to delegate this problem to a psychiatrist, midwife, or counselor (perhaps useful avenues to explore later), for the time being *you are the doctor she has chosen to come and see because she is unable yet to make any connection between her distress and her symptom.* You are therefore in a unique position to help her make that connection.

Now set aside the fact that her symptoms make no biological sense, and try looking for psychological "sense" in them, by switching from the rational into the imaginative part of your mind. Ask yourself what her main symptom could be the literal expression of, and wonder (if it feels appropriate, aloud, with the patient) if that has any connection with another part of her life. Is vaginismus about "keeping something out"? Nausea and vomiting about "getting rid of something"? Overeating as "feeling undernourished," or "pelvic pain" as "pain in her femininity"? And if so, in what way?

Your intuition and imagination, however sensitive a tool, will not in itself give you the diagnosis, nor will it cut through the resistance of a patient who is determined not to see what her underlying distress is really about. What it can do is point you in the right conversational direction to help the patient remake her own broken connection between mind and body.

To reach this point of insight, your patient needs to be able to trust you to take her physical well-being and the possibility that there may be some organic pathology, seriously. It may be helpful to demonstrate this by explaining your diagnostic thinking, much like looking explicitly in your driving mirror during a driving test. It will also be important not to get too attached to your own psychosomatic hypotheses and try and force them on her; instead, simply use your careful observation to inform the conversation. Remember that the ultimate authority and responsibility for a psychosomatic diagnosis is never wholly with the doctor, but between the doctor and the patient. If the patient senses that you accept this, she is likely to be more trustful and forthcoming about her hidden distresses.

4.4. Defenses

We are used to the word "defensive" as a description for someone who seems unjustifiably edgy or hostile—as though that person were warding off an imaginary attack. We rarely face or think about these defenses in their most extreme manifestations. Psychoanalysis thinks of defenses as the means of maintaining psychic equilibrium (8). All of us have, and need, ego defenses to maintain our sense of self—a kind of homeostasis or stability in our internal world. Defenses are what we employ to restore lost balance, when something or someone threatens our sense of self. We all quite naturally and healthily seek to protect ourselves from anything we perceive as undeserved hostility, and rebuff such insults with defenses such as sharp tone or a withdrawal from contact with the person whose behavior we feel has insulted us. These are examples of a flexible, adult form of defensiveness, which respond to the "real" level of threat. They are aimed at re-establishing a sense of fairness and are likely to be amenable to negotiation—e.g., if the other persons were to explain their behaviors in a way which offered us a different view or were to make a conciliatory gesture.

BOX 3

In dealing with defenses, remember

- We all need defenses and are entitled to them.
- Mature "on a good day" defenses are flexible and reasonable.
- Extreme pressure can trigger primitive " life and death" defenses laced with terror and/or aggression.
- Obstetrics and gynecology is rich in situations which can evoke traumatic memories, and therefore you are likely to meet patients' primitive defenses.
- Maintaining compassion for yourself will help you maintain compassion for your patient.

4.4.1.   Mature Ego Defenses

Familiar examples of defenses of the mature ego include denial (choosing to ignore a painful feeling, such as grief), repression ("banning" a feeling completely from consciousness), sublimation (using an inconvenient feeling to fuel a constructive activity such as a creative or career goal), regression (returning to an earlier psychological age in the face of a threat), intellectualization (using thought as a means of avoiding feeling), or reaction formation, which might manifest as being assiduously polite to someone we particularly dislike.

4.4.2.   Primitive Defenses

In addition to these adult defenses, we all have more or less hidden primitive defenses, which respond to a perceived attack on our very existence, and are aimed at warding off a sense of annihilation. These defenses, when activated, look much more like the uncontrolled distress and rage of the infant and can be fearsome to deal with in a grown person.

It is important to recognize that any of us could reach this "snapping point" of feeling not merely aggrieved, but broken or annihilated, if pushed far enough, e.g., via emotional or physical cruelty. Beneath the distresses and anxieties we feel able to "manage" with our adult defense systems, we all have a level of distress we could no longer manage and which would constitute trauma. For most people, it would take an extreme insult to provoke this, but the more fragile a person's sense of self, the more prey they are to feeling threatened by small triggers. Primitive defenses, unlike adult defenses, are desperate and heedless, and the person will often seem quite literally "beside herself."

A person whose primitive defenses have been thoroughly activated—e.g., by pain and fear—can no longer be reasoned with because she is no longer in touch with the "adult" part of herself. She is unable to deal with anyone else's needs or thoughts because her whole psyche is flooded with the life and death struggle to prevent herself from being psychologically "broken" or traumatized. We see this occasionally in the labor ward and learn intuitively that this is no moment for rational conversation, but instead for kind containment.

4.4.2.1.   What to Do with Primitive Defenses

If a woman in labor is "beside herself," perhaps screaming and warding off all interventions, we need to access a different level of awareness in ourselves. As her carers, we need to hold in mind both the panic-stricken small child and the grown woman that she is in the same moment and seek to address the needs of both parts of her rather than prioritizing the need we feel more competent to meet. If we can achieve this, we help her to "hold herself together" in a moment where she might otherwise become traumatized, "broken," and a candidate for postpartum posttraumatic stress disorder. It can be tempting, especially as a litigation-aware obstetrician, to side with the woman's rational, biological need for a safe delivery and a healthy baby—over her immediate, inarticulate infantile needs, which, however desperate, are much harder to discern or feel confident that we can begin to address.

4.5.   Trauma and Psychological Space

Trauma occurs where the degree of emotional pain exceeds our ego defenses' ability to cope, and we feel shattered, or annihilated, or psychologically "railroaded." Trauma is neither a feature of the event itself nor of the person, but of the interaction between the two. One person's passing distress—a difficult forceps delivery, being shut in a lift, or witnessing a terrorist attack— is another person's lifelong trauma. We therefore cannot ultimately know what will traumatize a patient because it depends on too many imponderables, including her psychological maturity and traumas (such as sexual abuse) she may have suffered in the past.

4.5.1. How to Help Prevent Trauma

What we can do is to notice the difference between the kind of inevitable distress or pain which is commonplace in the labor ward or medical emergency and that other "beside oneself" quality which might signal the risk of trauma; and to take whatever steps we can to restore a sense of control to the woman and psychological space to the situation.

Awareness of psychological trauma matters to the practicing obstetrician because of the increasing interest in obstetric posttraumatic distress disorder (9) and the key preventive role of the clinician managing the delivery. Other professionals can, at best, hope to offer post hoc "debriefing," as secondary prevention or treatment of the subsequent mental health problem, and the efficacy of these post hoc interventions in obstetrics is questionable (10). It is tempting to think, during a difficult delivery on a busy labor ward with a woman who is beside herself with anxiety, that there is "nothing I can do, beyond getting on with the job as quickly as possible" or that "the midwife will offer psychological care, while I deliver the baby." But to delegate psychological management wholly to someone else is to underestimate your own power to make a difference to the psychological experience, in apparently small but crucial ways.

Think of the exhausted primigravida in a prolonged second stage, with a possible malposition, distressed and refusing all interventions. Instead of bustling into the room and announcing from the other side the need for vaginal examination while you wash your hands to don the sterile gloves, take a moment to come close to the bed, perhaps bending to make eye contact or nonintrusive physical contact, such as a hand on her arm. Address her by name, let her know that you are aware of her distress, and what you have come for: "Anna, I can see you're struggling. Can I talk to you for a moment?" Already you are creating psychological space.

If she says "Wait a minute, I've got another contraction coming," then do so, if possible. Even if you are busy and anxious, brief patience is an excellent investment in her cooperation with the next step. Address her clearly, warmly, honestly, and briefly. Do not tell her "what is going to happen," but ask her permission for what you propose and why. Do not exaggerate or try and scare her, which may feel bullying and backfire, but simply be honest: "I'm worried that your baby is getting distressed. I need to know how far down the birth canal the baby is, so that I know. Will you let me examine you?"

Very rarely, a woman will refuse examination or treatment point-blank, despite your best efforts. You will rightly try and persuade her and, if a real impasse develops, involve a senior colleague. But for the most part, a woman who trusts her obstetrician and feels that her rights over her own body are being respected will consent, however reluctantly, to what you clearly and earnestly recommend.

You can create further space, and trust, during the feared examination by telling her honestly what you propose to do and offering her some control over what she can bear: "I'm going to have to push quite firmly to be sure which way round the baby is lying, and it might hurt for a moment" (try to avoid the dishonest use of the word "uncomfortable"). "If you say 'stop,' I'll stop. But bear with me if you can." Far from inviting resistance, these goodwill gestures are likely to invite cooperation.

This kind of awareness, coupled with a small amount of self-discipline, can bring compassion and cooperation into the psychological emergency which sometimes accompanies an obstetric emergency. With luck, you have achieved a safe delivery, prevented avoidable psychological trauma, and both you and your patient know that—however painful the experience—you were her ally, and not her persecutor.

Clearly, you have neither time nor responsibility nor permission to investigate your patients' deeper distresses in the manner of a psychotherapist. But like it or not, there are times when those distresses will claim your attention willy-nilly. In learning to recognize their symptoms and signs, you may find you can return to your primary clinical purpose sooner. You may even find you enjoy the challenge of bringing space to a claustrophobic discussion, thinking laterally where thinking has got lost, and bridging the gap between mind and body.

References

1. Klein M. The origins of transference. *Int J Psychoanal.* 1952;33:433–438.
2. Balint M. *The Doctor, His Patient and the Illness.* New York, NY: International Universities Press; 1957.
3. Heimann P. On counter-transference. *Int J Psychoanal.* 1950;31:81–84.
4. Ferenczi S. In: Dupont J, ed. *The Clinical Diary.* London: Harvard University Press; 1988.
5. Hinshelwood R. *A Dictionary of Kleinian Thought.* London: Free Association Books; 1989.
6. Bion W. A theory of thinking. *Int J Psychoanal.* 1962;43:306–310. Reprinted in *Second Thoughts,* 1967.
7. O'Dowd T. Five years of heartsink patients in general practice. *BMJ.* 1988;297(6647):528–530.
8. Spitz RA. Some early prototypes of ego defenses. *J Am Psychoanal Assoc.* 1961;9:626–651.
9. Reynolds JL. Post-traumatic stress disorder after childbirth: the phenomenon of traumatic birth. *CMAJ.* 1997;156(6):831–835.
10. Small R, Lumley J, Donohue L, Potter A, Waldenström U. Randomised controlled trial of midwife led debriefing to reduce maternal depression after operative childbirth. *BMJ.* 2000;321:1043–1047.

5
Sexuality

Kevan R. Wylie

Few commentators would argue that puberty and the change from a girl to a woman is possibly one of the most challenging transitions within the life cycle. The various demands of school, home, peers, and for many the frustration in the delay of puberty compared to their friends mean that the excitement and uniqueness of becoming a woman is lost amongst many of the other life stressors. As a consequence, in modern day life, this transition has become an ordeal rather than a transition of anticipation and bewilderment. Many cultures go further to circumvent the process of adolescence and puberty with sexual emancipation and potential.

It is hardly surprising therefore that the transition to adult sexuality is complicated and the potential pleasure attainable as a young woman is lost amongst many of the social and cultural taboos which attempt to distance all pleasure from sexuality. The consequence is not just the potential of sexual dysfunctions but also a number of psychosomatic presentations where listing sexuality as the token problem is far from the root cause of the symptoms.

Imagine the scenario then when such symptoms appear and the young woman is able to share with her mother her concerns of being different from her friends. When this is brought to the physician, one response would be to dismiss it with the suggestion that such pathology is a variation of normality. Such a dismissal may be due to embarrassment or difficulty for the physician in being able to deal with what is being talked about within the room. Even if it is "normal," there are clearly concerns and these need exploring. An increasing number of women are choosing to share their concerns with a female physician. This may be due to less embarrassment or knowledge assumed because of the same gender or may reflect the natural communication style of women doctors being more sharing.

However, there is a secondary consequence on male physicians in their confidence in obtaining and dealing with sexually related problems. This is not fair on good male doctors; this culturally inhibits women from good help which can be provided by male doctors; and this is not helpful in providing a service. Their consultations are further hampered by the need for chaperons (*note*: RCOG guidelines advise chaperons for all physicians, not just men), which inevitably changes the doctor–patient relationship. Just because you are a woman does not make you an expert either! Moreover, many female doctors feel undertrained and inadequate in this area as well.

All doctors practicing in the O&G field should have enough knowledge and confidence to start to help with sexual problems, as sexuality is inevitably bound up in this specialty. We must ask if the problem of confidence rests with the physician or within modern society. Embarrassment, lack of awareness of comorbid conditions, lack of emphasis on enhancing quality of life, fear of longer consultations are just some of the factors which may be as important as lack of knowledge or skills about talking to patients about sex or actually using strategies to avoid talking about sex. Asking open questions and confirming that it is acceptable to speak about such problems can be very helpful for women. Perhaps the key to solving this conundrum is the recognition that regular clinical supervision by a peer group is essential in modern day health care.

So what are the problems that may present themselves to a typical gynecological or general practice consultation that may be labeled as a psychosomatic, dysmorphophobic, or dysfunctional presentation? Some clinical conditions would include dissatisfaction with the size or shape of the labia, the smell or discharge emanating from the vagina, and issues around menstruation or potential pregnancy. There appears to be no evidence to counter the argument that early discussion and acknowledgment of sexual matters for young adolescents is beneficial.

More common conditions involve pain that is associated with sexual activity and will invariably bring patients to physicians seeking explanation and assurance. However, many clinicians will have no training or understanding of how to deal with such problems, and a negative or embarrassed response is likely to be further detrimental and damaging to the woman. Dyspareunia and the related pain syndromes are some of the most challenging clinical areas for physicians and sexologists to come to terms with and provide validated and, where possible, evidence-based information and guidance.

Broaching the subject of sexual matters with patients can sometimes be difficult. It is necessary for the clinician to approach such matters in a sensitive yet confident manner. By normalizing the possibility of sexual problems with statements such as "I just wanted to mention to you that several of my patients have remarked about sexual problems during their care. If this is something that is troubling you, we should talk about it sometime." It may be worth remarking that "I note that it is commonly the case that patients with gynecological matters can also have some problems in their sexual lives. Is this the case with you?" or the matter can be broached by a sentence such as "Tell me how things are for you at home." If necessary, it may be worthwhile specifying that you want to know about their intimate relationships, particularly in women who have had interventional procedures affecting the pelvis. Such intervention could be surgery, irradiation, or drugs which are known to affect sexual function such as tricyclic antidepressants for pain syndromes or SSRIs for late luteal phase dysphoric disorder or depressive conditions. A third approach would be to ask "What is bothering you? I wonder if this is something that is so personal to you that you feel it is difficult to raise this with me?" or "Many patients feel that it may be wrong to talk to their physician about sexual problems, but I want to assure you that many of my patients have told me about these kind of problems before and it is entirely appropriate for you to tell me about these so that we can try and help you." If time runs out in the normal consultation, then offer to make a second appointment or even a longer double appointment in the near future. This is particularly important when patients themselves raise the subject. If you feel it inappropriate or uncomfortable about offering such a session within the clinic, then the offer to seek alternative advice and to refer to specialist services is important. Remember that on some occasions, a sexual problem may be the primary purpose for seeking the advice of a gynecologist even if the presenting symptom is some other urogynecological problem.

Many would argue that the underlying problem is a failure to sufficiently educate patients and the population at large. Self-reassurance from some baseline knowledge will allow the woman to exchange with her clinician in an informed and mutually cooperative way.

Invariably some clinical scenarios will develop where the physician has no previous experience or confidence to deal with the problem. Examples may include persistent sexual arousal syndrome or pain in the clitoris or at the time of orgasm. Importantly, identification of local resources that may be available and accessed in these more difficult cases will help both the patient and the clinician. Similarly, membership of a supervision group to explore not only the detail and content of the problem but also the processes, emotions, and rationalization that take place—in order to appear a competent and informed clinician—is an ideal opportunity for the professional development of clinicians.

In certain circumstances, there may actually be a sexual concern, dissatisfaction, disorder, or dysfunction (SCDDD) of the sexual processes. Whilst criticized by some, to clinicians this term describes a number of defined problems. It is then possible to try and understand these and offer interventions.

Sexual dysfunction in women is, according to many studies, a common experience. Whilst the definition of the dysfunction may vary widely, prevalence rates of 43% (1) and 41% (2) among women are cited. However, these rates are questioned by many, most vociferously by Moynihan (3). Many of the symptoms are commonly experienced in comorbid conditions such as depressive mood disorder and premenstrual dysphoric disorder(PMDD) as well as perimenopausal depressive disorder. Often the problem is more of sexual satisfaction and communication within interpersonal relationships, and these, alongside environmental factors, can make the correct detection and diagnosis of these conditions difficult.

5.1. Normal Female Sexual Response

The first accounts of female sexual response by Masters and Johnson (4) reported a linear progression from excitation, arousal reaching a plateau stage, orgasm, and resolution. Kaplan's model (5) introduced the concept of desire bringing about arousal. More recently, Basson (6) has proposed that the spontaneous sexual arousal experienced by women, where recognized, will in favorable circumstances bring about a desire for sexual activity and behavior, especially when this is focused on enhancing intimacy and pleasurable outcome.

5.2. Classification and Diagnosis

The diagnosis of sexual dysfunction in women is defined as a disorder of one or more of sexual desire, arousal, orgasm, and/or a sexual pain (dyspareunia or vaginismus). The condition must result in significant personal distress and have a negative impact on the woman's health and her quality of life. The coexistence of two or more of these disorders must be recognized in any assessment process and an evaluation of both the interpersonal relationship and the sexual well-being of the partner recorded. The diagnosis of one or more of these conditions is made primarily on the clinical history and by careful enquiry into each of the clinical areas. Many women will use euphemisms when discussing sexual issues until the patient and clinician are comfortable in using more specific and explicit enquiry and language. Simple questions such as "Are you happy with your sexual life?" can be used in general consultations as an opening opportunity for patients to raise specific matters. With hypoactive sexual desire disorder (HSSD), it is important to establish the biological motivational (emotional and affective matters and the need for intimacy) as well as the cognitive (wishes and fears about sexual behavior) components.

The existence of any endocrinological disturbance, in particular of sex steroids, prolactin, and thyroid disease, is important, particularly with hypoactive sexual desire disorder. Other chronic medical conditions including cardiovascular disease, anemia, and postsurgical menopause following bilateral ovariectomy will need specific enquiry. Mental health problems, especially depression and substance misuse, are common contributors to HSSD. Psychological experiences, life events including work stresses and previous trauma and abuse are important factors. In arousal disorder and anorgasmia, specific enquiry around vascular and neurological disease is essential. For example, diabetes mellitus can bring about a sensory and autonomic neuropathy as well as small blood vessel disease. This can affect both the possibility for vasocongestion to occur and the perception by the woman of this physical change. In the case of vaginismus, which is a specific contraction of the muscles around the entry point into the vagina, a history of difficulties of using tampons or having cervical inspection for smears may be recalled. In cases of dyspareunia, the numerous gynecology etiologies must be considered for introital, vaginal, and deep pelvic pain.

The role of questionnaires as an adjunctive tool in diagnosis and assessment of severity and trouble caused by sexual problems in women is advocated by clinicians in the field. Some examples would include the Female Sexual Function Index (7), the Sexual Satisfaction Scale for Women (SSS-W; (8)), and the Scale for Quality of Sexual Function (QSF) which has been developed specifically as an outcome measure for therapies in men and women (9).

5.3. Examination and Investigation

There are few situations where a clinical examination would be contraindi-cated. An assessment of general constitution and cardiovascular status is essential. General inspection of the introital area and mons pubis is essential for localized pathology or evidence of local infection. The timing of any genital examination should be carefully considered and may be carried out by the general practitioner during routine screening procedures or as part of a specific therapeutic process (e.g., using the method employed by the Institute of Psychosexual Medicine).

Sexual aversion is often accompanied by autonomic symptoms, the patient experiencing a feeling of fear and anguish. It may not be evident to either the patient or the clinician until a routine vaginal examination (or gynecological examination) is attempted.

Assessment of androgen function, estrogen function, as well as prolactin and thyroid levels is a baseline measure in cases of HSSD and arousal disorder. For anorgasmia, evidence of autonomic neuropathy may be detected by a full blood count and folate/B12 and testosterone levels. In all cases, blood glucose estimation should be taken. The acidity of the vagina should be assessed with the normal pH less than 4.5. Assessment of vascular function using photoplethysmography and vaginal thermal clearance are more specialized procedures available only in secondary services. The reader is referred to a review by Nappi et al. (10).

5.4. Treatment Options

In most cases, the opportunity for individual psychotherapeutic work and couple psychotherapy will often be welcomed and useful in any package of care. Concurrent techniques of sex therapy including sensate focus are often beneficial. Information about sexual arousal, function, and treatments is easily available now with various self-help sites on the Internet and books, as well as instructional videotapes and DVDs. In HSSD where there is evidence of androgen deficiency, with the testosterone levels being within the lower quarter of the normal range (usually less than 0.9 nmol/l), consideration of androgen therapy may be appropriate, especially in the postmenopausal state. Adequate estrogenization is necessary with localized therapies equally helpful for vaginal atrophy and dryness where systemic effects are not desired. Androgen replacement is typically given in the form of subcutaneous pellets or more recently low doses of androgen gel although this is currently unlicensed. DHEA tablets are another source of precursor androgens. Other medications that may be beneficial include bupropion apomorphine and, in a postmenopausal woman, tibolone.

In arousal disorder where there are problems with lubrication and concomitant dryness with pain, the use of lubricants is highly recommended. There are a number of these that mimic the nature of vaginal fluid rather than using agents such as KY gel, which can be sticky. A more recent personal lubricant KY warming liquid is the first lubricant to be approved as a medical device by the FDA in the USA. Estradiol therapy may be appropriate (usually topically). Off-license medication may be useful to enhance congestion including PGE5 inhibitors, apomorphine, ephedrine, phentolamine (all off license). Sex aids and vibrators may be useful as may pelvic floor exercises, using the classic Kegel techniques (or modified). The Eros-CTD has also been shown to be beneficial in increasing blood flow to the genital area.

In orgasmic disorder, medications which may help lower the threshold for orgasm include ephedrine, bupropion, yohimbine and bethanecol (all off license). Where there is specific antidepressant-induced anorgasmia, cyproheptadine has been found to be helpful (as has yohimbine). The use of vibration and modified Kegel exercises may be beneficial. The role of cognitive behavioral therapy, particularly in promoting changes in attitudes in sexually relevant thoughts, is very relevant in this condition, as is self-exploration with desensitization and guided sexual self-stimulation.

In dyspareunia where gynecological conditions have been excluded or are managed concurrently, topical local anesthetics, estrogen therapy, and lubricants may be beneficial. Vaginismus is usually treated using sexual therapy and vaginal trainers and dilators.

It should also be noted that in the small number of women where there are intersex states, or at a later stage during adolescence where gender dysphoria is clearly identified and diagnosed, referral and provision of services within specialist care may be crucial to care.

Despite all this, it may be impossible with short consultation times or with limited clinical experience to feel confident to approach such matters. The physician–patient relationship is essential to uncover sexual difficulties and it is crucial for physicians to be aware of the importance that sexual well-being has for the quality of life and health for all women. Many problems will continue to be underdiagnosed or recognized. There are training opportunities available to clinicians (11) but recent surveys (12) would suggest that attempting to persuade clinicians, other than the interested few, would be counterproductive at least in delivery of care to patients. Raised awareness is important and clinically necessary. With the development of regional clinical services, this may become something less commonplace in the future, but at the moment many patients end up seeking help in primary clinical health care.

It can be seen from the above that there are occasions when clinicians, and in particular gynecologists, may need to refer to more specialist services. This may be when there are persistent sexual concerns, dissatisfaction, disorders, or dysfunction which the attending physician is unable to deal with. Certain interventions or psychological interpretations may be rejected or considered unhelpful by patients. This is not to say that the treatment offered is not correct or potentially effective, but just that the appropriateness or acceptability to the patient in the current clinical setting is less than optimal.

In order to ensure onward referral is successful, it is necessary to discuss with the patient your intention to refer. This may be by letter to established services or by encouraging the patient to make a self-referral to those agencies that will accept such. Self-referral agencies may include family planning services and genitourinary medicine services where there are psychosexual clinicians working within the service. Referral within the National Health Service (NHS) to sexual problem services will depend on local availability and awareness of such services. These may traditionally be based within gynecological, urological, or psychiatric health settings. Where no local services exist, the clinician is faced with either out-of-town referrals or recommendations to seek psychosexual and relationship therapy in the independent sector (through BASRT, http://www.basrt.org.uk, or the Institute of Psychosexual Medicine (IPM), http://www.ipm.org.uk).

Patients can usually expect to receive a letter from these services, regardless of where they are based, inviting them to attend for an appointment, which usually lasts 45–60 minutes. A leaflet outlining the services and the extent of services provided should be offered, and the invitation to attend with their partner is often encouraged. The promise of a nonjudgmental and empathic listening clinician, providing services which are private, confidential, and at a convenient time, is most likely to lead to high attendance rates. Whilst the various treatment options and effectiveness of clinical interventions across the field of sexual medicine is somewhat limited (outside the clinical field of erectile dysfunction and to a lesser extent rapid ejaculation), patients need to be assured that however personal they may feel their problems to be, all clinicians working within the NHS and affiliated to national associated groups such as IPM and BASRT adhere to a strict code of ethics and practice and regularly undertake supervision of their work. Such reassurance is often beneficial in ensuring patients keep their first appointment.

An ideal future development would forge closer links between experts in sexual medicine and psychosexual therapy and gynecologists, with the development of provision of services within one clinical setting that could facilitate interdisciplinary clinical care.

References

1. Laumann E, Paik A, Rose R. Sexual Dysfunction in the United States: prevalence and predictors (published erratum appears in JAMA 1999; 281: 1174) *JAMA* 1999; 281: 537–44.
2. Dunn KN, Croft PR, Hackett GI. Sexual problems: a study of the prevalence and need for health care in the general population. *Family Practice* 1998; 15(6): 519–524.
3. Moynihan R. The making of a disease: female sexual dysfunction. *BMJ* 2003; 326(7379): 45–47.
4. Masters WH, Johnson VE. *Human Sexual Response*. Boston: Little Brown; 1966.
5. Kaplan HS. *Disorders of Sexual Desire and Other New Concepts and Techniques in Sex Therapy*. New York: Brunner/Hazel Publications; 1979.
6. Basson R. Using a different model for female sexual response to address women's problematic low sexual desire. *J Sex Marital Ther* 2001; 27(5): 395–403.
7. Rosen R, Brown C, Heiman J, Leiblum S, Meston C, Shabsigh R, Ferguson D, D'Agostino R Jr. The Female Sexual Function Index (FSFI): a multidimensional self-report instrument for the assessment of female sexual function. *Journal of Sex and Marital Therapy* 2000; 26: 191–208.
8. Meston C, Trapnell P. Development and validation of a five-factor sexual satisfaction and distress scale for women: the Sexual Satisfaction Scale for Women (SSS-W). *Journal of Sexual Medicine* 2005; 2: 66–81.
9. Heinemann LA, Potthoff P, Heinemann K, Pauls A, Ahlers CJ, Saad F. Scale for Quality of Sexual Function (QSF) as an outcome measure for both genders? *Journal of Sexual Medicine* 2005; 2: 82–95.
10. Nappi R, Salonia A, Traish AM, van Lunsen RH, Vardi Y, Kodiglu A, Goldstein I. Clinical biologic pathophysiologies of women's sexual dysfunction. *Journal of Sexual Medicine* 2005; 2: 4–25.
11. Wylie K.R (2005) Becoming a sexologist in the United Kingdom. BMJ Careers, 15th Jan 2005, 23–24.
12. McFarland R., Wylie K.R. & Ridley J. Self help therapies within the NHS – providing a service for patients suffering with relationship difficulties. *Sexologies* 2005, 16, 29–37.

6
Disability, Normality, and Difference

Tom Shakespeare

> The use of the word normal poses a semantic problem. No end of misconceptions and lax thinking is caused by the belief in something called "normal man" or "normal human nature."
>
> *Theodosius Dobzhansky, 1962*

This chapter explores social and psychological aspects of disability, in the context of obstetrics and gynecology. First, I discuss concepts of normality and disability, exploring how values and contexts determine how those ideas are defined and experienced. Second, I look at three areas of practice: sexuality, parenting, and genetic screening. The field of disability studies has developed considerably in recent decades, primarily due to the activism of disabled people themselves (1–4). The world of medicine has, perhaps, been slow to engage with this new agenda. The assumption that disability is an individual health problem continues to dominate. While disabled people will often need medical intervention, a new relationship between disabled people and professionals is required in which disability is seen holistically, and disabled people are accepted as experts of their own lives.

6.1. Normality and Difference

Normality may be a "taken-for-granted" concept, but it is more complicated than it might at first appear (2). For example, normality might be taken to mean average, in the sense of a statistical mean. It could equate to what is conventional or common, in the sense of a statistical mode. It could mean "not extreme," in the sense of a statistical median. Broadly, "normal" conveys an idea about what is acceptable and natural—the status quo.

Normality is a concept with a history. The word "normal," in the sense of "standard, regular, or usual" was coined in 1840, followed by "norm" (1855), "normality" (1849), and "normalcy" (1857). Before this period, people sought perfection, rather than normality. For example, from Classical Greece, Plato's conception of "the forms" implied an ideal which people might aim at but would always fall short of. For example, Venus was the ideal of beauty.

A famous 1789 painting by Francois Andre Vincent in the Louvre Museum depicts the painter Zeuxis choosing as his model the most beautiful girls from the town of Crotona. It was thought that no woman was perfect, and therefore the painter chose the face of one, the hair of another, the body of a third, and so on, to represent the ideal.

The birth of statistics in the nineteenth century gave impetus to the notion of normality. Adolphe Quetelet (1796–1847) offered the notion of "l'homme moyen" or average man. This reflected the emergence of the bourgeoise, the middle class between the aristocracy and the workers or peasants, and their values. Whereas the ideal had been unattainable, the notion of the average implied that the majority of the population could be part of the norm. In Britain, the Royal London Statistical Society was founded in 1835, and the General Register Office in 1837. Statisticians such as Francis Galton, Karl Pearson, and R.A. Fisher were associated not just with the new mathematical concepts such as the bell curve and standard deviation, but also with ideas about eugenics. Social and scientific concern centered on outliers from normal distribution, in particular subnormal individuals and populations.

Understanding this history helps in deconstructing ideas about normality. First, it is clear that "normality" is a moving target. Looking at Anne Hathaway's cottage or medieval suits of armor or indeed the late twentieth century expansion in women's dress sizes demonstrates that Britons have had different physiques over the last 500 years. Second, many average values are in fact pathological. The average weight, blood pressure, and blood cholesterol values are unhealthy in many Western countries. It is clear that "normal" does not mean "healthy," and indeed that there is variability in how individuals attain health. Nor does "normal" equate to "natural": it is becoming "normal" for women to delay reproduction until mid or late thirties; it is becoming "normal" to have elective cesarean in some countries; it may even become "normal" to use assistive reproductive technologies. Normal is always a cultural and historical concept, and bodily normality differs for different individuals.

This counsels us to be careful in our thinking about "normal" people. In Western thought, it is taken for granted that normal human beings are healthy, independent, and rational. Many theories in politics and philosophy, as well as medicine rely on this assumption. Normality is defined as able-bodied. Yet perhaps this is a myth.

Within every life, there are periods of dependency. Typically, children and older people rely on the support of others. Those with responsibility for children or older people may themselves need the support of others. Everyone, when they are ill or injured, may require support and help. In complex modern societies based on division of labor, no one is fully independent. We rely on shops and buses and all sorts of other assistance every day of our lives. In other words, dependency or at best interdependency is normal for human beings. The good life depends on caring solidarity, in which families, neighbors, and local services are able to care for each other and provide necessary support to those who need help and those who help them. Over a lifetime, everyone finds themselves in both roles (3).

The polar distinction between normal and abnormal bodies and minds is misleading. People have a range of abilities and body types and personalities. Everyone has limitations. Everyone is vulnerable to injury and disease, and we will each inevitably die at some point. The term "temporarily able-bodied" reminds us that everyone is vulnerable to becoming disabled, through accident, disease or ageing. Impairment is a continuum, along which people move in both directions, not a matter of two separate groups of disabled and able-bodied people. Disability is a highly complex and diverse phenomenon, not a unitary concept. People are limited in different ways, through physical, sensory, intellectual limitation, and through mental illness; these states can be congenital or acquired, stable or fluctuating or degenerative, visible or invisible. Disability is complex and scalar, not absolute and unitary (5).

It is dangerous to generalize about disabled people, because impairment comes in so many forms, and because each individual reacts differently to their experience of impairment. The extent to which disability is a problem depends on the complex interplay between the individual's impairment and their personal resources for dealing with it, and the wider context of the social and physical environment in which they live. For many people living with impairment, particularly those born with their condition, disability is normal: they cannot imagine living in any other way, and they do not see their disability as a problem. There are many studies which demonstrate that disabled people very often rate themselves as having a good quality of life, even though to others they may appear to have a low quality of life.

6.2. Disability as a Human Rights Issue

Over recent decades, disabled people have mobilized to challenge the idea of disability as deficit or deviance. Political action to achieve civil rights has established disability as an issue of equal citizenship and equal opportunities, not as an individual problem to be solved by medicine (1).

In particular, disabled people have objected to the medicalization of their lives. Often, the solution to the problems which disabled people face is best achieved through barrier removal, not through treatment, rehabilitation or counseling. Clearly, disabled people often need medical interventions, but these will not always be related to their impairments, because disabled people have the same medical needs as nondisabled people.

Doctors are not the experts on disability, disabled people are. Histori-cally, disabled people have often not been consulted about their treatments, or their living choices, or other aspects of their daily lives. Parents, carers or professionals have dominated the lives of disabled people. Listening to disabled people is a very important principle. Almost all disabled people are capable of understanding options and expressing preferences. For example, there has been extensive work to support people with learning difficulties to express their views, and to turn written material into simple language or pictograms (6).

Disabled activists and academics argue that disabled people are not abnormal. They have normal needs—housing, education, employment, health, relationships—only these ordinary needs are not normally met or are met in ways which are "special" or segregated, not mainstream and ordinary. The goal for disability rights activists is independent or integrated living. In other words, disabled people want to live in the community and have control over their lives. This does not mean being able physically to do everything for oneself. It may mean employing personal assistants to help you achieve your own goals, in the way you prefer.

The problems which disabled people experience often do not originate in their impairments or illnesses. They usually arise from the way society fails to meet their needs, or places barriers in their way. This has led many disabled activists to argue that people are disabled by society, not their bodies. This approach is known as the "social model of disability." Others argue that it is important not to lose sight of the predicament which impairment itself presents. From this perspective, people are disabled by society as well as by their bodies. Disability operates at different levels and requires a range of responses: medical, psychological, social, and political.

One set of barriers which disabled people may face results from the attitudes or prejudice of others. These may be family members, who perhaps overprotect the disabled person; they may be professionals, who do not listen to the disabled person or impose their own solutions and values; they may be members of the public, who are ignorant, fearful, or hostile about disability. Disabled people can sometimes face abuse and mockery, as well as neglect.

Another set of barriers arises from lack of access to environments or services. People may have specific needs resulting from their sensory or mobility impairments. Lack of a ramp or lift or failure to provide information in different formats or sign language interpretation can unnecessarily disable people. Legislation such as the Disability Discrimination Act (1995) mandates barrier removal, yet still schools, hospitals, leisure and transport facilities often make it difficult for disabled people to use them.

Finally, there are barriers and difficulties arising from poverty. Discrimination in employment means that many disabled people, even disabled graduates, find it much harder to find work than nondisabled people. Those disabled people who are in work are often in jobs for which they are overqualified. Lack of flexibility makes it difficult to work part time or to move between living on benefits and mainstream employment.

Disabled people, particularly those who are unemployed, are consequently disproportionately likely to be living on low incomes and to be vulnerable to poverty. Disabled people often have extra costs as a result of their impairment or illness, such as equipment, heating, taxis, or assistance. Unlike older people, disabled people are not entitled to extra winter fuel payments, for example. Whereas other disadvantaged groups have improved their economic position over the last decade, disabled people have fallen further behind. Poverty makes people more vulnerable to disability, but it is also a consequence of disability.

Health professionals may be limited in what they can do to improve the wider situation for disabled people, outside the immediate clinical encounter. But they can learn to listen to disabled people and to talk directly to them, rather than their parent/carer/partner. Professionals can avoid the assumption that the disability is the problem which has led to the consultation. They can avoid being patronizing, instead treat the disabled person as they would any other patient, with respect and recognition for their individuality and humanity. Professionals can learn from disabled people as well as by sharing their own clinical expertise with them.

6.3. Disability and Sexuality

Turning to practical issues within obstetrics and gynecology, sex and gender may be an important starting point. There is a dominant and incorrect cultural assumption that disabled people must, as a consequence of their impairment, be either asexual or sometimes sexually deviant. This may arise from the tendency to infantilize disabled people. It may also reflect an older historical fear of disabled people reproducing their own kind, dating back to the eugenic movement of the late nineteenth and early twentieth centuries. Ideas about eugenics cast a long shadow over the disability/obs and gyn encounter. For example, people with learning difficulties continue to be at risk of involuntary sterilization.

The literature and practice which does engage with disabled sexuality tends to take a rather medicalized view. This focuses on the biological deficits or functional inabilities of disabled people and remedies such as Viagra or other medications or aids. Yet a social model perspective would suggest that the problem of disabled sexuality is less "how to do it" and more "who to do it with." A social barriers' approach would highlight social and psychological issues such as

- Lack of information and particularly sex education
- Confidence, self-esteem, and body image
- Venue access, transport, and social inclusion
- Money to pay for clothes, drinks, and socializing

In particular, many people make friends through university or employment. If disabled people are excluded from these settings, they may remain isolated and lonely. Abuse, and the legacy of abuse, remains a problem for many disabled people, particularly those with communication difficulties or who live in residential schools or institutions.

If professionals and policies are to enable sexuality, then new ways of thinking may be required. For example, ideas about normalization might suggest that the key is to enable disabled people to access gender and sexual roles in the same way as everyone else. But this obscures the possibility that disabled people might live their gender and sexuality rather differently from others. It may be preferable to respect and accommodate these differences.

For example, disabled people may have different, less stereotypical, ways of being men and women. One respondent to our survey of disability and sexuality (7) reported:

I think disability is a breed on its own, neither masculine or feminine.

Others felt that their masculinity was different due to their impairment: they were less macho and had closer relationships with women friends. Disabled people may also challenge mainstream ideas about body image and beauty. James Patridge, founder of the Changing Faces charity, has been quoted as saying:

I am never going to conform to society's requirements and I'm thrilled because I am blissfully released from all that crap. That's the liberation of disfigurement.

In some cases, disabled people may have different ways of having sex. Just as the threat of HIV forced gay men and others to think more imaginatively about sex, so the limitations of impairment mean that some disabled people have to reorient their sexual lives, perhaps away from penetrative sex and toward more adventurous and varied ways of achieving and giving pleasure. Others may rely on personal assistants to get them ready for sex and sometimes even need to use sexual surrogates or prostitutes to achieve sexual expression.

Acceptance of difference means being open to these variations in the way that some disabled people perform gender and sexuality or achieve intimacy or family life. Rather than imposing normality or normal expectations on disabled people, openness to difference offers a potential expansion of what is possible for all in these areas. The challenge to normality offers advantages as well as disadvantages.

6.4. Disabled Parents

For many disabled people, their aspirations can be summed up as "a job, a partner, and a family." In this, disabled people are exactly like everyone else. However, there may be medical and social barriers to reproduction. For example, people with some genetic conditions are infertile. Some disabled women may have problems during pregnancy or labor.

Yet possible medical problems are only part of the picture. After all, reproductive technology, donated gametes, cesarean section, or adoption can overcome many of the practical barriers to becoming a parent. What causes more problems for many would-be disabled parents is the ignorance and prejudice of others.

Despite extensive research showing that disabled women and men can operate safely and successfully as parents (8,9), health and social services agencies—and sometimes family members—sometimes fear that disabled people might put their children at risk or even inappropriately rely on or exploit their children in caring roles. But given appropriate support—for example, aids and adaptations or personal assistance—almost all disabled people can potentially care for children. There is no reason why disabled people cannot love and cherish their children, even if they find different ways of performing caring roles. Children themselves are very adaptable to different situations and love and value their parents, regardless of their disabilities.

6.5.   Disability and Screening

A third area where disability is an issue in obstetrics and gynecology is genetic testing and prenatal screening (10). This pertains both to clinical responses to disabled people who wish to reproduce and to nondisabled people who may be offered screening to detect pregnancies affected by genetic or developmental conditions.

Here too it is necessary to challenge assumptions about normality. There is no "normal" human genome, for example. It is the ubiquitous variation in genetic endowment that creates individuality. Mutation is the engine of natural selection. Each person has several hundred mutations in their genome and is a carrier of several recessive genetic conditions. The vast majority of disabled children are born to nondisabled parents. Moreover, even harmful genetic variations may depend on context: a single copy of the sickle cell allele is protective against the effects of malaria. Understanding the imperfections and variations in human genetics and human reproduction includes remembering that many conceptions result in abnormal chromosomes, leading to figures of 50–75% for early stage pregnancy loss. It also suggests that despite understandable ambitions to achieve the "perfect baby," there is no such thing. All babies, and people, are both perfect and flawed. The quest to eliminate disability through screening is ultimately doomed to failure. After all, while 1–2% of births are affected by congenital abnormality, between 12 and 20% of the population is disabled in some way.

Disabled activists and commentators have drawn attention to two linked issues in prenatal diagnosis (1,3,10). First, there is a danger of resurgent eugenics. This may arise from the failure to support informed consent. Maternity services have been effective in reducing maternal and infant mortality, but sometimes at the cost of a routinization which deprives prospective parents of the counseling and support they need to make fully informed decisions about testing and termination in pregnancy. Prospective parents should be supported to decline testing and to continue affected pregnancies, as well as to choose testing or termination. Families with disabled children should be welcomed and supported at every stage. Second, there is a linked argument that screening can express a negative message about disability and disabled people's lives. Scientific and medical language and cultural representation about disability and genetics have sometimes been discriminatory, inaccurate, or offensive.

The new knowledge which genetics offers has potential harms as well as benefits. In addition to information about congenital conditions, it is also possible to learn clues about late onset problems such as cancer, heart disease, and dementia. This raises questions about how much we want to know and where we should draw the line. Every individual is potentially at risk, which blurs the traditional division between disabled and nondisabled people. Genetic information is, in this sense, toxic knowledge, not least because it could potentially lead to discrimination. Faced by this brave new world, the idea of genetic solidarity may have value as a response to genetic reductionism or to any future eugenic drive to overcome difference and disability through genetic cleansing. Disabled people can take a lead in showing that people matter—and can contribute—regardless of their physical or intellectual endowment.

6.6. Summary

- "Normality" should be deconstructed to reveal its history and the context which informs judgments.
- Disability is a matter of equality and human rights: people are disabled by society as well as by their bodies.
- Listening to disabled people is essential for the partnerships which can ensure effective health improvement.
- Disabled people are sexual beings: services need to recognize sexual rights and help people develop intimate relationships in a safe and healthy context.
- Disabled people can be parents too: services need to be imaginative and constructive in supporting disabled families.
- Genetics will not solve the disability problem: informed consent is vital in screening, and genetic solidarity is necessary to combat potential discrimination.

References

1. Albrecht GA, Seelman K, Bury M, eds. *The Handbook of Disability Studies*. Thousand Oaks: Sage; 2001.
2. Davis L. *The Disability Studies Reader*. New York: Routledge; 1997.
3. Priestley M. *Disability: A Life Course Approach*. Cambridge: Polity; 2004.
4. Thomas C. *Female Forms*. Buckingham: Open University Press; 1999.
5. Shakespeare T. *Disability Rights and Wrongs*. London: Routledge; 2006.
6. Atkinson D, et al. *Good Times, Bad Times: Women with Learning Disabilities Telling Their Stories*. Worcester: BILD; 2000.
7. Shakespeare T, Gillespie-Sells K, Davies D. *The Sexual Politics of Disability*. London: Cassell; 1996.

8. Booth T, Booth W. *Parenting Under Pressure: Mothers and Fathers with Learning Difficulties*. Buckingham: Open University Press; 1994.
9. Olsen R, Clarke H. *Parenting and Disability: Disabled Parents' Experiences of Raising Children*. Bristol: The Policy Press; 2003.
10. Kerr A, Shakespeare T. *Genetic Politics: From Eugenics to Genome*. Cheltenham: New Clarion Press; 2002.

Web sites

Antenatal Screening Web Resource, http://www.antenataltesting.info.

Disability Parenting and Pregnancy International, http://www.dppi.org.uk.

Disabled Parents Network, http://www.disabledparentsnetwork.org.uk.

Partners in Practice (Disability Equality in Healthcare Education), http://www.bris.ac.uk/pip/.

Sexual Health Network, http://www.sexualhealth.com.

7
Cross-Cultural Issues in Gynecology and Obstetrics

Pittu Laungani[†]

> If you were to destroy in mankind the belief to immortality, not only love but every living force maintaining the life of the world would at once be dried up. Moreover, nothing then would be immortal; everything would be permissible.
>
> *Dostoevsky, Brothers Karamazov*
> *(Pt. 1, Bk. 1, Ch. 6)*

If for some inexplicable reason, no children—not a single child—were to be born for the next 100 years or longer, the human race would come an end. The earth would become a barren planet. No traces would remain. But short of a meteor the size of our planet crashing onto the earth, such an eventuality is unlikely to happen, unless of course a supremely powerful megalomaniac, of which there are quite a few scattered round the world, were to order nuclear weapons to be dropped all over the world, which would inevitably lead to *The End of History and the Last Man*—the chilling title of Francis Fukuyama's book (1). It is a possibility that does not bear consideration.

But children might well turn out to be our saviors. So long as children continue to be born there is hope. Children are the inheritors of the earth and, with it, their own future and the future of the world. By carrying the genes of their parents, children also perpetuate at a symbolic level—the immortality of their parents. For the parents know that even after their death, a part of them—a genetic "template"—will remain in their children who in turn will leave part of themselves in their children and so on. From among several motives for having one's own children, one of the strongest motives, if not the strongest, is *the desire for immortality*. The primeval fears and terrors of death that lurk in one's unconscious are so overwhelmingly powerful, as Becker (2), Kasterbaum (3), Kubler-Ross (4), Laungani (5), and several others have reminded us that *no one* likes to die and be forgotten, as though one had never existed. One wishes to live and be remembered forever—if not in body, certainly in spirit. We all, each in our own way, wish to leave "our footprints on the sands of time."

[†] Dr Laungani's post was honorary (he is now deceased)

Although the wish and the desire to have children is fairly universal, cultural norms and expectations play a major role as to whether a child shall be born out of wedlock or within it or aborted; the age at which it is acceptable for a woman (or a teenager) to conceive; whether the expectant mother should be examined and delivered by a male or a female gynecologist or by a trained midwife (or by an unqualified but experienced *dai*); whether it is preferable, within family expectations to have a male or a female child; and so on. In several Eastern cultures, including Pakistan, India, Bangladesh, Sri Lanka, Malaysia, and Indonesia, the notion of "auspicious" (*shudh kal*) and "inauspicious" (*ashudh kal*) time of birth is also given very serious consideration. Beliefs in astrology and the malevolent and benevolent influences of planets on one's life are strongly ingrained in the psyche of people from most Eastern cultures. A careful record of the exact time of birth is maintained, which then forms the basis for casting a detailed and meticulous horoscope of the child, which "maps out" so to speak the present and the future of the infant. The readings from the horoscope often serve as a guide to a variety of related factors: what name the infant shall be given, how the infant shall be looked after, by whom, and the kinds of religious rites, rituals, and ceremonies that would need to be undertaken to propitiate the gods to ensure a healthy growth and development of the child. In some instances at the behest of the family priest (whose power over the parents is not inconsiderable), the infant may be brought up for the first few years not by the mother but perhaps by the grandmother, until such time as is deemed necessary.

(In the case of my own family members, my oldest sister delegated the care and the bringing up of her son to my mother because her first two children had died soon after their birth, and it had been prophesied by our family priest that the next child, if it were to survive, would need to be brought up by a close family member but not by the mother of the child. In accordance with religious dictates, the child was looked after and brought up by my mother until he reached puberty. The child survived and is now in his late fifties, a grandfather. It should be noted that regardless of any hard evidence to support the truth of such prophesies it is difficult for believers to be convinced otherwise.)

I would dearly love to consider the salient cultural beliefs, attitudes, and values of parents from different cultures toward marriage, dowry, pregnancy, prenatal care, delivery, the child's gender, abortion, IVF treatment, and so on. Given the constraints of space, such an action would take me beyond the scope of the chapter. To incorporate the unique features of a variety of Eastern cultures, I shall focus on *India*—the largest multicultural and democratic country in the world.Its present population hovers at around 1.1 billion. It is best to describe India as a conglomeration of small countries within one large country. To an untrained eye, India might seem like a vast monocultural country but a closer examination reveals a different picture. One is struck more by the differences than by the similarities! To the 40 officially recognized languages spoken, one might add over a 1000 dialects, making easy communication difficult, to say the least. The differences also extend to climate, geographical terrain, skin color, physiognomy, food preferences,

social relationships, levels of education, affluence, poverty, religious differences and groupings, patterns and styles of worship, and so on. But despite
the vast differences what unites the country and its people are their salient
beliefs, attitudes, and values, their family and extended family structures, their
network of social relationships, and the politico-legal system codified in the
written Indian Constitution.

Let us now turn to a few culture-specific issues, which have a strong bearing
on the gynecological problems with which this chapter is concerned.

7.1. Marriage in Eastern Cultures

Marriages in general are arranged in India, Pakistan, Bangladesh, Nepal,
Malaysia, Sri Lanka, Indonesia, Thailand, and other South Asian countries.
The emphasis in most of these countries is on *early marriages*, which is in
keeping with the cultural expectations that the girl will remain a virgin until
her marriage. A marriage is seen as "destiny" for nearly all women in these
cultures. Women who never marry are seen as an oddity. In orthodox Hindu
and Islamic families, the prospective bride and bridegroom are seldom *allowed
to* question parental decisions. It is their duty to obey. In the past, the bride
and the bridegroom were not even allowed to see or talk to each other until
after the marriage ceremony had been performed. The idea of courtship was—
and still is—frowned upon, but *modernity* has led to a reluctant acceptance
among the educated classes in many of the countries.

Hindu marriages are considered to be sacred and binding. Muslim marriages
are seen as a contract, a covenant (*mithaq*), which can be easily revoked by
the husband but not by the wife because her right to a divorce is limited.
Ali (6) points out that although a marriage is referred to as a contract, it is
according to the Koran a union of two souls which are one in essence.

7.2. What the Stars Foretell

The arrangement of a marriage in general is based on a careful matching
of horoscopes of the prospective "boy" and the "girl", and of course their
individual social standing and their caste status. Beliefs in astrology are
strongly ingrained within the Eastern psyche: the belief that one's life is influenced by the nine planets, referred to as *grahas*, headed by the sun is widely
prevalent in India (7). A carefully cast horoscope reveals a person's fate (8).
The heavenly configuration of planets at the moment of birth is seen as a
determinant of one's life chances. Such astrological formulations permit explanations and the "acceptance" of untimely deaths and sudden deaths, including
suicides and murder.

The expectation that the bride will be virgin is taken as given. It might
be of interest to learn that among many orthodox Muslims in Pakistan and
India and in some other Arab countries, on the day following the nuptial

night a white bedsheet is paraded through the streets amid much rejoicing provided of course the bedsheet contains blood stains, which indicates not only the consummation of the marriage but, *more importantly*, establishes the virginity of the bride. But the custom is practiced more in its breach than in its observance.

In many villages in India, particularly those in North India, the parents do not shy away from arranged betrothals of their very young children, and in some instances even infants! And barring any unforeseen events or mishaps, the betrothals are binding and the marriages are solemnized when the children reach marriageable age—or even earlier. Child marriages too, although banned in India, are still practiced particularly in parts of North India, including Rajasthan, Madhya Pradesh, Bihar, and Haryana.

The priest or the Imam involved in casting horoscopes remains in an impregnable position, regardless of the future outcome of the arranged marriage. If the marriage "succeeds" within the accepted norms of the social and cultural system, the priest takes the credit for his accurate predictions. If the marriage fails—and sad mishaps occur within the couple's family, the priest merely attributes factors such as an evil eye, a curse, past karma, bewitchment, unforeseen factors, such as sudden death in the family, that account for the mishap.

7.3. The Dowry (Dahej) System

Dowries—euphemistically referred to as "bride-price" (9,10,11), play an important role in arranged marriages. Among the middle and upper class and caste Hindus, dowries have a strong religious sanction. In recent years, dowries have also extended to groups such as peasants, artisans, and other lower castes. Dowries may be in the form of land, clothes, jewellery, household goods, and cash. The girl's parents are expected to provide the dowry, which is often negotiated in advance. In many cases, the demand is so high that it leads to the financial ruin of the girl's parents. Even after the agreed dowry payments have been made, further demands are made upon the bride's parents soon after the marriage. The demand for dowries has increased significantly in the last 25 years or so, and naked, unashamed greed has replaced common human decencies (12). In extreme cases, the discontented parents of the son wreak vengeful vendettas on the young bride, often leading to her death. Cases referred to as "dowry deaths" or "accidental deaths" of women generally through burning are by no means uncommon in India. Sadly, such monstrous crimes do not always come to light because of conspiracies of silence among the family members and, in extreme cases bribery, which prevents any serious investigations.

One might have wished to believe that the iniquitous dowry system at least in the West might have shown a decline. That, sadly, is not the case. There is a mistaken belief among Westerners that as a result of living (or being born) in Western countries, the second or even the third generation settlers would have imbibed Western values and as a result discarded the dowry practice. If anything, it has been known to increase both in England and in other Western countries. While a villager in India or in Pakistan might have settled for a cow, cash, and a few items of jewellery as part of dowry, in England the demand for dowries has taken a different form: a furnished apartment, a luxury car, a wardrobe crammed with designer clothes, cash, and jewellery are not uncommon demands made upon the bride's parents.

7.4.   Parental Attitudes Toward Male and Female Children

Among Hindu parents, the birth of a male child in a family is considered to be a blessing, for a variety of reasons. First, it ensures the perpetuation of the family name. Second, the son is seen as an economic asset and upon marriage would "bring in" a handsome dowry. Third, he would also be expected to support and look after his parents when they become old and frail. Fourth, it is the son, who on the death of his parents, is expected to perform all the funeral rites and also light the funeral pyre, to ensure the safe passage and the eventual repose of their soul (13). While boys are pampered, given more food, and accorded more privileges, girls are often brought up on a relatively strict regime, and in some cases may be given leftovers. Such gender differentiation extends into the area of food, nutrition, the quantity and quality of the food apportioned to the boys and the girls. In many parts of North India, even milk is generally given to boys and not to girls.

The birth of a daughter is treated with mixed feelings and even with some misgivings. As Kakar (14) points out, the daughter in a Hindu family hardly ever develops an identity of her own. Upon birth, she is seen as a daughter; she is expected to remain a virgin, chaste, and pure; upon reaching marriageable age she may be seen as an economic liability because of the dowry she is expected to take with her to her husband's home.

Girls, right from an early age are socialized into becoming virtuous. Virtue consists of obedience (initially to parents and then to the husband and the husband's family), doing one's duty, truthfulness, prayer, and ensuring the health and security of the husband and the family—and producing male heirs in the family. However, in educated and enlightened families, parents bring up their children without any gender differentiations; they see it as part of their religious duty—their *dharma*—to ensure that their daughters are cared for, educated, and handsomely married.

7.5.   Infant Mortality

Rates of infant mortality in Eastern countries in general tend to be much higher than those in Western countries, as listed in Table 7.1.

What emotional and psychological effects do such high infant mortality rates have on the parents? And how do they cope with such traumatic experiences?

TABLE 7.1. Deaths per 1000 births in the first year

USA	6.30	Pakistan	91.86
UK	5.78	Bangladesh	69.68
Sweden	3.91	India	60.81
Germany	5.14	Indonesia	57.30

There are several culture-specific factors, which come to their assistance and enable them to cope with the death of their child (or children):

1. For a variety of reasons, not the least of which is poverty, people in Eastern cultures are brought up with the expectation that not all the children born to them will survive and that many will die within the first year of birth.
2. Death in Hinduism and Buddhism is explained in terms of the Law of Karma, and in Islam in terms of the Will of Allah. It is preordained. Destiny plays an important part in life and death. Illness and disease are explained not only in medico-legal terms but also in religious and spiritual terms. The two sets of explanations, religious and scientific, exist side by side, impervious to logical contradictions.
3. Most marriages, as has been pointed out, take place when the couples are barely out of their teens. The death of a first or second child, or even a third child, within the first year of its birth does not make it impossible for the female to conceive and have more children subsequently.
4. The bereaved couples often find comfort and solace within their close-knit family and extended family network.

Given the limitations of space a comprehensive exposition of contrasting worldviews, though desirable, is not possible. However, a few points need to be made before we examine the problem from a Western perspective:

1. It is not always recognized—least of all by politicians—that when people emigrate to another culture they do not jettison their imbibed cultural values at the airport, acquiring overnight the ones of their host country. No one in that sense ever travels light. Like the prisoners in Plato's cave, one is handcuffed to one's culture by socio-historical forces.
2. Lessons from past history teach us that any attempts to enforce a rapid change on values is unlikely to succeed. One might, in this context, recall the naïve and absurd proclamations made by the Home Secretary of UK that immigrants to the United Kingdom would need to learn the National Anthem as a test of their loyalty to Britain. One wonders how many of the native-born British would be able to recite the National Anthem! Besides, one could teach a parrot to recite the National Anthem! The fact that the pronouncement was in serious conflict with liberal notions of multicultur-alism and cultural diversity was ignored. Luckily, saner counsels prevailed and the idea evaporated in paroxysms of hilarity.

3. The value differences, which separate Westerners from Easterners, are far—far greater than the similarities that might enjoin them. They have been discussed in great depth elsewhere (5,13,15). One might at a superficial level acquire the "trappings" of another culture, but the core of one's personality or one's psyche remains stubbornly resistant to rapid changes. We carry our culture as a tortoise carries its shell. When danger threatens, like tortoises we withdraw into our shell. But if you break the shell, you destroy the tortoise.

4. The second and the third generation immigrants have learned to make the necessary adjustments to acquire what Roland (16) refers to as a bicultural personality, which often acts as a survival strategy. But at the same time, they succeed in retaining their inherited cultural norms and values.

Let us now consider how a Western doctor might relate to a patient in the following situations.

1. **Examination of the patient**

   For a *male* doctor to carry out a vaginal examination of a patient from Eastern cultures is likely to be met with strong resistance, for such an examination would involve an infringement of strongly ingrained cultural taboos. No outsider, other than the woman's husband, is permitted to see her body. Whether the woman concerned is a Hindu, a Muslim or a Buddhist, whether she is a young bride or a middle-aged woman, she would be extremely reluctant to permit a male doctor to carry out an intimate bodily examination. Such taboos are very strong and are not easily discarded.

   In this connection, you might recall the hilarious opening scene in Salman Rushdie's novel, *Midnight's Children*, where a Kashmiri doctor, Dr Aadam Aziz, is hastily summoned to examine the daughter of a rich landowner—only because the female doctor is on holiday. Much to the doctor's astonishment he is asked to examine only the affected part of the girl's body, which is displayed through a 7 in. perforated gap in a curtain! Under no circumstances is he allowed to see the patient. Over several visits he gets to examine several parts of her body, but never the whole person. It is only after Dr Aadam Aziz marries her that he is able to feast his eyes on her in her pristine purity.

   Among the Chinese too, a similar system prevailed. To prevent an examination of a naked female body, the Chinese carved beautiful models made of ivory (now seen as expensive collectors items) of the naked female body, which the woman took with her when she went to see the doctor. The model allowed her to pinpoint the exact location of the pain in the body. They were known as *Doctors Ladies* or *Dames de Medecin* (Pawson, personal communication).

2. **Attitudes to contraception and sterilization**

   In most countries in South East Asia, particularly among the poorer sections of the population, there is considerable ignorance related to the use of condoms and other contraceptives; consequently their usage is both limited and haphazard. At any rate the desire to have a male child overrides economic, social, and health-related considerations. Several initiatives by various governments over the past 50 years have failed to control the rapid growth of population in Eastern cultures. Both contraception and sterilization come into play only *after* the couple has succeeded in having two or three *male* children, not before. Having more than two or three male children is seen as a hedge against infant mortality. Female sterilization is the most popular method of birth prevention, despite the fact that male sterilization is safer, quicker, and less expensive (17).

3. **Attitudes to premarital sex**

   The very idea of premarital sex is considered sinful and abhorrent among Hindus, Buddhists, Jains, and even Christians. In keeping with Vedic teachings, the lives of three upper-caste Hindus in ancient times were structured around four distinct stages: (1) the celibate student (*brahmachari*), (2) the married householder (*grahasti*), (3) the accumulator of wealth (*artha*), and (4) the retired, detached individual (*vanaprasthya*) devoted to spiritual pursuits. Among Muslims too the notion of premarital sex is seen as being reprehensible and, depending on the orthodoxy of the family concerned, severe and even inhuman chastisements (e.g., stoning) may be perpetrated upon the "miscreants"—particularly upon the female who has strayed away.

4. **Sexual taboos related to intercourse**

   The issues of premarital sexual relations have already been discussed above. Restrictions to sexual intercourse usually come into play under a few conditions, one of them being when the woman is menstruating. A menstruating woman is seen in many cultures as being in a state of hygienic and spiritual "impurity." Despite unwarranted pressures from her husband, she is at great pains to avoid any sexual intercourse during that particular period. The fact that she is menstruating becomes known to virtually all the members of the household because her state of impurity excludes her from participating in all the domestic activities, including cooking, cleaning, and more importantly in religious activities at home or outside. In many orthodox Hindu homes, she remains isolated from all domestic activities. The care of her own children is delegated to other members of the family. Since the burden of work is taken away from her, she looks forward to her periods because it allows her to have a few days of complete rest at home. It does not take long for all the members of the household, including the children at home, to acquire an understanding of menstruation.

   Much to the chagrin of the husband, further taboos also come into play when the woman becomes pregnant. A tussle of wits and wills occurs between the spouses. What the outcome of such tussles has been I have never been able to discover.

5. **Abortion and feticide**

   In India, it is estimated that about 6 million abortions take place every year, of which 2 million are spontaneous and 4 million are induced. Of the induced abortions, between 500,000 and 600,000 are legal and the rest are estimated to be illegal abortions. The preference for boys has also skewed the gender ratio in India. The number of girls per 1000 boys declined in the country from 945 in 1991 to 927 in 2001, according to government figures.

Contemporary research in medical science has now made it possible to determine, among other things, the gender and any abnormalities of embryos. Such facilities are also available in large private hospitals in major cities in India. What is even more distressing is the fact that many private commercial diagnostic organizations with ultrasound scanners and other equipment which detect the sex of a child advertise their services with brazen confidence:

SPEND 500 RUPEES NOW AND SAVE 50,000 RUPEES LATER

The 500 Rupees refers to the cost of the abortion and 50,000 Rupees, as one would have guessed, refers to the dowry, which the parents would be expected to pay if their daughter were to live and reach marriageable age. These methods are becoming increasingly available in rural areas of India, fuelling fears that the trend toward the abortion of female fetuses will continue to increase dramatically. The ethics of such practices, to say the least, is questionable.

7.6. Conclusion

This chapter does not claim to offer a comprehensive account of the cross-cultural issues related to women's health, gynecology and obstetrics. There are several areas, for example, female circumcision, unplanned adolescent pregnancies, attitudes to IVF treatment, HIV and AIDS, detection of genetic abnormalities, which remain untouched. The research literature in all these areas is fairly extensive. To do justice to all these issues, which would also include the ethical and moral factors, lies beyond the scope of the chapter.

The purpose of the chapter has been to provide a platform from which gynecologists and obstetricians, unfamiliar with the cultural problems of Asians living in Britain, will acquire a fundamental background into their beliefs, attitudes, and values. It is hoped that such knowledge will enable them to work more effectively not only with their patients, but in tandem with the Asian gynecologists and obstetricians in Britain.

References

1. Fukuyama F. *The End of History and the Last Man*. New York: The Free Press; 1992.
2. Becker E. *The Denial of Death*. New York: Free Press Paperbacks; 1973.
3. Kasterbaum R. *The Psychology of Death*. 3rd ed. London: Free Association Books; 2000.
4. Kubler-Ross E. *On Death and Dying*. London: Tavistock Publications; 1969.

5. Laungani P. *Understanding Cross-Cultural Psychology*. London: Sage Publishers; 2006.
6. Ali MM. *The Religion of Islam*. Delhi: Motilal Banarasidass Publishers; 1961.
7. Madan TN. *Non-renunciation: Themes and Interpretations of Hindu Culture*. Delhi: Oxford University Press; 1987.
8. Fuller CJ. *The Camphor Flame: Popular Hinduism and Society in India*. Princeton, NJ: Princeton University Press; 1992.
9. Dube L. *Women and Kinship: Comparative Perspectives on Gender in South and South East Asia*. New York: United Nations University Press; 1997.
10. Srinivas MN. *Some Reflections on Dowry*. London: Oxford University Press; 1984.
11. Upadhyay CB. Dowry and women's property in coastal Andhra Pradesh. *Contrib Indian Sociol*. 1990;24(1).
12. Uberoi P. *Family, Kinship and Marriage in India*. Oxford: Oxford University Press; 1993.
13. Laungani P. Family life in India. In: Jaipaul L, Roopnarine, Uwe Gielen, eds. *Families in Global Perspective*. Boston: Aylln & Bacon; 2005.
14. Kakar. S. *The Inner World: A Psychoanalytic study of Children and Society in India*. Delhi: Oxford University Press; 1981.
15. Laungani P.*Asian Perspectives in Counselling and Psychotherapy*. London: Bruner-Routledge; 2004.
16. Roland A. *Cultural Pluraliism and Psychoanalysis*. New York: Routledge; 1988.
17. Bhatia JC. Ideal number and sex preference of children in India. J Family Welfare. 1978;24:3–16.

8
The Family

Ken Daniels

8.1. Introduction

How does a chapter on the family come to be included in a book designed primarily for obstetricians and gynecologists? Given that the primary focus in obstetrics and gynecology is the female patient and assisting her to "have" a child, consideration of the family may seem tangential and therefore not a high priority for the busy professional. Of course, it is the female who is seeking to conceive and subsequently to give birth, but in order for this to occur, a male must be involved. The degree of involvement may vary and for some lesbian couples or single women there may be a desire to minimize this involvement, but the sperm of a male is always a necessary prerequisite for conception. When a male and a female decide to "have" a child, it is a joint decision and it is they, as a couple, who are wishing to have a child. All the issues that arise from that decision are issues for both of them, although they may well experience and respond to those issues differently (1). Recognizing the role and psychosocial significance of the male will contribute to more holistic and effective intervention with the female partner (2). Such recognition requires professionals to extend their boundaries and thinking to look beyond the person in front of them, the so-called "patient." This chapter argues for extending the boundaries and thinking even further by taking into consideration the family that will be created as a result of medical intervention. This is because in most societies "having" a child means a change of status from couple to family. Equally, not being able to "have" a child and become a family raises important issues for the would-be parents and for the social networks of which they are a part. In almost all societies family status is accorded to those who are a parent/s and their child/ren. Greater knowledge of infertility and its psychosocial impact and knowledge concerning developments in assisted human reproduction (AHR) designed to overcome infertility are an increasingly important part of gynecology and subsequently obstetrics. AHR interventions not only "treat" the female "patient" and her partner, where there is one, but also lead to the creation and building of families in different ways (3). Different should not imply better or worse, but simply difference. Factors associated with building families in different ways are important to reflect on, as they impact not only on the treatment stage, but also very significantly on the health and well-being of the family. Extending the boundaries from female patient to the couple who would be parents to the family that will result is challenging. It requires an understanding of what is meant by family, who is regarded as family, and how notions of the family are changing. There is also a need to consider how developments in AHR and particularly the use of donated gametes or embryos impact on our understandings of family. All of these areas are discussed in this chapter, which will conclude with a consideration of some implications of this knowledge for professionals working in this field.

8.2. What and Who Is a Family?

Archard (4) has said, "The family is one of the great, enduring institutions of organized human life. Indeed, it has persisted over history across extremely different kinds of society and culture" (p. 65). Despite its endurance, readers of this book will be very aware of how families now come in a variety of forms. From a traditional view that a family consisted of two heterosexual parents and one or more children who were biologically or genetically their offspring, there has been a move to embrace within the notion of family parents who are not heterosexual, one parent only, and children who are not biologically or genetically the offspring of one or both parents. This movement from the traditional to what might be described as modern has been the focus of much debate. Some of the debates focus on moral considerations, namely that the traditional family is the only "right" family form and that for some this is the God-given plan and those who seek to change or modify this are "wrong." In other debates the focus is on whether the traditional family form is "better" than any alternative. This extends particularly to concerns for the welfare and best interests of the children. It has been argued that children who are born as a result of AHR procedures are likely to be harmed or damaged in some way. A central focus in the commissions of enquiry that were set up around the world following the first birth as a result of in vitro fertilization (IVF) was a concern for the health and welfare of the resultant children. A third set of debates centers on what I would describe as the "normal" versus the "abnormal" or "natural" versus "unnatural." Because of the emphasis on normality and natural—with their positive overtones—anything that differs or diverges from these positions is seen to be "less than natural/normal" and a less-valued position.

Behind these debates lies the issue of the relative importance and relationship between the biological and the social as the base for family. Early anthropologists who have studied families and kinship for long used the biological relationship as the starting point for their studies (5). It was Scheinder (6–8) who began to challenge biological connectedness as the basic assumption/premise of family and kinship. The variety of family forms, now so much a part of Western societies, shows that families need not be biologically related. Finkler (9) has said, "...a good argument could be made that the new reproductive technologies have done more than anything else to call into question our traditional understanding of family and kin" (p. 236) and hence we return to the involvement of medicine, and particularly gynecology, with the family.

Elsewhere (10) I have written that "A common and traditional assumption is that being a 'family' means that a 'blood tie' exists and that such blood ties imply that family members will be closer and their relationships more significant than the relationships they have with non-family" (p. 265). A common saying "blood is thicker than water" symbolically reflects this viewpoint. It was difficult for anthropologists to move from this position, often described as the natural position, to acknowledge that many families not linked genetically were functioning as families and carrying out the tasks of being a family. The recognition of a social, in contrast to a biological, basis for "being family" and understanding family connectedness has been slow to emerge. The slowness may in part be due to the debates discussed earlier, and particularly the emphasis on the natural (biological connectedness) being morally superior. What is clear is that families in this generation are formed in many different ways from previous generations. Such new forms of the family continue, however, to fulfil the traditional functions of families, namely loving and nurturing their children. The family tasks have not changed, but the family forms have.

8.3. The Impact of Developments in Medicine on Family and Kinship

Grace and Daniels (under editorial review) have said, "Just when families in the west are becoming more diverse, more 'blended', less reliant on the assumed biological precursor of 'blood ties' throughout the latter part of the twentieth century this liberal pluralism is being challenged by an increased emphasis on the medical importance of genetic connectedness." The emphasis on genetic connectedness has arisen from the research and information that is now available (and increasing at a rapid rate) concerning the importance of genes in the alleviation of disease. The discovery of a new gene related to a particular illness/condition is frequently portrayed by the media as having the potential to eliminate that illness and therefore to extend the life span. Genes are inherited and it is therefore increasingly important to know one's family history. That family history is of course the biological family history and not the social history. One of the implications of this move is that genetic connectedness is seen to be very significant. Every time doctors ask patients if there have been other family members who have been treated for or died as a result of a particular illness they are emphasizing the importance of the biological connections as the foundation of family. For those patients who are in a family that is not at all or only in part genetically connected, there is likely to be the feeling that they are "different," they do not fit the norm and therefore are deviant. For those persons who have been deceived about their genetic connections—those conceived as a result of their parents receiving infertility treatment which utilized third party gametes, those children who were born as a result of a relationship that has not been declared to the child or perhaps to the partner— they will almost certainly give the history of the parents they understand to be biological parents, when this is not the case. This may well place them at considerable risk. Parents of a DI-conceived adolescent once told me of their dilemma when their son lay seriously ill in hospital from an unknown cause. They had not disclosed the DI to their son. In front of the adolescent the doctor asked for the family history. The parents experienced great conflict, partly because they did not have medical information about the semen donor and partly because to share this information with the doctor in front of their son would, they felt, have been damaging to the family relationships.

It is the emphasis on genes and biological connectedness that has led Finkler and colleagues (9,11) to argue that we are seeing the medicalization of family and kinship in the West. Family and kinship have moved from a biological base only to the recognition of a biological and social base, and now with these new developments the emphasis is swinging back to a recognition of the biological as dominant and by implication the "natural" and "right."

The field of gamete and embryo donation within AHR provides an interesting example of the dilemmas associated with biological and social constructions of family and kinship. This field of AHR has been traditionally characterized by secrecy with parents not sharing their use of DI with their children or their families and social networks (12). Parents were usually advised to adopt this position of secrecy by medical practitioners. One of the reasons for taking this stand was that by doing so parents could appear to be "normal," that is pretend that their child was the genetic offspring of both parents. In this connection the matching of the physical characteristics of the donor with the infertile partner (in the case of gamete donation) was designed to avoid physical differences being observable, as such differences could have to be explained. The effect of this was to reinforce the view that biological was the natural and valued way of being family and that social connectedness was of less value. It needs to be noted that the stigma associated with infertility was also a contributing factor (13).

Those who have challenged the secrecy surrounding family building using gamete donation (14,15) have argued that secrecy has negative impact on all the involved parties. Part of the means of changing this culture of secrecy has been to encourage parents to see this means of family building as valid, rather than deviant (16). There have been attempts to normalize family building using third party gametes (17). This challenges the dominance of the biological as the only and legitimate means of family building. This is not to deny that there are significant and powerful differences between family building with parents' own gametes and with gametes supplied by someone outside the committed partners. An Australian parent once sought to sum this up when he said, "It wasn't our ideal way of having a family but it is our ideal family" (3).

The major arguments for changing the culture concerning gamete donation have been psychological ones: the rights and needs of the children (18), the negative impact of family secrets, and challenging the stigma associated with infertility (19,20). What is now intriguing is that with the increasing importance of knowing one's genetic history, another argument—a biological one—can be added to the calls for a more open approach to third party reproduction. In the example of the parents with the seriously sick child quoted earlier, there was a need to have access to the family history of the semen donor. Because this was not available (it is almost always available in New Zealand now with the donor's family health history being given to the parents), the child was placed at significant risk. Whereas many doctors at conferences and symposia argued that the psychological reasons for being open about DI were not based on research or that the likely psychological damage from openness was greater than from secrecy, it is hard to imagine, in the light of the increasing importance of knowledge concerning genetic history that such doctors would argue for placing offspring deliberately at risk because of a lack of knowledge.

Within third party reproduction the debates between doctors (and others) advocating secrecy, and counselors (and others) advocating openness and sharing of information lies a difference of views concerning how family and kinship are viewed. Secrecy can be equated with pretending that there is a biological connection because this is seen to be the norm, natural, and valued. To use third party reproduction is therefore classified as deviant and of less value. Openness and the sharing of information on the other hand can be equated with viewing families that are partially or not at all genetically linked as being as valued as biologically based families.

The growing emphasis on the importance of genes in health and illness is a major challenge to doctors involved in gamete and embryo donation and those other procedures, for example, IVF and surrogacy that utilize donated gametes or embryos. Such doctors are confronted with the need to think beyond the female "patient" in front of them and the couple, if there is a partner, to the child and family that will hopefully exist because of their intervention/treatment.

The way in which the doctor talks to the patient/patient couple especially concerning the sharing of information with future offspring will almost certainly reflect their view of what type of family is natural, normal, accepted, and valued. Do they view this form of family building as inferior, because the child will not be related genetically to one or both parents, or do they see this as a different way of family building—not one, however, that heterosexual couples would normally choose—which recognizes that the social basis of family and kinship is a legitimate partner to the biological basis enjoyed by most families.

The procedures of AHR are designed to respond to and overcome infertility. Infertility of course pre-dates AHR and it is interesting to consider Finkler's (9) views regarding the medicalization of family and kinship from this perspective. Prior to AHR, adoption was the chief means of responding to infertility.

Families who adopted children were of course socially rather than biologically based. They were accepted as families, in that they functioned as families, providing love and nurture for the children. Adoption has, however, never provided the challenge to the biological dominance of family and kinship that AHR has. I would suggest that this is in part due to the respective systems within which adoption and AHR fall. Adoption policy and practice falls within the domain of the health services. Finkler (9) is almost certainly correct when he asserts that the new reproductive technologies have done more than anything else to question the traditional understanding of family and kinship. Why is it that the new reproductive technologies achieved this, when adoption—which was also a response to infertility and led to socially based families—did not have this impact? Why did we not see writers arguing that adoption has led to the questioning and traditional understandings of family and kin? After all the outcome, in terms of families, has been the same. Two explanations seem possible. The first relates to the relative status of health and welfare services. Health and medicine have always enjoyed a higher social status than welfare, social work, and counseling. The second is the extensive publicity and with it a mixture of fascination and anxiety, that has accompanied the scientific and medical developments associated with AHR. The medicalization of family and kinship, not only in relation to AHR but also, and perhaps more powerfully, in relation to the significance of new findings in relation to genes, means that every member of society is potentially affected. The new findings and developments are almost certainly shaping thoughts about kinship and family. We now turn to how this may impact on health professionals and particularly doctors.

8.4. Some Implications for Professionals

The concluding section of this chapter seeks to raise some practical implications arising from the foregoing discussion. Three major implications are outlined.

The first of these is the need to address the issue of who is the patient. Traditionally it has been the person who has been referred and is being seen. Most referrals will be of an individual. However, in the case of infertility it is increasingly likely that it will be a couple who is being referred. The challenge of extending the boundaries from the female to the couple and then to the family that will exist if a child is born requires a "mind shift" on the part of the professional. The inclusion of a consideration of the family that may be created means that account is being taken of the welfare of the child or best interests of the child that is now an established dimension of social policy and legislation concerning AHR. A child's welfare can only be assessed in the context of the family of which it will be a part. Such an approach also means that the professional is considering past, present, and future. No professional considers intervention without gathering information concerning past history.

A consideration of the potential family also means actively considering a future perspective. What implications and issues will arise, from this particular intervention, for the family becomes a matter for consideration.

The second implication is to consider how the changes in understanding of family are likely to impact on interaction with those whom the health professional is working with. If some doctors, for example, hold the view that a biologically based family is natural and therefore superior, their attitudes to an infertile couple who need to use third party gametes, may be one of proposing this form of treatment as being of less value. If they encourage the would-be parents to keep the use of donated gametes a secret, they are in effect encouraging the parents to view this as a shameful treatment, something they have to hide. The stigma of infertility is added to by the stigma of a treatment that is not really acceptable to the doctor.

Finkler et al. (11) says, "It could be said that the medicine of the future will not be the medicine of the individual but of the family" (p. 409). The implications of this at the intervention level is that the professional will have to be circumspect in seeking information concerning family history. It cannot be assumed that the persons being seen are aware of the biological and/or social origins of their family creation. If they are aware of being part of a socially constructed family, they may well feel embarrassed or upset that the professional sees them as being "different" with the negative values that are frequently associated with difference.

It also needs to be noted that issues concerning confidentiality arise when moving from an individual to a family focus. The person who has an illness and is asked/told by the doctor to contact other family members to see if they know of the existence of the illness in their family history may not want other members of the family to know. Where family members are estranged, such a request may create or add to tension and stress. How the health professional manages such situations will have considerable impact on the psychosocial functioning of the designated patients and potentially their networks.

The third major implication is the consideration of how to assist, from a psychosocial perspective, the would-be families who are going to use alternative ways of becoming a family. Recognition of the psychosocial issues associated with not being able to conceive in the way that had been expected is now well accepted by most health professionals. Those psychosocial issues do not end or disappear when a conception occurs. Consideration needs to be given to the responsibility of the health-care team to provide preparation that will, as far as possible, prepare those who are to be treated with different procedures. To take the example of those using third party gametes, there will be a need to explore with the parent/s the issues associated with information sharing with the child/ren and the social networks. In a research undertaken in Germany Thorn and Daniels (17) have found that attending preparation seminars leads couples to feel increased levels of confidence about using DI as their way of building their family. This increased confidence leads them to talking with others in their social networks (therefore being able to receive support and encouragement) and deciding to share this information with their children. If they have already made the decision to share the information the research shows that attending the preparation seminar increases their confidence about doing this. Part of this growth in confidence is a reflection of the shift from a marginal and stigmatized position to one which they can feel that although this was not the way they would ideally become a family, it was their choice and they were fully committed to it. Such a position is likely to form a solid foundation for the health and well-being of the family.

References

1. Edelmann RJ, Connolly KJ. Gender differences in response to infertility and infertility investigations: real or illusory. *Br J Health Psychol.* 2000;5:365–375.
2. Leiblum S, Aviv A, Hamer R. Life after infertility treatment: a long-term investigation of marital and sexual function. *Hum Reprod.* 1998;13(12):3569–3574.
3. Daniels K. *Building a Family: with the Assistance of Donor Insemination.* Palmerston North, NZ: Dunmore Press; 2004.
4. Archard D. *Children, Family, and the State.* Burlington, VT: Ashgate; 2003.
5. Lowie R. *Social Organisation.* New York: Rinehart; 1948.
6. Scheinder D. Kinship and biology. In: Coale A, Fallers L, Levy M, Scheinder D, Tomkins S, eds. *Aspects of the Analysis of Family Structure.* Princeton, NJ: Princeton University Press; 1965.
7. Scheinder D. What is kinship all about? In: Reining P, ed. *Kinship studies in the Morgan centennial year.* Washington, DC: Anthropological Society of Washington; 1972:32–63.
8. Scheinder D. *A Critique of the Study of Kinship.* Ann Arbor, MI: University of Michigan Press; 1984.
9. Finkler K. The kin in the gene: the medicalization of family and kinship in American society. *Curr Anthropol.* 2001;42(2):235–263.
10. Daniels K. Is blood really thicker than water? Assisted reproduction and its impact on our thinking about family. *J Psychosom Obstet Gynaecol.* 2005;26(4):265–270.
11. Finkler K, Skrzynia C, Evans JP. The new genetics and its consequences for family, kinship, medicine and medical genetics. *Soc Sci Med.* 2003;57(3):403–412.
12. Brewaeys A, Golombok S, Naaktgeboren N, de Bruyn J, van Hall E. Donor insemination: Dutch parents' opinions about confidentiality and donor anonymity and the emotional adjustment of their children. *Hum Reprod.* 1997;12(7):1591–1597.
13. Miall CE. Community constructs of involuntary childlessness: sympathy, stigma, and social support. *Can Rev Sociol Anthropol.* 1994;31(4):392–421.
14. Blyth E. Secrets and lies: barriers to the exchange of genetic origins information following donor assisted conception. *Adoption Fostering.* 1999;23(1):49–58.
15. Daniels KR, Taylor K. Secrecy and openness in donor insemination. *Polit Life Sci.* 1993;12(2):155–170.
16. McWhinnie AM. Gamete donation and anonymity. Should offspring from donated gametes continue to be denied knowledge of their origins and antecedents? *Hum Reprod.* 2001;16(5):807–817.
17. Thorn P, Daniels K. A group-work approach in family building by donor insemination: empowering the marginalized. *Hum Fertil.* 2003;6:46–50.
18. Daniels KR, Blyth E, Hall D, Hanson KM. The best interests of the child in assisted human reproduction: the interplay between the state, professionals, and parents. *Polit Life Sci.* 2000;March:47–58.

19. Daniels K. New Zealand: from secrecy and shame to openness and acceptance. In: Blyth E, Landau R, eds. *Third Party Assisted Conception Across Cultures*. London: Jessica Kingley Publishers; 2004:148–167.
20. Edwards J. Donor insemination and 'public opinion'. In: Daniels KR, Haimes E, eds. *Donor Insemination: International Social Science Perspectives*, 1 edn. Cambridge: Cambridge University Press; 1998:151–172.

9
Research in Psychosomatic Obstetrics and Gynecology

H.B.M. van de Wiel and W.C.M. Weijmar Schultz

Within psychosomatic obstetrics and gynecology (PsOG) two paradigms can be distinguished, the realistic and the ideological, both which have a long history in medicine. With the rise of the quality revolution, the need arose to bridge the fundamental gap between both approaches. In this chapter a proposal of a research paradigm is outlined that combines these two visions.

9.1. Introduction: The best of Both Worlds

The eclectic or holistic approach to women's health and its problems, here referred to as PsOG, has become popular over the last decades. About 25 years ago it was quite common to treat patients without putting much effort neither into criteria such as quality of life and patient satisfaction nor into activities such as patient education and counseling. Only on rare occasions were ethical questions raised about the need to treat patients with highly sophisticated technology. More and more these core characteristics of PsOG have been accepted worldwide as parameters of the quality of (gynecological) health care. This upgrading of criteria for evaluating medical care went hand in hand with the widely accepted notion that man is more than just a *soft machine* and that within the boundaries of biological possibilities we construct our own psychological and cultural reality. It is the great strength of PsOG that it takes into account the existence of different (cultural) realities, putting the patient's experiences and her needs first. Illustrative of this patient centeredness is the pluralistic domain of medical treatments. Sometimes it is better to look at symptoms from a physiological perspective; sometimes a psychological approach is more appropriate. In most cases several perspectives can be used, whether or not in a multidisciplinary mix. Everyone can accept the fact that in France a patient with vague complaints about an aching stomach may be diagnosed as suffering from liver crises (crise de foie), whereas the same patient in the USA probably would be treated for an allergic reaction to food and in the Netherlands or Great Britain for a virus infection (1). In fact this medical diversity may be seen as evidence for the assumption that man is not just a biological but also a cultural and historical entity. The view that man is a result of cultural and historical lines is described in science as an *ideological* or *constructivist* approach. An important illustration of this way of thinking is the concept of holistic or biopsychosocial medicine postulated by Engel (2). Alongside the ideological tradition, another development has influenced modern medicine to a large extent: the use of a physical approach or more precisely *reductionistic materialism*. In terms of discoveries especially, and in combination with the Darwinian concept of evolution, this approach has been very successful. It has enabled us to overcome infectious plagues and given us a grip on our own reproduction. Until now in Western modern medicine reductionistic materialism is the gold standard in research.

9.2. One World Standard

Until recently, there was a fine balance between evidence-based medicine and patient centeredness. This balance is now disturbed by a new way of looking at professionalism, namely *the quality revolution*. Historically, professionalism comprised qualities such as the use of consensus in clinical practice, the way a discipline is organized, the use of an educational framework, the way one deals with complaints and errors, and so on. Today the emphasis is more and more on *assimilation*: the use of narrower standards, thereby eroding differences between professionals. The McDonalds and Holiday Inn approach now also holds for health services: "All around the world, the same products and services at the same quality level." This so-called quality revolution is nowadays the mantra in medicine and is based on concepts such as benchmarking and accountability. The difference with more traditional research in medicine lies in its nonmoral use of empirical studies. There is an old urge to be evidence based in order to be able to distinguish real medicine from alternative medicine and charlatanism. Because PsOG embraces a number of disciplines, at the same time having some specific characteristics including its claim to be holistic, it is difficult to fit PsOG research into the classical reductionistic materialism paradigm. If we look back into the recent past, we see two types of discussions dominating the research agenda:

- A methodological discussion reflecting the benchmarking principle, based on the outcomes of different therapies. Investigators, and in their trail governments, insurance companies, and so on, attach importance to the merits of these therapies and, to a lesser extent, their underlying theories.
- A fundamental scientific philosophical discussion, based on more general developments in science, especially in fundamental disciplines like physics on the one hand and philosophy on the other hand. New objects of research and new ways to study them are defined.

Both developments will be discussed here briefly; for more extensive information, see recommended literature.

9.3.   BenchMarking: The Methodological Approach

The main issue in this type of research is the question of how to select an appropriate therapy and to differentiate effective from ineffective treatment. In order to answer this question, medical research leans heavily on developments in reductionistic methodology of which the main features will be commented upon here briefly.

After it became clear that the question "does it work?" was too simple and had to be replaced by the question "*what* does work for *which* patients, for *which* purposes?,*" an era of methodological progress began. An interesting pallet of research strategies has been developed over the past decades (for a more elaborate description, see (3)):

- *Treatment package strategy*: this strategy evaluates the effect of a particular treatment "in toto" (package), which is in fact as often as that treatment ordinarily is used.
- *Dismantling treatment strategy*: this strategy consists of analyzing the components of a given treatment package.
- *Constructive treatment strategy*: this method refers to developing a treatment package by adding components that may enhance outcome.
- *Parametric treatment strategy*: this principle refers to altering specific aspects of a treatment to determine how to maximize therapeutic change.
- *Comparative treatment strategy*: two or more different treatments are compared in order to answer the question, which treatment is better among various alternatives for a particular clinical problem.
- *Process research strategy*: this strategy traditionally has addressed questions about transactions between patients and physicians, the type of interactions, and their interim effects on patients' or physicians' behavior. Nowadays, process research, including process redesign, is related to outcomes more and more.
- *Patient and physician variation strategy*: where other strategies emphasize the technique as a major source of treatment variance, given the great impact of placebo on medical outcomes, one could focus on the role of patient and physician variables.

One of the most important ways to reduce this enormous amount of information was to put research in order in respect of level of evidence. This led to an emphasis on what is now known as randomized clinical trials (RCTs) and in its trail the meta-analysis (MA). Clinical trials refer generally to outcome investigations conducted under clinical settings. This requires methodological compromises and sacrifices to meet practical, administrative, and ethical demands. Based on design, a distinction is made between case studies, true experimental designs and quasi-experimental designs, varying from case reports (the least amount of evidence) to RCTs as the top of the evidence pyramid. However, when the amount of results based on RCT became so overwhelming, a further reduction or condensation of effectiveness had to be developed: the meta-analysis. Although very important and useful for a limited number of themes and patients, this reductionist approach with the meta-analysis as the summit of level of evidence has its limits in terms of PsOG. To put it clearly, in order to meet the conditions for RCT and MA, the patient has to be deconstructed from a cultural, historical agent into a somewhat sophisticated laboratory mouse. These limitations are also found in the statistics on RCT and mutatis mutandis in meta-analyses.

9.4.   The Scientific Philosophical Approach

Another line of reasoning is to see PsOG as more than just a broad area to investigate; it is a way of thinking, a philosophy with all the resultant problems of definition. The use of different theories and corresponding definitions and wide variations in application does not make it open to systematic testing or even to systematic comparison as is so typical for the benchmarking principle. If, nevertheless, we want to leave the arguments, opinions, and presumptions behind us, we can also look at the route PsOG-R should take in order to enter the domain of what is agreed upon as true science.

9.4.1.   Reductionistic Materialism

One of the core aims in science is the principle known as *Ockham's razor*: to reduce and unify as much as possible. With regard to PsOG, there are problems with this. The most important problem is probably a phenomenon which lies right at the center of PsOG: human consciousness and the experience of man as an intentional being, driven by cultural and historical influences. According to reductionistic materialism, pain and pleasure are purely physical processes which take place in the brain. As long as the mental processes, for example, the pain experience, correlate perfectly with the condition of the brain, we may assume equality between both entities and reduce them to the simplest explanation. This perfect correlation, also known as *supervenience*, however is seldom the case. And because of that imperfection, other philosophical perspectives have developed, of which Descartes' dualism is one of the most influential examples.

9.4.2.   Dualism

According to traditional dualism, mind and body were so different that they were mutually exclusive, thereby making the concept of monism impossible to hold. However, in order to explain our normal experiences of a complete entity, nobody experiences his/her mind apart from his/her body or vice versa: dualism hypothesizes all kinds of causal relationships between the physical and the mental world. This hypothesis, that mental and physical events can be part of the same causal chain, violates one of the fundamental laws in physics. If a physical event happens at a point at time T, there has to be a physical cause for that event at time point T. To put it in other words, how can something nonphysical lead to changes in a physical world or system? Applied to PsOG, in the case of vaginismus, it is assumed that fear is a mental and, therefore in former philosophical terms, a nonphysical process, which nevertheless leads to physical reactions, that is, involuntary contraction of the vaginal sphincter. According to the laws of physics, this is impossible. In order to solve the problem with monistic as well as pure dualistic models, a number of mixed approaches were developed under the term *dualism of characteristics*. This point of view denies the monistic idea of two perspectives describing basically the same (physical) world. On the contrary it hypothesizes that mental descriptions are referring to an autonomous domain of reality: the mental world. Therefore they are not reducible to physical laws and theories. Within this type of dualism, two parallel ways of thinking can be distinguished: *functionalism* and *emergentism*. Whereas functionalism focuses on the mental domain, primarily on cognition (that is the way we process information by learning, perception, problem solving, etc.), emergentism focuses primarily on consciousness. For a more extensive description, see (4). In summary we can conclude that there is a temptation to say that there is the body, which is a physiological system, and there is the psychological mind. Between them lies what is sometimes referred to as an ill-defined no-man's-land occupied by something called psychosomatic medicine. The question is whether this no-man's-land exists, especially in view of the recent work of people like Damasio (5). Briefly stated, the results of studies in which PET scans and MRIs play an important role, the investigation of the human brain, emotions and feelings, makes clear that emotions and feelings, formerly hypothesized as mental concepts, in fact can be regarded also as physiological concepts. What we experience as consciousness appears to be no more than *an epiphenomenological (concomitant of something else not regarded as its cause or result) echo of our biological systems.*

9.4.3. Toward a Humanistic Monism

Although the discussion above may evoke the reaction that psychological and social factors are no longer interesting for physicians, the opposite is the case. In everyday life, including the perception of pain, emotions, and feelings, psychological and social mechanisms still play the same important role as they always did. The discovery of quarks did not change our operating theaters much, nor the work done there. The idea of psychosomatic refers not only to the interaction of body and mind but also to a description of good clinical practice, in which patients, including their social context, are taken seriously. We therefore would like to end this chapter by presenting the concept of a theory that not only takes into account the above-mentioned scientific monism but also permits us to look at behavior as an ordered evolution from some less organized state to some more organized state. This dynamic system provides an explanation as to why low correlations are often found between mental and physical processes. The research question that arises is, how to get a grip on these complex relationships? By regarding the development of object and subject together, we can see interesting parallels between individual growth, as described by the dissimilation theory of Piaget (6), and scientific developments, as described by Kuhn (7). Like any other growth, scientific growth may progress, regress, fixate, or change. It is assumed that there is something of an inherent scientific nature in man which is triggered by one or another further scientific system by certain life circumstances. Also, it is assumed that as a growth phenomenon, scientific behavior develops naturally through definable but overlapping stages. This is an orderly progression from a less complex to a more complex stage. This concept is that of epigenesis, a concept in the field of embryology: the theory that the germ cell is structureless and that the embryo develops as a new creation through the action of the environment on the protoplasm. In other words, all which grow have a ground plan, not always achieving its final form, yet if achieving this final form, still infinitely variable. Like others did for ethical behavior (8), we can combine these notions into a theory of PsOG. The theory is summarized in 10 postulates, in order to serve as signposts for psychosomatic research in the near future.

9.5. Ten Postulates

1. The scientific system of a group of men is a function of the dynamic system triggered by the life circumstances in which that group is living.
2. Normally the system of scientific behavior by which this group lives changes in an orderly determined manner as broader dynamic systems are triggered by more humanly favorable life circumstances.
3. There emerges a scientific theme of what is true or false in science, which is appropriate to each level of dynamic emergence.
4. Within each theme, certain specific values of right and wrong will be expressed by one group because of variations in the components of a dynamic system, while another group may accentuate certain other values because of a different arrangement in the dynamic system.
5. There is a natural drive in man to proceed from a lower to a higher level dynamic system and thus a concomitant natural drive to move from a lower, more humanly restricting conception of true and false to a higher, more humanly freeing conception.
6. As man moves from a lower to a higher level of scientific behavior, some values by which man judges true from false are discarded as no longer appropriate to his changed status; this dynamic emergence resembles human cognitive emotional development, which can be summarized as dualism, pluralism, relativism, and moral choice.
7. The scientific systems by which men live may progress, fixate at an over- or underdeveloped level.

8. The movement, lack of movement, or abnormality of movement is a function of the conditions which affect man's psychological dynamic system.
9. Lower level dynamics produces a more rigid scientific system, thus making it impossible for those living by lower science to comprehend the meaning of living by higher level sciences.
10. It requires a higher system of science than the human mind to understand the meaning of the human mind.

References

1. Payer L. *Medicine and Culture: Varieties of Treatment in the United States, England, West Germany, and France.* New York: Holt Company; 1988; see also Payer (1996).
2. Engel GL. The need for a new medical model: a challenge for biomedicine. *Science.* 1977;196(4286):129–136.
3. Bergin AE, Garfield SL. *Handbook of Psychotherapy and Behavior Change.* New York: Wiley; 2003.
4. Dennet DC. Evolving the mind. On the nature of matter and the origin of consciousness. *Nature.* 1996;381(6582):485–486.
5. Damasio AR. How the brain creates the mind. *Sci Am.* 1999;281(6):112–117.
6. Piaget J. *Biology and Knowledge.* Chicago: University of Chicago Press; 1971.
7. Kuhn TS. *The Structure of Scientific Revolutions.* Chicago: University of Chicago Press; 1962.
8. Graves CW. Lecture. Senectady. New York; 1959.

Part Two
Obstetrics

10
Coping and Adjustment in Pregnancy: Giving Babies a Better Start

Michelle Sowden, Nigel Sage, and Jayne Cockburn

From a psychological perspective, even a healthy pregnancy is a challenging time. To be prepared emotionally and practically for the arrival of a baby, a number of psychological tasks need to be addressed. These include

- Accepting the reality of the pregnancy
- Facing the consequences of being pregnant
- Coping with physical changes
- Coping with uncertainty and unpredictability
- Coping with change in role and relationships
- Managing unexpected or untoward events and minor pregnancy complications (major complications are beyond the scope of this chapter and will be addressed elsewhere)

Individuals will vary in how they set about dealing with these tasks. Some will seek as much information as is available, whilst others will be comfortable accepting what the "experts" tell them. Some will barely register that the pregnancy is happening, whilst others will immerse themselves in the experience of being pregnant right from the positive test result or even before. The fact that the pregnant woman does cope effectively is usually rather more important than how she does it.

So what does it mean to cope with pregnancy?

In general, we can quite reasonably assume that the women we perceive to be mastering the tasks of pregnancy in the way we expect are coping well. These women are likely to be the ones we feel reassured about when they attend clinic. They generate little anxiety for us as clinicians and we feel no need to make special arrangements. We perceive them as initiating contact with health services in a timely way, following reasonable health-care advice, seeking information, and making rational decisions; they cooperate with us in planning their care.

In contrast, there are other women attending clinic whose responses do not fit our expectations for mastering one or more of our psychological tasks list.

They may not engage in health-care services, may fail to adapt their lifestyle to accommodate the pregnancy e.g., continue to smoke or drink alcohol, and they may make decisions and changes that we are concerned that they will regret (including traveling in late pregnancy or following unconventional advice). Alternatively, perhaps we perceive them as failing to address issues or to make decisions at all (such as when a partner or parent dominates consultations). They may seem to be unable to discriminate between events that they can change or influence and those they cannot (perhaps seeking excessive reassurance or overplanning for worst case scenarios). We might perceive these women to be coping less well. But are our perceptions of who is not coping correct? How can we determine who is and who is not managing pregnancy well and how can we begin to help?

In this chapter we aim to provide an introduction to how clinicians can review patients' coping and identify those who need further help. Many women who struggle with pregnancy have at their disposal effective coping skills, having previously mastered other challenging life events but for some reason their coping has broken down at this point in time. Often, whilst these women are in need of additional support, they cause us to feel pushed for time, lacking in skills and fearful of "opening a can of worms." It is this group of women that the present chapter will focus on. These women may well be able to make use of relatively brief discussions aimed at enabling them to identify what needs to change or it may be necessary to refer some one for other expert help.

The material presented in this chapter draws heavily on psychological theory and techniques that have a solid evidence base. However, what is presented here is a translation of this evidence base into what we hope will be a more accessible framework for the practitioner who has little or no formal training in psychological therapy and who has limited time in which to identify and address difficulties in coping. As such, the material presented is not intended to be either definitive or prescriptive but rather an introduction and pragmatic guide that the interested reader could expand upon through further reading and training. What this chapter does aim to do is to equip the busy practitioner with sufficient psychological tools and techniques to improve the psychological health of the women attending routine obstetric services. We will first define what we mean by coping and then explore what can go wrong, together with signs of difficulties in coping that may present in clinic. We will go on to discuss strategies for psychological change and when to refer to.

10.1. Defining Coping

Coping can be defined as an effective response that diminishes distress and serves the person's best interests, even taking into account the adverse conse-quences generated by the coping response.

Whenever people are distressed, they behave in ways that attempt to ameliorate or manage that distress. We call these responses coping strategies. Coping strategies are anything someone is doing to try and manage distress.

Two main types of coping strategy have been identified. These are problem-focused strategies and emotion-focused strategies. Problem-focused strategies are those strategies that are concerned with managing or changing the problem that is causing the distress. Emotion-focused strategies are those that are concerned with managing distress directly.

Coping strategies can be further categorized by whether they attempt to confront and tackle problems or emotions or attempt to avoid and minimize these problems or emotions. The four main types of coping strategy that will be referred to in this chapter are presented in Table 10.1.

To understand more about the different coping strategies, we will leave the theme of pregnancy for a moment and imagine, for example, the plight of a parent whose child's beloved budgie dies during its first day at school. How could the parent manage this situation? The parent could avoid the child's distress by quietly buying an identical budgie and hoping the change goes unnoticed. Alternatively, they could confront the situation after school by explaining what has happened and encouraging the child to have a good cry. Both solutions could effectively resolve the situation. However, both also have consequences. Buying an identical budgie avoids the child becoming distressed in the short term but gets expensive for the unfortunate parent if faced with a succession of pet bereavements. More seriously, it is not allowing the child opportunity to learn to cope with normal feelings of loss. However, confronting the situation will undoubtedly lead to a miserable few days for the child who then has to struggle with complex issues around life and death and might even start to worry that the parent too could die during school time.

So what should the parent do? Deciding to avoid or confront the situation might be influenced by whether the parent feels able to cope constructively with the child's distress at this point in time and whether there is time to go and find an identical budgie. Weighing the relative importance of different possible outcomes will also influence the parent. If highest priority is given to settling the child at school, then the parent is likely to choose an avoidance strategy. If teaching the child to cope with loss is perceived as more important, then a confronting strategy will be chosen. However, the anguished parent may feel both of these outcomes are important in which case they could employ firstly avoidance coping strategies (perhaps by sending the budgie on holiday for a few days) and then switch to confronting coping strategies at the weekend (when the news is broken that the budgie died on its way home).

But what does coping with the death of a budgie have to do with understanding how women cope with pregnancy?

It highlights three key points.

TABLE 10.1. The four main types of coping strategy

	Confronting it	Avoiding it
Problem focused	Problem solving	Problem avoidance
Emotion focused	Emotional regulation	Emotional avoidance

TABLE 10.2. Examples of confronting and avoiding problem-focused and emotion-focused coping strategies and the resources required for their application

Coping issue	Responses and resources	Problem solving	Problem avoidance
Problem focused—managing or changing the problem	Cognitive—the way we think	Identifies the problem	Postpones making decisions
		Identifies possible solutions	Delegates decision making to others
		Seeks information about options	Ignores the issue
		Weighs pros and cons of change	Keeps opinions to self
		Makes a plan to change the situation	Declines to discuss issues
		Makes changes	Reassures self that it will turn out alright
		Makes decisions	Remains optimistic that no action needs to be taken
	Behavioral—the way we act	Monitors threats/risks/symptoms	
		Sets and works toward goals	Withdraws from the source of the stress, e.g., walks away from an argument
		Makes use of aids and equipment	Avoids entering situations where has encountered difficulties before
		Asserts self to bring about change	
		Takes action	
		Seeks reassurance	
	Other resources required	Access to information	Access to others to whom to defer or delegate decisions
		Aids and equipment	
		Time	
		Energy	

Emotion focused—managing emotions directly	**Emotional regulation**	**Emotional avoidance**
Cognitive—the way we think	Thinks/reflects on the situation Actively triggers painful emotions through reminiscence	Distances self emotionally Avoids thinking about the situation (cognitive avoidance) Thought suppression Minimizes emotional response
Behavioral—the way we act	Cries Talks Writes/draws Actively triggers painful emotions through looking at photos, visiting grave of deceased, maintaining contact with people who remind of loss or fears Behaves in accordance with the changes	Avoids situations that trigger distress (behavioral avoidance) Behaves as if nothing has changed Laughs it off (emotional blunting) Distracts self
Other resources required	Access to social support Time Energy to manage heightened emotions	Alcohol/substances Energy to repress/suppress emotions

Firstly, there is no such thing as a good or a bad coping strategy; rather different strategies fulfill different functions. In pregnancy, women need to use a range of strategies to address the psychological tasks in our list. For example, emotional regulation strategies (allowing expression of a full range of emotions) help acceptance of the reality of the pregnancy; but emotional avoidance (such as "It's not a big deal") may serve an important protective role for those who fear the unknown and need to come to that acceptance gradually.

Secondly, all coping strategies require resources (such as time, energy, money, cooperation of others, information, expertise), and availability of those resources will determine strategy selection. Getting more information from the midwife about the birth experience, for instance, may be a helpful problem-solving strategy to alleviate anxieties about high probability outcomes such as labor pain, but if access to the midwife is delayed, then problem avoidance as an immediate strategy is of value in reducing distress in the short term.

Thirdly, all coping strategies have consequences. Those strategies that yield the greatest benefits in the short term may have costs in the longer term and vice versa. A patient who routinely allows her partner to dominate consultations may maintain marital harmony by using this problem-avoidance strategy of non-assertiveness. However, ultimately this strategy may result in her receiving health care that does not properly meet her needs.

Examples of the different types of coping strategy and the resources required to apply them are presented in Table 10.2. These are described in terms of cognitive strategies (which are to do with the way we think) and behavioral strategies (which are to do with the way we act).

As stated at the beginning of this section, coping can be defined as an effective response that diminishes distress and serves the person's best interests even taking into account the adverse consequences generated by the coping response. In Section 10.2 we will consider what can go wrong to create difficulties in coping and how to distinguish between those who are and are not coping.

10.2. What Can Go Wrong to Create Difficulties in Coping?

Having defined what we mean by coping, we now turn to the issue of what can go wrong to create difficulties in coping. We will look at two case scenarios, the first of which will leave us feeling reassured about the patient and the second of which will raise concerns about the patient. Exploring what concerns and what reassures us about these patients will enable us to develop a framework for distinguishing between those who are and are not coping.

Mary is pregnant, having lost a baby early on in a previous pregnancy. Her coping strategies have included planting a tree to mark the loss of the dead baby. Caring for the tree triggers intensely painful feelings of loss, sadness, and guilt, but these feelings are reducing in intensity over time. In spite of her grief, she appears to be behaving in accordance with our expectations of a pregnant woman; she attends appointments, makes decision in a timely way, seeks information, and is planning ahead for the future.

Janice is also pregnant and also lost a baby early on in a previous pregnancy. In contrast to Mary, she has coped with the pain of the loss and the possibility of further loss by distancing herself emotionally from her pregnancy and by behaving as if she was not pregnant. She appears to be functioning well in daily life, but whilst she attends routine appointments, she has done virtually nothing to prepare for the baby's arrival. When questioned, she declines to discuss the previous pregnancy loss, saying that it does not help to dwell on the past and her husband gets angry if you say things that might upset her.

So what is it about Mary that reassures us and what is it about Janice that raises concerns?

In the first scenario, Mary's way of coping fits with her longer-term needs and objectives, which is to be able to prepare for having her baby. Whilst confronting her loss intensifies her distress, she is progressing in resolving her grief, and her coping strategies are not creating any further difficulties for her.

In contrast, Janice's coping response is not congruous with her long-term needs and has potentially serious consequences. It is not enabling her to prepare for motherhood and this may increase her anxiety in the perinatal period. It is also not enabling her to resolve her loss, and her unresolved feelings could surface after the arrival of the baby, when she is likely to be more emotionally labile. She might manage these unresolved feelings by distancing herself from her newborn baby and avoiding contact with other new mothers.

If Janice were not pregnant, there would probably be no need for concern about the way she is coping. She could continue using this strategy for years without any serious consequences. The problem arises because she now needs to prepare for a very high probability outcome—the arrival of her baby. So, in distinguishing who is and who is not coping, it is important to look at the consequences of the coping response in the context of the individual's life circumstances. To enable the reader to consider the potential consequences of each of the various coping strategies, the short- and long-term advantages and disadvantages of each type of coping strategy are presented in Table 10.3. If short-term use of any one particular strategy can generate adverse effects, then potentially over reliance on this strategy could have very serious consequences indeed and the problems associated with over reliance on each of the strategies are also included.

In summary, difficulties in coping are not defined by the use of a particular coping strategy per se but in terms of the consequences of using that particular strategy to manage a given situation. If, at the point at which the coping response generates unacceptable consequences, the individual is able to switch to a more helpful coping response then the individual is unlikely to need help. However, some individuals become stuck in a particular coping response, even when this is no longer helpful to them or possibly even harmful. It is in these cases that there may be scope for making changes. Difficulties in coping might be presented to us directly in clinic or might need to be inferred

TABLE 10.3. Short- and long-term advantages and disadvantages of different coping strategies and problems associated with over reliance on a particular strategy

Strategy	Advantages		Disadvantages		Problems associated with over reliance
	Immediate	Subsequent	Immediate	Subsequent	
Problem solving	↑ sense of control and mastery	↓ problem	↑ awareness and distress	Neglect other issues	New problems caused
		Learn new skills	↓ energy Time consuming		Hypervigilance to risk Overreactions Impatience Nonacceptance of the unchangeable Demanding
Problem avoidance	↓ awareness and distress	No errors of judgment	↓ sense of control and mastery	Unresolved problems may persist, worsen, or repeat	↑ sense of being out of control
	No burden of responsibility	No failed strategies			↓ belief in coping skills
		No self-blame			↓ self-confidence ↑ use of avoidance Passive aggressive responses
Emotional regulation	Some control over when and how distress experienced	Releases emotions	↑ distress experienced and displayed	Others may judge critically	Depends on social support

	Allows friends and family to give support	May resolve issues	↓ normal functioning during distress	Others may become distressed Relationship may be strained Privacy may be forfeited	"Compassion fatigue" in social support May deflect from effective problem solving
Emotional avoidance	↓ distress	Postpones distress until more suitable time or increased ability to cope	Need to avoid potential emotional triggers in daily life Prevents family and friends from being supportive	Intrusive distress at unexpected or unsuitable times Vulnerable to future triggering of distress	↑ avoidance causing restricted lifestyle Adversely affects close relationships Cold, callous, uncaring demeanor Important changes not made Poor engagement with support services Emotional distraction and suppression strategies employed, e.g., alcohol misuse, abrupt lifestyle changes

from an individual's behavior. In Section 10.3 we consider the ways in which difficulties in coping with pregnancy might be presented in clinic.

10.3.   Signs of Difficulty in Coping with the Psychological Tasks of Pregnancy

In order to optimize the chances of a healthy pregnancy, a pregnant woman would ideally initiate contact with health-care services, follow up-to-date medical advice, and plan ahead to accommodate the baby. However, we must not assume that failure to do so signals difficulty in coping. In other words we must be careful not to make value judgments of how a good patient should behave. Rather, it is important when patients behave in ways that are counter to a healthy pregnancy or that may create issues further down the line, to see them as a possible sign of difficulty in coping and to explore with the patient what motivates these behaviors. We must carefully distinguish poor coping from active decisions to not adhere to medical advice. In particular, we must assess the extent to which the woman is making informed decisions and behaving in a way that is consistent with her longer-term goals and wishes.

However, as we have seen, coping strategies have adverse consequences. As a pregnant woman struggles to master the psychological tasks of pregnancy, her attempts to cope may inadvertently generate problems. For instance, when faced with uncertainty and unpredictability, a woman who overrelies on problem-solving strategies may try and plan for all possible outcomes, even ones that have a low probability of occurring. This could increase her anxiety as she remains focused on what might go wrong and seeks expert reassurance or advice to reduce distress. It could also deplete her resources (energy, consultation time) and detract from her enjoyment of pregnancy. The signs of her difficulty in coping with the psychological task that would be presented in clinic might include frequently asking "what if" questions and repeatedly seeking reassurance or confirmation of test results.

In Table 10.4 we present the signs of difficulty in coping with each of the psychological tasks of pregnancy that might be presented in clinic. We include in Table 10.4 a suggestion as to how the difficulty in coping may have arisen and a guide to the alternative coping strategy that might be more helpful. In Section 10.4 we discuss how, once a difficulty and possible alternative solutions have been identified, one might set about shifting patients into more helpful ways of coping.

10.4.   Shifting People into More Helpful Ways of Coping

Returning to Janice, she is struggling with one of the items on the pregnancy task list: accepting the reality of being pregnant. Whilst she is not completely in denial, her fears of losing another baby are leading to her distancing herself from the pregnancy experience to the extent that she is not behaving as if this pregnancy is really happening. She is employing emotional avoidance strategies that enable her to avoid or at least minimize her distress about her loss and her fear of further loss. In order to cope better, she needs to more fully resolve her grief for her dead baby and to develop strategies for actively managing the anxiety she feels about losing this baby too. In doing so, she needs to act as if the present pregnancy is a reality, and this is very likely to provoke an intense grief reaction that she will then need to talk and cry about. If she is to achieve satisfactory adjustment to being pregnant, Janice will need help to shift from strategies that are avoiding her distress into strategies that are about facing up to it.

To do this a clinician could simply confront Janice with the "realities" of the situation and offer advice that she needs to take action to change things. However, this is unlikely to be a successful strategy with someone who has used a coping strategy, which, to them, seems to work effectively. The most probable outcome is that Janice will reject the advice and (conforming to the avoidance of distress coping style) possibly the clinician as well.

As in psychological therapy, a more successful approach is often to invite the person to re-examine all the possible options before them and choose the one that best meets personal needs. Using this method, the clinician helps Janice discover the best coping strategy for herself. She will be committed to it because it is her own advice and her own decision. The clinician has been an ally, assisting rather than challenging her.

The method used in this approach is often referred to as "guided discovery.". Whilst essentially a simple technique of asking questions that encourage Janice to think things through, it requires the clinician to exercise a lot of self-discipline in resisting offering advice and solutions. The questioning encourages Janice to identify alternative ways of thinking and behaving, exploring the implications and consequences of each alternative, weighing the advantages and disadvantages of different coping styles, and working out which one is likely to be most suitable. Examples of the types of questions one might ask are summarized in Table 10.5.

If as a result of this re-examination of coping, Janice is now intending to face this emotional pain to help her cope with her present pregnancy, she will also need to have some preparation for how she can manage the adverse consequences (e.g., prolonged bouts of crying). There may be a need to consider what other resources she will need to have at her disposal (such as time off work, comfort, and understanding from her partner) or whether she would be helped by acquiring new skills and techniques (such as new ideas for "letting off steam," learning to relax or thinking about things from a different angle). Again, careful use of the guided discovery questioning by the clinician can help Janice to address these issues constructively, coming up with a plan of action that is relevant to her personal circumstances and to which she is committed.

Writing it all down as the "guided discovery," progresses will help Janice recall the train of thought that led her to her new perspective and remind

TABLE 10.4. Signs of difficulties in coping with the psychological tasks of pregnancy

Psychological task	Signs of difficulties in coping with the psychological task of pregnancy	Difficulty arises from excessive/unhelpful application of	Coping strategy to try (see Table 10.2)
Accepting the reality of the pregnancy	Continues to behave as if not pregnant	Emotional avoidance	Emotional regulation
	Presents in clinic at a late stage		
	Acts in ways that may be regretted at a later stage		
	Avoids other pregnant women		
	Avoids talking about pregnancy		
	Denies or distances self from pregnancy		
	Does not plan for or prepare for baby		
	Fails to follow health-care advice		
Facing the consequences of being pregnant	Indecisive	Problem avoidance	Problem solving
	Changes her mind frequently		
	Has difficulty following through a long-term plan		
	Relinquishes responsibility for her own decisions and care		
	Fails to address problems that have a high probability of occurring		

Source of stress	Manifestations		
Coping with physical changes	Continues with pre-pregnancy levels of activity Reluctant to modify activity Hides bump Reports extreme methods of controlling weight gain	Emotional avoidance	Emotional regulation
Coping with uncertainty and unpredictability	Repeatedly asks "what if" questions Formulates plans to cover all possible scenarios Repeatedly seeks reassurance, investigations, and test results Hypervigilant to risk Anticipates worst possible outcomes	Problem solving	Problem avoidance
Coping with change in role and relationships	Absence of partner Dominance of consultation by others Concerns about time off from work Reluctance to start maternity leave	Problem avoidance	Problem solving
Managing unexpected or untoward events and minor pregnancy complications	Highly distressed by minor abnormalities Behaves as if the worst case scenario is happening Requests unwarranted investigations/admission	Emotional regulation	Emotional avoidance

TABLE 10.5. Examples of "guided discovery" questions

A sequence of questions described by Padesky[a]

Have you ever been in similar circumstances?
What did you do?
How did that turn out?
What do you know that you didn't know then?
What would you advise a friend who told you something similar?
Other useful questions could be
Do you have a friend who you think is good at coping with difficult situations?
How do you think your friend would deal with a situation like this?
Is that something you could try?
What might be the worst that could happen?
And if that happened, what effect would that have on you?
What alternative ways would there be to cope with that?
How does thinking that make you feel?
Is there any other way of seeing the situation?
Is there something else you could say to yourself that might be more helpful?
What do you think you could change to make things better for you?
What might you tell a friend to do in this situation?

[a]Padesky CA. *Socratic Questioning: Changing Minds or Guided Discovery?*
http://www.padesky.com

her of her decisions and the actions she has planned. The written summary is an important and powerful tool for consolidating change, which can be so easily overlooked. It can be prepared by the clinician or the patient, but to be effective, it should be immediately available (a neatly typed copy 2 weeks later is less valuable than the scribbled scrap of paper at the end of the consultation) and in the terms and structure that the patient understands and identifies as the product of her own thinking.

10.5. Important Personal Considerations for Clinicians

Although the emphasis of this chapter has been on tools and techniques to assist the clinician in identifying and modifying poor coping strategies, it is important not to overlook the role of the clinician's own emotional reactions and personal style in this process.

In the introduction to this chapter, we referred to clinician experiences of "feeling reassured," experiencing "little anxiety," being "concerned," and sensing a "can of worms." We have subsequently discussed ways in which we can evaluate coping strategies more precisely. However, we should not dismiss the value of these feelings described above. Gut-instinct alone would never be a satisfactory clinical tool, but sensitive clinicians will often detect patient unhappiness or anxiety through their own emotional reactions in the presence of the patient. These personal warning signals can often indicate when and where to make a more detailed assessment. Patient nervousness is particularly infectious, but so too are feelings of hopelessness. Clinician frustration may reflect distrust or resentment from the pregnant woman. An urge to "mother" the patient is likely to be provoked by a child-like helplessness in the woman herself. Whilst resisting the temptation to act out these emotional experiences, the clinician can use them as clues for further paths of enquiry.

Turning to style, clinicians who project a sensitive and supportive manner will more quickly gain patient confidence and fuller information than those who are more "business-like" in their style. Patients will decide what and how much to disclose together with how long to spend talking to the doctor from a range of environmental cues (e.g., waiting-room "turnover," degree of privacy) to clinician cues like body language signals (such as posture, body orientation, and eye contact), speed, and tone of speech. The effective interviewer manages to put the patient at ease, makes the interview seem the entire focus of attention and interest, and resists bombarding the interviewee with hasty advice and opinions. This encourages openness, trust, and confiding in return. By contrast, even the most troubled mother-to-be is likely to clam up when the clinician faces her with a noisy and rather public room, a rushed and critical set of questions and comments, and body language that suggests distance and superiority.

10.6. When to Refer to

If coping strategies are failing to work and in her own way the pregnant woman is not effectively addressing the psychological tasks we have listed, then she is likely to benefit from prompt action to help her adapt and adjust. The clinician who first detects such problems is therefore best placed to assist.

However, constraints of role, time, and environment will limit the level of intervention possible for even the most experienced practitioner. Sometimes, it is possible to advise the general practitioner and primary health-care team to pick up and develop themes initially identified in clinic. On other occasions it may seem apparent that the woman is too rigidly adhering to unhelpful attitudes and strategies that will require careful examination by mental health-care specialists who have the time and expertise to help bring about constructive change. Some of the women requiring this help may have a diagnosable mental health condition (such as clinical depression or generalized anxiety disorder), but others needing this extra input may have "adjustment difficulties" that do not warrant a diagnostic label as such.

Many women with a history of depression or anxiety cope very well from an obstetrics perspective and would not require more guidance and support than other pregnant women. Assuming they need specialist help because of past history or other current events may undermine confidence in coping strategies that have been quite effective during the pregnancy so far and may damage the clinician's relationship with the woman. It is the fact that the woman seems to require sustained and highly skilled treatment and that sensitive questioning and advice has proved insufficient that should determine the need to refer to, not the diagnosis or past history.

10.7. Concluding Remarks

Relatively brief but skillfully delivered interventions can make a significant difference in enabling the pregnant woman to cope more effectively. Just as a small stone creates spreading ripples on the surface of a pond, these benefits will be carried forward as she enters childbirth from a more robust psychological position having made reasonable preparations for this and for life with a new baby beyond. With practice, the clinician who confronts and embraces this challenge will become

1. Increasingly adept at identifying difficulties in coping
2. Able to relate these to the psychological task that needs to be mastered
3. Able to consider alternative, more helpful coping responses
4. Able to conduct consultations in a way that engages pregnant women in the process of change

This process is likely to increase satisfaction with the consultation and may alleviate some of the more unpleasant feelings engendered by challenging consultations.

Regardless of how skilled the clinician, working in close contact with human suffering takes its toll. If we are to remain engaged rather than adopting our own avoidance strategies in the face of this stress, we need to attend to our own emotional needs. For example,

1. Whilst clinicians often lack control over the logistics of their clinics, it may be possible to schedule more psychologically demanding consultations at those times of day when we are at our best.
2. Access to clinical supervision can also be of benefit, enabling us to process and gain an intellectual understanding of patients who elicit a particularly strong response in us.
3. Establishing effective routes for onward referral may enable us to focus our energies on those patients that we feel able to help within the constraints of our role, time, and resources.

Recommended Reading

1. http://www.padesky.com which includes access to training videos.
2. Snyder CR. *Coping: The Psychology of What Works.* Oxford: Oxford University Press; 1999.

For an Alternative Perspective

1. Raphael-Leff J. *Pregnancy: The Inside Story.* New Jersey: Jason Aronson Inc.; 1995.

11
Psychosocial Aspects of Prenatal Diagnosis: The Challenges for Doctors and Patients

Josephine M. Green and Helen E. Statham

11.1. Introduction

Over the past 30 years, techniques for detecting fetal abnormality have become a major influence on the antenatal care timetable. Some structural abnormalities can be detected via ultrasound and all pregnant women in the UK are offered an anomaly scan at 18–20 weeks and many are also scanned in the first trimester. Other abnormalities require the use of invasive tests—either amniocentesis, which is generally performed at 15–16 weeks, or chorionic villus sampling (CVS) which is performed at 11–12 weeks of pregnancy. Both of these techniques carry a risk of causing a spontaneous miscarriage, the risk being cited as between 1 and 2% from early randomized controlled trials to between 0.5 and 1% from more recent observational studies. It is therefore not considered appropriate for everybody to have these tests. Rather, pregnant women are screened to identify a higher-risk sub group for whom the costs and risks are thought to be justified. The screening may be done on the basis of a woman's age, ethnic group or family history, or it may involve a screening test (e.g., measuring markers in maternal serum and/or nuchal translucency). Either way, screening *per se* cannot tell us that the baby definitely does or does not have an abnormality, only that there is a relatively high or low likelihood of that being the case. It is therefore in the nature of screening tests that they "get it wrong," that is, some people with a "high-risk" screening result (or "screen positive") have babies that are fine ("false positive"), and some with a "low-risk" ("screen negative") result do in fact have affected babies ("false negative"). Methods of screening and cut-offs are usually chosen to minimize the number of false negatives, but that often means a high proportion of false positives.

Current guidance in the UK from the National Screening Committee demands that the screening test offered for Down's syndrome should detect 60% of cases with a 5% false-positive rate; by April 2007, the test offered must detect 75% of cases with a 3% false-positive rate. In either scenario, the vast majority of women who get a positive (high risk) result will have babies who will not have an abnormality.

Ultrasound can also serve as a screening test if "markers" are found (although the relevance of single markers in low-risk women is currently under discussion) and the woman will have to make decisions about further tests. It can also be diagnostic if a definite abnormality is found, but even then some women will have to decide about invasive testing.

11.2.   Women's Experiences of the Screening-Diagnostic Process

The screening-diagnostic process has been likened to a roller coaster—once you are on, it is very difficult to get off. Most women accept routinely offered screening tests because they want the reassurance that all is well and because they cannot see why they would want to refuse. The fact that tests *are* routinely offered carries a powerful message that the default position should be to accept them. Once a screening test comes back positive, however, the scenario changes and parents find themselves having to cope with a very high level of uncertainty that can only be resolved by having further (diagnostic) tests.

11.2.1.   Supporting Parents After Positive Screening

Parents who receive a high-risk screening result may need help and support in deciding whether or not to have invasive diagnostic testing. The support group ARC (Antenatal Results and Choices) have produced a number of excellent booklets, one of which is called "Supporting Parents' Decisions: A Handbook for Professionals" (see http://www.arc-uk.org)(1). This will be of assistance throughout the prenatal diagnosis process, including when an abnormality is detected by ultrasound. Apart from useful references it includes suggestions for forms of words to use and ways to respond to some of the difficult questions that parents ask. One particular question that challenges health professionals is "What would you do?" and there is a helpful discussion about the conflict between the principle of non-directiveness and the need to assist parents in their decision-making useful references as well.

11.2.2.   Stress and Anxiety

Despite considerable methodological variation, the psychosocial literature is very consistent in demonstrating the stressful nature of the period waiting for diagnostic test results and parents' worries about potential miscarriage (2,3). While there is no evidence that giving women more information *increases* anxiety, provision of information alone does not necessarily *remove* anxiety (3). Knowledge that is needed for improved decision-making may not be the same knowledge as would reduce anxiety. Furthermore, some anxiety is an appropriate response to a perceived threat to the health of a baby and anxiety might aid coping and decision-making. Management of anxiety is often difficult for health professionals, but the goal of removing it entirely is unrealistic. However, the doctor can validate their anxiety by acknowledging it as an issue, by discussing it and letting them talk about it rather than leaving them isolated and alone with their deep concern

Anxiety levels generally drop after receipt of reassuring results but some women remain anxious. We should not under-rate the anxieties that parents experience before that moment, especially with emerging evidence that maternal stress in pregnancy may have implications for the developing fetus (4).

11.2.3.   CVS and Amniocentesis, the Choice

It is often assumed that CVS is less stressful for parents than amniocentesis because

- They do not have to wait so long to have the test done (11 weeks after their last period instead of 16).
- They do not have to wait so long for results (1 week versus 3 weeks for conventional karyotyping).
- Termination of pregnancy, if requested, can be carried out in the first trimester and thus by dilatation and evacuation rather than by inducing labor at 14/15 weeks or more.

The first two assumptions are, on the whole, supported by the literature. The third assumption—that earlier terminations are less distressing—will be revisited later in this chapter.

Whether a woman is offered CVS or amniocentesis is likely to be a function of her gestation at the time, but some women are offered a choice and they may have to balance the advantages of CVS outlined above against a higher likelihood of miscarriage. This is partly because CVS does actually cause more miscarriages than amniocentesis and partly because there is a higher rate of spontaneous loss at this earlier stage of pregnancy. However, no woman can know whether her particular miscarriage was a consequence of the procedure or was one that would have happened anyway. Robinson et al (5) found that women who miscarried after CVS experienced a great deal of guilt and blamed their loss on their selfish desire for an earlier test result. They, in fact, had even less reason for feeling this way than might be supposed because they were part of the randomized trial and had not actually chosen to have CVS. There are no more recent data concerning this issue, as miscarriages are infrequent occurrences within individual studies. It is, however, an important point which should be taken into account when counseling women for prenatal diagnosis.

Key Points

- Most women having prenatal diagnostic tests are doing so as the result of a screening test.
- Positive screening test results cause a great deal of anxiety and some parents will find it difficult to decide whether to go on to have an invasive diagnostic test.
- The period of waiting for the results of diagnostic tests is particularly stressful.
- Most women having prenatal diagnostic tests will not have an abnormality detected.
- Women who miscarry after having an invasive test may blame themselves.
- Health professionals find many aspects of this process difficult, particularly managing women's anxiety and aiding decision-making.
- Ask them about their anxieties.

11.2.4. Women Who Have a Fetal Abnormality Detected

The women who have a fetal abnormality detected are few in number compared to all those with false-positive results and there is a much smaller research literature concerning their experiences. The most comprehensive study carried out in England was in the late 1990s, funded by the NHS R&D Maternal & Child Health Initiative (6,7,8), and the rest of this chapter will draw on its findings.

The study involved 247 mothers and 190 fathers who were interviewed approximately 2 months after the diagnosis of their baby's abnormality and then followed up with postal questionnaires for a further year; 148 women terminated their pregnancy and 72 continued. In the remaining 27, the diagnosis of abnormality was not made until the baby was born, although it could, in principle, have been made antenatally. These parents were included for comparison with those who continued their pregnancies in order to address the question of whether it is helpful for parents to have foreknowledge. Parents were recruited through four Fetal Medicine Units, seven District General Hospitals, and two voluntary organizations.

11.2.4.1. Getting the Diagnosis

Despite the distressing news that parents received, they were able to appreciate when it was handled well. Both the content of what they were told and its manner of delivery were important. The information given needed to be adequate and accurate; parents preferred a health professional to declare lack of knowledge rather than tell them something they later discovered was incorrect. Information also needed to be given in a way that made it clear to the parents that the health professional recognized the impact the diagnosis would have on them. The diagnosis of abnormalities perceived by health professionals and parents as "less severe" than others and that were usually treatable, for example, cleft lip and palate, still caused significant distress for parents. "Belittling" the abnormality was not a strategy that parents found helpful.

What to Say and How to Say It

- Parents will be in shock: follow the rules for "giving bad news."
- Be honest: admit the limits of your knowledge.
- Refer on to someone who can help.
- Give sources of information that can be accessed later, for example, a written summary of what has been found, leaflets, contact details for support groups.
- Don't make assumptions about what decision the parents will make.
- Don't belittle less severe abnormalities.
- Show you care but don't let your own distress get in the way.

Getting a diagnosis was, for most parents, a process, and there was a need for coordination of services so they could progress through the system as easily as possible, and so that all the health professionals who needed to be aware of the situation were well informed. There was a need for good communication between local and specialist hospitals and the community health professionals. This aspect was mentioned frequently and was often the area that was seen as "not good enough." The doctor at the hospital must take on the responsibility of communicating results personally; poor communication of such important information will let down an otherwise excellent service.

Health professionals need to be aware that parents' perceptions of what was said to them, and how it was said, remain with them. Sensitivity to parents' feelings is of major importance at all times. Many parents realized that this was a difficult job for health professionals and appreciated when it was done with kindness, sensitivity, and competence. As the father of a baby diagnosed with hydrocephalus said:

F: There's two bits of it [satisfaction with getting a diagnosis]. There's compassion, their ability to handle a problem even if it's unknown to you, which is a skill which every doctor should have....And there's the next bit, which is, OK, we know you've got a problem, neither you nor us know really the extent of it. But we're not going to stop there. We're going to make sure that we get you in touch with somebody else who knows about it, based on our diagnosis so far, and you can ring them whenever you want to and get this cleared up.

We asked parents to rate how satisfied they were with the process of getting a diagnosis. We asked for a satisfaction rating for their booking hospital and a separate rating (or ratings) if they had been referred to one or more specialist hospitals (referral hospitals). Multivariate analyses of these measures showed that.

- Satisfaction tended to be higher for referral hospitals.
- Parents who continued pregnancies and whose baby had been diagnosed with a non-lethal abnormality were more satisfied with the care they got at referral hospitals.
- Parents who felt pressurized to make a decision after the diagnosis, or to make it quickly, were dissatisfied with their care while they were undergoing a diagnosis.

11.2.4.2. Deciding to Continue or to End the Pregnancy

Some parents had thought about what they might do before becoming pregnant, others had never contemplated that they could have a baby with an abnormality. Whichever position parents started from, most found making this decision immensely difficult. Some parents make their decisions quickly while others take time to reach what is the right decision for them at that time. Parents take account of many factors including the impact of the abnormality on the baby, the impact on themselves and other children, and their personal and moral beliefs. Accounts in the media of how different parents make their different decisions and live with the consequences of that decision can be helpful or can raise challenging questions. Supporting parents through the decision-making period appears to be an area that is difficult for health professionals.

One of the things that a number of parents found valuable at this time was the handbook produced by the support group ARC (Antenatal Results and Choices) (9). ARC was originally called SATFA (Support Around Termination for Fetal Abnormality) and the intention of the handbook is that all hospitals have it available to give to parents who might want to consider terminating the pregnancy. Where parents were dissatisfied with the handbook, it was usually because they had been given it too late. The best time to be given it was at the time of diagnosis so that parents could find out what they would face and what questions they might want to ask. Since the study was completed, and as a result of the findings on the needs of women who continue pregnancies (see Section 11.2.6.1) a subsequent handbook addresses the issues that will face parents if they are contemplating continuing with the pregnancy (10).

11.2.4.3. Parents' Experiences of Undergoing a Termination of Pregnancy

It is only since stillbirth has been recognized as bereavement that health professionals have begun to understand that parents who terminate a wanted pregnancy after the diagnosis of an abnormality are also bereaved and will grieve for the loss of their baby. Accounts from parents in support group newsletters appear to show that many aspects of care have changed for the better, but prior to our study there had been little formal documentation of what does happen to parents and how they feel about aspects of the care they receive.

Satisfaction with care in hospital was high: only 12 mothers and 8 fathers scored less than 3 on a 0–5 rating and some would have wished to award a score higher than 5:

> F: ... from the moment we hit that labour ward, five doesn't even come into it, it's ten, a hundred, because they never left my side or [Mother]'s side the whole time, and anything we needed doing, they tried to do for us.

As this quotation suggests, perception of the staff was the major determinant of overall satisfaction. In many cases this surpassed expectations and many instances of extreme sensitivity were reported. However, some staff were less helpful and an unhelpful person had a relatively greater impact on parents' reported level of satisfaction than a helpful one. Staff attitudes to fathers were also important and on the whole men were well cared for, being given food and beds and helped to feel part of the process. Many individual midwives, doctors, nurses, and chaplains were given special recognition for their sensitivity.

Satisfaction was *not* related to how many weeks pregnant a woman was when the termination was carried out. However, women having a termination under general anesthetic spent less time in hospital and were more likely than those who had an induced labor to report dissatisfaction with staff attitudes and to be less satisfied overall with their care in hospital.

Satisfaction was not influenced by whether the termination was carried out on a labor ward or on a gynecology ward. Parents gave advantages and disadvantages for both places. It was often mentioned that hearing and seeing new babies was very hard for parents whose termination took place on labor wards.

Issues around seeing the baby seem to have been handled well and a number of couples who had not expected to want to do this were pleased that they had. Not being able to see and hold the baby was a source of regret to some women who terminated under a general anesthetic. However, in the current climate where seeing the baby is deemed to be the norm, it is important to remember that others who had chosen not to see their baby did not regret their decision.

Looking back, most parents felt that the right decisions had been made about how the termination was managed in terms of the method of termination (under general anesthetic or through induced labor), where it took place (on a labor ward or gynecology ward) and the decision about whether or not to see the baby. Most of the parents who would have liked something different mentioned a preference for general anesthetic over induced labor; to have been admitted to a gynecological rather than a labor ward; and regret over not seeing their baby.

11.2.5. Feticide

When termination takes place late in the second trimester or early in the third (as is legal in the UK) it is necessary to ensure that the baby is not alive at delivery. This procedure, feticide, is usually carried out in Fetal Medicine Units by means of an injection of KCl into the fetal heart. Parents talked about this in a variety of ways: for some it was the worst possible moment and the moment at which they felt they killed their baby, whereas for others it was a distressing part of a distressing experience. Mothers could not usually see the screen whereas fathers could and for some this was a source of deep regret, whereas for others it provided some comfort and reassurance that the baby was no longer going to suffer. As with all of the events around a termination, parents are very upset and require sensitivity to their particular needs.

11.2.6. Aftercare

Parents were generally much less satisfied with after-care: over one-fifth of the women who terminated their pregnancy had no contact with any health professional, community or hospital based, after leaving hospital. Overall, satisfaction with aftercare was higher if women saw health professionals than if they did not. There were, however, a small number of women who did not want follow-up care and who were very satisfied if they did not see any health professionals.

Parents had different expectations of different health professionals. GPs were not necessarily seen as someone to talk to, but parents wanted to know that the GP was aware of their situation and recognized the importance of what they had been through. Most women thought that at least one home visit from a community midwife was an appropriate expectation. As women who had just given birth, many expected a physical check-up, although care that consisted only of physical checks was often not seen as particularly satisfactory.

Many women would have liked, but did not have, contact with a counselor. Other things that parents would have liked but did not always get included: someone to talk to; knowing that someone cared; and contact with other parents. Fathers, as well as mothers, expressed these views. A number of parents expressed anxiety about contacting other parents whose names had been given by ARC. This was because they did not wish to cause upset or intrude into these befrienders' home lives.

Many women were not warned in hospital about the physical and emotional problems they might experience after discharge from hospital. Even with warning, prolonged bleeding and lactation were physically and emotionally distressing.

There seemed to be an assumption that women having early terminations were less in need of care and support afterwards than other women. The responses of these women, their low satisfaction with care and their expressed wish, a year later, for having had more contact with health professionals suggest that this may be a false assumption.

Key Points—Termination of Pregnancy

- Earlier diagnosis is welcomed but the grief of parents terminating early is no less than that of those terminating later.
- Parents need information about how and where the termination will take place.
- The handbook from ARC will help parents make important decisions about whether or not to see the baby; postmortems; how to dispose of the body.
- Women need accurate information about lactation; post-delivery problems, whether physical or emotional, and they should know who to contact if they need someone.
- It is normal for parents to be deeply sad for many weeks or months after a termination—they have made a difficult decision, they do not have the baby they had hoped for and may have limited support from family and friends.

11.2.6.1. Parents' Experiences of Continuing a Pregnancy Following a Diagnosis of Abnormality

Seventy-two couples who received an antenatal diagnosis of a fetal abnormality did not terminate the pregnancy. In some cases they made a definite decision not to terminate; in others, either termination was not offered as an option or the baby died before a decision could be made. Whatever abnormality had been diagnosed, parents entered a world of significant uncertainty. Parents described very graphically feelings of being *"in limbo"* and of the strangeness they felt once they knew they had a baby with something wrong:

> M: I don't actually feel like a pregnant person. I feel like I've got a baby with a problem.

11.2.7. Antenatal Care

Parents talked a great deal about how care was, or more often was not, coordinated. Care could be based in a local hospital or a specialist hospital or in the community, or in all three places. Often, parents found that communication between health professionals working in different places was not efficient. This was a source of distress and anxiety—it could mean that a woman had, repeatedly, to explain her situation to yet another health professional or be given an appointment (sometimes at a distant hospital at great financial cost) for no clear reason. What parents appreciated was care that was supportive both physically and emotionally, which gave them the information they needed about their baby, and which recognized the woman as a pregnant mother-to-be.

Not all health professionals, family, and friends were able to recognize the emotional impact for parents of being pregnant with a baby with an abnormality. This was particularly true when the abnormality was seen as something less serious. Parents were given little opportunity to talk about how they felt about the baby and the future; the focus was usually on the medical aspects of care. It was possible for parents to have doubts and worries about the future, but perhaps not easy to express such mixed feelings in case this was perceived as "having second thoughts" about continuing the pregnancy.

11.2.8. Preparing for Birth

Preparing for birth was difficult. Many parents did not attend antenatal classes and could not look forward to the birth as anything other than a means to deliver the baby. For mothers in particular this was sometimes yet another loss. They had lost the healthy baby they had hoped for, the normal pregnancy that other women had, and a pleasurable anticipation of birth.

Many parents were concerned during their pregnancy about very practical issues: how to get to the right hospital for the birth and would an ambulance take the mother there if necessary; costs of antenatal care, including child care and transport; car parking at distant hospitals which were often in inner cities; whether the special care unit would be full when their baby came to be born. It appeared that addressing these concerns was not the responsibility of any one health professional. It was therefore difficult to obtain reassurance or practical help.

Overall, the impact of remaining pregnant was similar for all parents, regardless of the abnormality that had been discovered. Whether treatment was an option and the outcome for the baby likely to be good, or there was no treatment available or where treatment was a very risky procedure, parents were upset, anxious, and grieved the loss of the healthy baby they had been expecting. Health professionals, family and friends sometimes undermined the emotional impact of the less serious abnormalities and talked only about the "wonderful things that could be done." The ARC handbook for women continuing pregnancies can be helpful to parents and health professionals (10).

11.2.8.1. Are There Advantages in Prenatal Diagnosis in the Absence of Termination?

Cognitive consistency ensures that on the whole, parents are more likely to highlight the advantages of the path that they did actually follow and the disadvantages of the alternative. So parents whose baby was diagnosed postnatally could mostly see only disadvantages to knowing prenatally; similarly, very few of those parents who knew prenatally of an abnormality saw this as only disadvantageous.

There are, clearly, practical advantages in prenatal diagnosis for the baby where immediate treatment is going to be necessary. Though this is talked about as an advantage to the parents, it is of greater importance for the health professionals who will be caring for the baby after birth. But the impact on parents of prior knowledge, whether the condition is life-threatening or not, is distressing, just as it is when the knowledge is gained at birth. Parents talked about "being prepared" but it was not always clear that preparation was possible, given the uncertainty that surrounded all but a small number of diagnoses that were certainly lethal. While they may be prepared for "something" they cannot be sure quite what that something is. We were concerned that sometimes the appropriate preparations were not always made in hospitals after prenatal diagnosis, as in the provision of bottles for feeding babies known to have a cleft palate.

Some aspects of what happened to women after a postnatal diagnosis appeared to us at the time of interview to be particularly distressing, in particular the need to transfer to a distant hospital, knowing the baby was seriously ill and having just given birth, sometimes after a caesarean section. We anticipated that this would be seen with hindsight as a disadvantage of not knowing prenatally, but it was not raised by parents. If outcomes had been less successful for the babies that were transferred, the parents may have responded differently.

Key Points—Continuing a Pregnancy

- Parents may experience ambivalent feelings.
- Understand the practical difficulties that parents face—travel, cost, childcare.
- Communication between all health professionals involved in care is essential.
- Remember that the mother is still a pregnant woman who requires care for herself.
- Prepare parents as much as is possible about what will happen during and after the birth.
- The woman may be isolated from normal sources of community support like health visitors or groups of other mothers because of how the pregnancy was managed.

11.2.8.2. Emotional Well-Being 1 Year Later

We looked at a very wide range of variables across a wider range of parents than any other study has been able to do. Emotional well-being soon after the event accounts for much of the variance in mood one year later, but we have still only been able to account for a small proportion of the variance in initial mood. Parents who seek help initially are generally experiencing more emotional distress than those who do not and these differences persist a year later. Overall, mood generally improves with a supportive relationship and with another, successful, pregnancy. Older women with other living children who do not go to have another pregnancy, even if this is by choice, have low emotional well-being one year later.

A number of studies have tried to quantify women's grief by measuring psychological responses to termination after diagnosis of abnormality (11). Studies in that review showed great diversity, as do those published subsequently. What is constant across all studies is that psychological distress is high in the immediate aftermath of termination; it falls over time for most women. Some women remain distressed and, even for those coping well, aspects of the loss remain troublesome. It is in establishing the predictors of more adverse psychological responses that there is considerable inconsistency in the findings of different studies. Obstetric, demographic and social factors have been indicated in some studies but not all, with social support as the factor most consistently associated with mood disturbance after perinatal bereavement.

It is clearly important to know what is a normal response and hence what is pathological so that interventions can be offered to try to alleviate distress. It is particularly important to know if there are factors that can be identified, which place women at increased risk for an adverse psychological response. However, caution is needed in the interpretation of the findings of these empirical studies including our own: perinatal grief is a complex emotion and we may be doing women a disservice if we focus on trying to measure it rather than taking account of the individual woman.

Clearly individual differences, such as coping style, are important although it is difficult to assess these formally in studies like ours. It is clear there is no "right way" to grieve. One notable finding of our study was that women who specifically did not want care and who rejected a ritualized approach to grieving had the highest emotional well-being, that is, the lowest scores. Both men and women who said that there was nothing they wanted to talk about as time passed since the termination, also had consistently lower scores. We should remember, though, it is only the coping style that is right for those parents—it does not mean that other parents should be denied the opportunities to remember their baby and seek care as they wish. Yet again, the issue for health professionals caring for parents at such times is that they should allow and encourage parents to consider what they wish to do and what care they would like but not impose on any individual a rigid regime about "the right way" to grieve. Informing distressed parents of the options available to them is difficult but the ARC handbook was found by many in our study to be supportive in this respect. It may be particularly helpful as an aid to health professionals since it is a way of saying, "Here are some things that other parents have done" rather than "Here are some things that I think that you should do." In other words it is a more neutral way of conveying options without expectations.

11.2.8.3. Provision and Coordination of Care

In our study report (6) we documented the care-paths that parents follow when in a range of circumstances. With so many professionals potentially involved, the need for services and care to be coordinated is clear.

Although most individual health professionals provided good care, it was a persistent finding that coordination of care was poor. Failures in communication between and within hospitals and the community were common. The impact of this on parents was a cause for concern. In particular, it sometimes meant that the pregnant mother found it hard to access care for herself once the focus of the pregnancy had become the baby with the abnormality, who appeared in almost all cases to be given all of the care that could possibly be needed. Similarly, women who had terminated pregnancies often met community health professionals who did not know of their situation. The community health professionals could have offered care and/or support to women if only they had known it might have been needed. But of equal importance is the fact that many community-based health professionals reported their own distress when faced with the embarrassing consequences of communication failure (8).

Some Useful Web Resources

- http://www.arc-uk.org
- http://www.dipex.org/endingapregnancy
- http://www.dipex.org/antenatalscreening
- http://www.antenataltesting.info/
- http://www.rcog.org.uk/resources/Public/pdf/aminiocentesis_chorionicjan 2005.pdf
- http://www.cafamily.org.uk

References

1. ARC. *Supporting Parents' Decisions: A Handbook for Professionals.* London: Antenatal Results & Choices; 2005.
2. Green JM. Women's Experiences of Prenatal Screening and Diagnosis In: Abramsky L, Chapple J, eds. *Prenatal Diagnosis: The Human Side.* 2nd ed. Cheltenham: Nelson Thornes, 2003.
3. Green JM, Hewison J, Bekker HL, Bryant LD, Cuckle HS. Psychosocial aspects of genetic screening of pregnant women and newborns: a systematic review. *Health Technol Assess.* 2004;8(33).
4. O'Connor, T, Heron, J, Golding, J, Beveridge, M, Glover, V. Maternal stress or anxiety in pregnancy and emotional development of the child. *Br J Psychiatry.* 2002;171:105–106.

5. Robinson GE, Carr ML, Olmsted MP, Wright C. Psychological reactions to pregnancy loss after prenatal diagnostic testing: preliminary results. *J Psychosom Obstet Gynecol.* 1991;12:181–192.

6. Statham H, Solomou W, Green JM. When a baby has an abnormality: A study of parents' experiences.Part 1 of the Final Report to the NHS Exec (Mother and Child Health Initiative) of Grant no . MCH 4–12; 2001.

7. Statham H, Solomou W, Green JM. Continuing a pregnancy after the diagnosis of an anomaly: parents' experiences. In: Abramsky L, Chapple J, eds. *Prenatal Diagnosis: The Human Side.* 2nd ed. Cheltenham: Nelson Thornes, 2003.

8. Statham H, Solomou W, Green JM. Communication of prenatal screening and diagnosis results to primary-care health professionals. *Public Health.* 2003;117(5):348–357.

9. ARC. *A Handbook to Be Given to Parents When an Abnormality Is Diagnosed in Their Unborn Baby.* London: Antenatal Results & Choices; 1999.

10. ARC. *Supporting You Throughout Your Pregnancy: A Handbook for Parents After Prenatal Diagnosis.* London: Antenatal Results and Choices; 2003.

11. Statham H. Prenatal diagnosis of fetal abnormality: the decision to terminate the pregnancy and the psychological consequences. *Fetal and Matern Med Rev.* 2002;13(4):213–247.

12
Premature Labor and the Premature Baby: Psychological and Social Consequences

Gillian Gill

12.1. Incidence

The preterm delivery rate has been stable at between 5 and 10% of births in developed countries. A recent study has shown that almost 50% of deliveries between 28 and 35 weeks were iatrogenic with hypertension and pre-eclampsia as the major pathologies. Other factors include multiple pregnancy, intrauterine growth restriction, maternal stress, and heavy physical work (1). Every one of these births would have caused some degree of emotional trauma to the parents, which is unavoidable. A majority of these mothers will be counseled and cared for, antenatally, by obstetricians in future pregnancies. The challenge is to respond appropriately so that the adverse effects on parent–child relationships are minimized.

12.2. Management

In the immediate psychological crisis of premature delivery of their baby (whatever the medical context) most parents will display the common responses to hearing bad news. Good explanations, repeated if necessary on later occasions, as to why labor cannot be inhibited or delivery is advised on maternal or fetal grounds, are obviously desirable. The news will cause instant transition to a state of threat with both global and specific fears, which may inhibit recall of the explanation and verbal responses. For some it is the culmination of weeks of anxiety engendered by fertility treatment or close ultrasound surveillance; others will be encountering the often-unrecognized threat of pre-eclampsia. Feelings of helplessness and hopelessness will exacerbate the anxiety over what lies ahead and fears of this loss of autonomy are the norm.

12.3. Guidance for Good Practice

When premature delivery is likely to be planned rather than a sudden spontaneous event, there is an opportunity to mitigate the mother's anxiety to some extent by talking to her with her partner (to answer his questions directly) and working in collaboration with her midwife as she is likely to be informed on particular social stressors affecting the couple.

Counseling about risks and outcomes should ideally involve the offer of contact with your colleagues in Neonatology if this is practical. A consistent opinion on risks, outcomes and resources is clearly desirable. The recent research data on outcomes at the earlier gestations is easily available in the EPICURE Study (http://www.epicure./home page}.

If a lack of suitable cots necessitates lengthy negotiations with different hospitals and a transfer, this will naturally increase anxiety which is increased further if the separation of mother and baby is unavoidable. An acknowledgment of this, particularly if the mother has experienced previous loss or other obstetric complications, is clearly required alluding to the consequent social/family stress. If the patient does need transfer elsewhere for delivery, all involved will be sensitive to the disruption that this entails. Discussions, which are likely to elicit distress, need to be held in the maximum privacy possible, and particular regard paid to those for whom English is not the first language by using interpreters.

The process of good counselling should allow time for the couple to share their responses with each other, on their own if circumstances allow, and for the obstetrician to return to answer further questions, or acknowledge the inevitable feelings of fear, failure, and loss of autonomy.

The parents' hierarchy of concerns is likely to be first for the baby's survival but also that the baby will be both healthy and "normal." Maternal feelings of inadequacy may be to the fore, but there may also be anger that adherence to all the guidance on diet, smoking, and drinking has not brought the deserved outcome and the emotional and practical investment in the pregnancy is in jeopardy.

None of these feelings may be articulated at the time but may be very relevant in future debriefing, so reassurance that there will be continuing care and interest after delivery is valued.

It is always good practice to record these discussions in hand held notes for continuity of care, and in recognition that anxiety will make accurate recall difficult.

12.4. Debriefing After Emergency Delivery

Clearly the process outlined above may be precluded by events. Parents may have moved on emotionally to concern for the baby and put their concerns about delivery on hold for a future discussion.

If there was severe pre-eclampsia, or other threats to the mother's survival, she may have gaps in her memory of events which need addressing and have the risk of intrusive flashbacks in the future (2). It is extremely common for her partner to have experienced feelings of utter impotence and exclusion, contrary to all his expectations to add to the obvious fear for the mother's survival. The partner also may have recurrent disturbing dreams over such events but subordinate their needs in the desire to be appropriately supportive.

The offer to go through the medical record may need to be repeated at a later date. Evidence of infection may trigger further maternal guilt and rational explanations may not have much impact. Parents may construct their own version of events and many will attribute preterm delivery to stress, a very imprecise term.

Evidence-based research indicates that "Not all women reporting high levels of psychosocial stress deliver preterm but exposure to high levels of chronic stress and infectious pathogens increases risk" (3).

If at all possible visit the baby on the Unit as part of your postnatal care of the mother, so that there can be an informed sharing of feelings regarding the baby and of transition to the care of the neonatologists. Parents rate such visits highly and respect the intention of the obstetrician and those involved in her care previously to remain informed regarding the baby's progress.

Finding time for emotional scars as well as the physical aftermath of delivery to be assessed is extremely important as unresolved issues may surface again in subsequent pregnancies.

It is common for parents to seek information from many sources as they try to make sense of their experience and wish to share it with others. The internet may be a helpful source in this respect.

Current Useful UK-Based Web Sites

- http://www.bliss.org.uk for premature birth
- http://www.tommy's.org.uk
- http://www.apec.org.uk for pre-eclampsia
- http://www.tamba.org.uk for multiple births including the loss of a twin
- http://www.gbss.org.ukfor Group B Strep Support
- http://www.sands.org.ukfor stillbirth and neonatal death
- http://www.infertilitynetwork.uk for those who have had assisted reproduction

  These sites are designed to inform professional practice through anecdotal accounts as well as research abstracts highlighting both good and not so good practice from the patient's perspective.

12.5.   Difficult Scenarios

12.5.1.   Extreme Prematurity

Clearly the psychological sequelae of decisions made and actions taken at the borderline of viability are potentially the most controversial and problematic. The survival of a baby with severe disability has profound effects on relationships and family life.

Parents need to meet the neonatal team to discuss options at delivery and make a joint agreement about whether full resuscitation is to be offered. This meeting can also outline the normal practice of reviewing on a regular basis the appropriateness of continuing intensive care in the hours or days to come. When delivery is indicated for the sake of one twin, the clinician and couple face an extremely difficult decision. There is no avoiding extreme emotional pain, as anticipating the survival of either one or neither twin evokes immediate feelings of impending loss and bereavement.

Many parents may not have a clear ethical stance based on religious belief. The concept, appropriately phrased, of the lesser evil, may enable them to manage this experience when they revisit decisions and fear the disapproval of family, friends, and society.

Some parents will wish to have other significant family members present as they face the painful dilemma as to whether to intervene or not. They should have this choice if time permits, although the process is inevitably more complex. Parents may need this support for fear of ill informed criticism in the future. It does expose the clinician to more emotional stress and time commitment so is often not considered. As with most emotional trauma in life, including bereavement, the first recourse for help is normally the family.

However clear the recommendation, however painstaking the making of the decision has been, it is not always possible to prevent the guilt felt by parents at the overwhelming sense of failure to produce a healthy baby. But parental guilt over whatever decision is made, can be mitigated by giving time, when possible, to exploring their fears; by reassuring them that rejecting the risk of suffering and a poor quality of life is not the same as rejecting the child.

Factors such as age, existing children, social support, or the fact that the pregnancy is medically assisted, will influence all parties. Severe pain and strong analgesia may affect the ability of the mother to make a decision. There may also be the problem of different views between the parents.

The young doctor needs to remember that such discussions, undertaken on a case by case basis are extremely demanding on all involved and the professionals need their own support through formal and informal means. Self-awareness and openness can be a challenge and may only be achieved in the relative safety of chosen colleagues. It is common to experience a personal feeling of loss or inadequacy if the pregnancy has involved much clinical care and the mother has suffered previous losses.

A detailed record of these discussions and decisions is required. This will assist postdelivery contact, as there may be gaps in the recall of the sequence of events and the rationale for the decisions. Parents may need to have their choice reinforced in this way.

12.5.1.1. Points to Consider

- Guidelines exist in making informed recommendations. http://www.bapm.org/documents/publications/threshold.pdf
  Recent research emphasizes the importance of clarity and consensus of advice given respecting individual choice (4).
- Refer to the EPICURE Home Page for survival and outcome risks designed to assist counseling.
  http://www.nottingham.ac.uk/human development.EPIcure/info

12.5.2. Transfer Elsewhere for Delivery

12.5.2.1. Preparing for the Transfer

Giving any expectant mother the news that she needs to be sent out by ambulance to another hospital with suitable resources for a high-risk delivery and intensive care cots will inevitably raise anxiety and the sterling efforts to secure such resources may not seem to be rewarded. Acknowledging the real but unavoidable psychosocial consequences is helpful.

These include

1. Dislocation from family and friends.
2. Care of siblings becomes more complex.
3. Fear of staying in an unfamiliar hospital/town and what accommodation is there.
4. Disruption in professional obstetric and midwifery care.
5. Disempowerment as the decision is based on resources not choice.
6. Depersonalization. It is common for a mother to be defined by gestation and complications and not by name. Her personal social circumstances may be omitted in the referral letter.

If it is possible to give information about the named consultant who will receive the referral and the neonatal unit this can be helpful in the transition process. A commitment to continuing interest and the wish to debrief in the future are also helpful at this time which feels like abandonment.

12.6. Psychological Impact of Premature Parenthood

Bonding with their baby is a matter of concern to most parents. It is a term in common parlance which is often much too simplistic, and the majority of mothers who do not experience a surge of love and attachment at delivery can cope with this as they have the freedom to touch and explore their baby as they wish. Parents need help in relating in very different ways to a tiny fragile baby "covered in wires and pipes" who elicits fear. Attachment feels very risky, as the outcome is so uncertain. Normalizing these reactions and discussing the roller coaster of emotions is supportive. These parents will not receive many birth congratulation cards.

12.7.   Helping the Process of Attachment in the Neonatal Intensive Care Unit

Pre-delivery visits to familiarize parents with the environment and to meet staff is emphasizing that they will be told at once of any significant change in their baby's condition and gives them opportunity to assist in the transition of care. Looking at the photograph taken soon after the baby is admitted with parents and discussing good pain relief if required to coincide with visits to the Unit is important as mothers will ignore their own needs, and become exhausted by the physical as well as emotional demands on them.

Staff on the Unit will need to adapt their practice and care to individual parents in order to give them the best support. This care is characterized by:

- Emphasis on physical touch and holding as soon as possible.
- Explanation of the monitoring, treatment and the baby's condition as often as needed.
- Reassurance that they will be told, wherever they are, of any significant change in their baby's condition.
- Encouraged to do at least mouth care and to change nappies in the incubator.
- Identifying reactions to parental voices as the sense of hearing is shown.
- Demonstrating containment holds to calm their baby.
- Supporting all efforts to supply breast milk and valuing any amount, however small.
- Offering kangaroo cuddles (skin to skin) even at times when the baby has ventilatory or CPAP support.
- Ensuring the progressive involvement of both parents and siblings in care.
- Identifying the individual stresses of parents and developing honest communication with regular updates on their baby's progress.

12.8.   Caring for Fathers

Recognition of their needs is viewed positively as they have been denied the role that they had anticipated at the birth and may have had to deal with the twin fears for their partner's physical and emotional well-being and the outcome for the baby. Many will describe their feelings of disempowerment and inadequacy on being thrust into a role of supporting their partner and the rest of the family in a crisis that was not envisaged.

Their rights to paid leave will usually be brief and are designed to help when the baby goes home. State benefit is modest and many will rely on the goodwill of employers to survive financially. The self employed are under greater stress.

The care of any other children will be even more demanding as they react to the absence of their mother and the general high levels of anxiety and disruption to routines.

The pressure on time to fulfill home demands and make hospital visits, perhaps at a distance, added to lack of sleep can lead to a state of exhaustion and there are circumstances when they will need to seek the advice of their GP. Often fathers will need explicit permission to share these feelings as they consider them trivial compared to the trauma their partner has experienced.

On a practical level a long NICU stay has considerable financial implications as only a small minority on specific benefits can claim any state help in the cost of visiting. Charitable help is very limited. These factors will add to the other financial pressure to return to work. Generally, compassion is forthcoming for a baby in intensive care but their NICU stay may be many weeks. If the baby is likely to have extra-care needs then there will be concern as to whether the plans for the mother's return to work will need revision.

12.9.   Neonatal Death

12.9.1.   Parental Fears and Reality

The risk of loss for the extremely premature baby in the first week of life appears to be higher if conceived by IVF (5). There will be ongoing risks of infection or intraventricular hemorrhage or other complications.

Parents are at times often involved in several difficult discussions with their neonatal consultant on the appropriateness of continuing intensive care, particularly if the ultrasound examination of the brain indicates a high risk of significant future disability or when treatment appears futile. The aim should always be for the parents to be prepared for the death. They should be supported if they wish to be present and it is extremely rare for the baby not to be cuddled by them at that time, even if fairly briefly.

These memories are usually of some psychological comfort in the future as death in these circumstances is usually a gentle and peaceful event.

The death of one twin is a complex challenge. The grief is not only for themselves but also for the surviving twin and its own loss of a sibling. Parents will sometimes interpret any change in the surviving baby's behavior to a sense of loss for the baby. Simultaneously their anxiety over the survival of the other twin increases and often postpones elements of their grief until the surviving twin is discharged. They then have a strong feeling that there should have been two. Continuing to visit the NICU up until discharge is very hard.

Staff need to accept that the impact of grief is individual. It is not helped by phrases such as "You are only young" or "At least you have.... ." Expressions of condolence and listening are the most helpful. Couples may want to de-brief at this point as to the reasons for the premature birth or postpone this to the future when further information may be available from a post-mortem. The parents' feelings of failure and guilt experienced at the delivery may be re-enforced at this time.

Most parents will be aware of the risks of multiple birth, particularly if they are the result of assisted pregnancy, but that in itself does not diminish the sense of loss and shock. Like all risks it is common to be optimistic until life proves otherwise. Twinning is reported to be 10 times more likely in IVF pregnancies (30% of IVF births) (5).

12.10.   Long Term Consequences of Premature Birth

Refer to the EPIcure data for the physical, cognitive, and behavioral outcomes for babies born very prematurely (6).

Many mothers describe enhanced levels of anxiety which are confirmed by research (7,8). The study by Auslander showed fathers to rate higher than usual on the Edinburgh Post Natal Depression Scale.

Immediately, post discharge parents may need to cope with extra-care needs such as oxygen dependence or feeding problems, but it is common for this to be helped by the empowerment which marks discharge from hospital, and an enhanced attachment to the baby. Overprotective behavior toward a medically vulnerable child at this stage would be normal.

Many parents will experience isolation after taking their baby home. Social contacts are selected and the parents avoid situations where their baby's difference in size or development is the source of comment. It is appropriate to correct for gestational age for the first 2 years. This can confuse parental expectations. Mothers would have spent a proportion of their maternity leave in NICU and may amend plans for their working lives with obvious economic consequences. This may lead to fathers having to work longer hours.

Social support from the wider family can be extremely valuable. Existing children may resent the high level of care needs of the baby. This level of care may have an impact on the timing of any subsequent pregnancy.

12.11.   Caring in the Next Pregnancy

All couples will value a plan, subject to amendment by mutual agreement, for care in the next pregnancy. They may seek prepregnancy counseling to re-visit the circumstances of their premature delivery and discuss the risk of recurrence.

Scans to establish dating of the fetus and serial scanning are usually an obvious source of support, although at times a mother may wish to label her pregnancy as "normal" and opt out of the pressures of many appointments. Most will inevitably experience a heightened fear of all the possible complications of pregnancy and even at term fear the outcome of delivery.

Hospitalization during the pregnancy is very stressful as it will mean separation from their ex-premature infant. This can re-arouse past events if feelings remain unresolved and there is not an obvious substitute carer.

The fear of prematurity again and the need for NICU care is ever present. Furthermore, parents are fearful that such anxiety is in itself stressful and therefore increases the risk of preterm labor. This is a vicious circle difficult to break. Staff should be alert to symptoms of Post Traumatic Stress Disorder and check for a history of postnatal depression. Anxiety will rise instantly if there is any recurrence of symptoms of the previous pregnancy. Most mothers will value open access to midwifery care where these fears and symptoms are taken seriously.

For parents themselves there is often the wish to make some kind of reparation for the previous pregnancy "to do it right this time."

12.12. Summary

Premature delivery creates premature parents both emotionally and practically unprepared.

- Most mothers will experience a traumatic loss of autonomy and the need to adjust to unwelcome dependence on authoritative professional advice and judgments.
- Acknowledgment of this transition to dependence and the concomitant fears by assurance of individual care is helpful.
- Counseling on risks and statistics will be subject to individual interpretation and often inhibited by time factors and analgesia [Zupanic 2002 op cit] .
- Acknowledging the paternal concerns lessens maternal anxiety.
- Debriefing after delivery is essential to address maternal feelings of guilt, failure and fears for the welfare of the baby. It is an opportunity to listen to the full experience from both parents not just to present the clinical facts, and should have the appropriate allocation of uninterrupted time.

References

1. Steer P. The epidemiology of preterm labour. *Br J Obstet Gynaecol.* 2005; 112(Suppl. 1):1–3.
2. Post-traumatic stress disorder after pre-eclampsia. An exploratory study. *Gen Hosp Psychiatry.* 2002;24(4):260–264
3. Wadhwa, et al. Stress, infection and preterm birth. *Paediatr Perinat Epidemiol.* 2001;15(Suppl. 2): 17–19.

4. Kaempf JW, et al. Medical staff guidelines for periviability pregnancy counselling and medical treatment of extremely premature infants. *Paediatrics.* 2006;117: 22–29.
5. Panel reviews Health Effects Data for Assisted Reproductive Technologies. *JAMA.* 2004;292:2961–2962.
6. EPIcure study, associations and antecedents of neurological and developmental disability at 30 months following extremely pre-term birth. *Arch Dis Child* (Fetal and neonatal edition). 2005;90(2).
7. The impact of very premature birth on the psychological health of mothers. *Early Hum Dev.* Aug 2003;73(1–2):61–70.
8. Auslander GK, et al. Parental anxiety following discharge from hospital of their very low birth weight infant. *Fam Relat.* 2003;52.

13
Posttraumatic Stress Disorder

Susan Ayers

Pregnancy and birth are naturally a time of great change and adjustment, and the postnatal period is associated with mental health problems such as the baby blues, postnatal depression, and puerperal psychosis. In the last decade, research has also shown that a proportion of women suffer from posttraumatic stress disorder (PTSD) after obstetric and gynecological events (1). PTSD has been identified after birth, stillbirth, miscarriage, and a variety of gynecological procedures. This chapter concentrates on PTSD after birth because this is where the majority of research has been carried out. For psychological outcome after stillbirth or miscarriage, see Chapters 17 and 21.

This chapter is divided into four sections. Section 13.1 explains what PTSD is, how many women suffer from PTSD, and uses case studies to illustrate how PTSD can occur and present clinically. Section 13.2 gives an overview of research into the causes of postnatal PTSD and subsequently how it might be prevented. Section 13.3 explores clinical implications. Section 13.4 deals with treatment for PTSD.

13.1. What is PTSD?

Diagnostic criteria for PTSD are given in Table 13.1. It can be seen that PTSD occurs when people believe their life or physical integrity is threatened or that there is a threat to the life or physical integrity of another significant person, such as their partner or baby. In addition to this, people have to respond with intense fear, helplessness, or horror. Both of these are possible during gynecological and obstetric events where there can be a real or perceived threat to the life of the woman or baby. Symptoms of PTSD fall into three clusters: (i) re-experiencing symptoms such as nightmares and flashbacks; (ii) avoidance and numbing symptoms, such as avoiding all reminders of the event and feeling emotionally numb; and (iii) arousal symptoms, such as hyperarousal, irritability, and aggression.

However, as with physical illness, individuals differ in their symptom presentation for PTSD. Some clinicians distinguish between simple PTSD, which tends to occur after an acute trauma and is usually characterized by

TABLE 13.1. DSM-IV criteria for PTSD (2)

Criteria	
Stressor	Trauma involves actual or threatened death/serious injury or threat to physical integrity of self or others
	Individual responded with intense fear, helplessness, or horror
Symptoms	
Re-experiencing: one or more	Recurrent and intrusive distressing recollections of the event
	Recurrent distressing dreams of the event
	Acting or feeling as if the event was recurring (e.g., flashbacks, hallucinations)
	Intense psychological distress at exposure to internal or external cues that symbolize or resemble the event
	Physiological reactivity on exposure to internal or external cues that symbolize or resemble the event
Avoidance and numbing: three or more	Efforts to avoid thoughts, feelings, or conversations associated with the event
	Efforts to avoid activities, places, or people that arouse recollections of the event
	Inability to recall an important aspect of the trauma
	Diminished interest or participation in significant activities
	Feeling of detachment or estrangement from others
	Restricted range of affect
	Sense of foreshortened future
Arousal: two or more	Difficulty falling or staying asleep
	Irritability or outbursts of anger
	Difficulty concentrating
	Hypervigilance
	Exaggerated startle response
Duration	1 month or more
Disability	Symptoms cause clinically significant distress or impairment in social, occupational, or other important areas of functioning

high levels of fear and avoidance of factors associated with the event, and complex PTSD, which is more likely after repeated or prolonged traumas and can involve symptoms of personality disorder and other comorbid problems. People with PTSD can also present with predominantly different emotions, such as fear, anger, shame, or guilt. This is shown in Boxes 13.1 and 13.2, which describe two women with postnatal PTSD who have different causes and symptom presentations.

Sarah (13.1)

Sarah was 35 years old. Her daughter was born 14 months previously as a result of a planned pregnancy. Sarah had a termination of an unwanted pregnancy when she was 19 years old, which she kept a secret for 16 years because she thought people would judge her negatively. Sarah was very anxious during pregnancy because she was scared of disclosing the abortion and worried that something might go wrong with the pregnancy as retribution for having an abortion. During her pregnancy, Sarah had frequent bleeding and a colposcopy was carried out to investigate.

Sarah's waters broke before term and her labor was induced 3 days later. There was confusion over the induction, and Sarah arrived at hospital for what she thought was a routine check and was immediately admitted for induction. At this point she panicked because she was unprepared, had no personal belongings with her, and her husband was not present. The midwife attending Sarah's birth was not sympathetic to Sarah's high levels of anxiety. Following a painful internal examination during which Sarah cried and asked the midwife to stop, the midwife said, "if you think that's painful, what are you going to be like giving birth?" From this point onward Sarah's labor and delivery was characterized by pain, very high levels of distress, and fear of the midwife who continued to be brusque and unsympathetic toward Sarah. Sarah said, "the midwife was barking at me...I brought my barriers up completely and was petrified... I didn't know what was right and what was wrong."

During a long labor, Sarah was given pethadine, which had a severe effect on her mental state—she said she was "off the planet"—and then an epidural despite a long-standing fear of epidurals because of risk of paralysis. After 25 h Sarah was only 1 cm dilated, so her daughter was delivered by emergency cesarean section during which Sarah thought she might die. Sarah reported starting to feel the surgeon cutting her half way through the cesarean and was given morphine. She reported dissociating during the cesarean and cannot remember anything for 12 h after the delivery. She said the first few months after the birth "are a blur" and it took her a year to bond with her daughter. The main themes of Sarah's birth experience seemed to be (i) feeling terrified, vulnerable, and out of control; (ii) high levels of confusion and later dissociation; and (iii) confirmation of her belief that others will judge her and hurt her through her experience with the midwife.

Four months after birth, Sarah was diagnosed with postnatal depression by her GP. She was treated with antidepressants and attended a local support group for postnatal depression. When Sarah first attended therapy, 14 months after birth, she was highly distressed because coming to hospital triggered memories of her birth experience. During this session she appeared to be reliving the birth experience and was frightened, crying, and shaking. She had the full range of PTSD symptoms in the form of flashbacks, nightmares, strong physical and emotional reactions to reminders of birth, feeling emotionally numb yet crying all the time. Her flashbacks were to seeing herself lying in the delivery room, feeling helpless, and terrified, with the midwife coming in through the door. Sarah had only mild symptoms of depression by this stage and was reducing her dose of antidepressants.

Juliet (13.2)

Juliet was 32 years old. Her daughter had been born 8 months earlier as a result of a planned first pregnancy. Juliet's pregnancy was straightforward. She had a spontaneous labor of 32 h during which Juliet experienced difficulty breathing because of her asthma. The midwife called the obstetrician as labor was progressing slowly, and Juliet was offered the option of a cesarean section "at some point in the next few hours if things do not speed up," Juliet felt that she was not coping well, and wanted a cesarean immediately, but lacked the confidence to ask. Her husband encouraged her to continue with a vaginal birth, and she felt very resentful about this. Eventually she was told a forceps delivery was necessary, and an episiotomy was performed in an effort to prevent tearing. Juliet was then rushed into the operating theater as the baby appeared to be in distress, and it was thought an emergency cesarean section would need to be performed. However, her daughter was born vaginally with forceps and Juliet sustained a third-degree tear. On the second postnatal day, Juliet experienced fecal incontinence, which she was extremely embarrassed and ashamed of and felt humiliated. She continued to experience incontinence for the first postnatal week and was discharged home on day 8. She was depressed by this time and spent the first 2 weeks at home in bed, refusing to get up. Her relationship with her daughter remained positive.

Although Juliet was coping better when she attended for therapy, there were still multiple problems. Juliet felt dirty most of the time. She blamed herself and her husband for the traumatic birth, believing that they should have demanded a cesarean section earlier in the labor. She additionally blamed the hospital staff for not intervening more quickly. Juliet and her husband Neil were fighting a great deal of the time, and the couple had not been sexually intimate since the birth. Juliet was still experiencing some incontinence of urine and wind. She was receiving regular physiotherapy and physically her symptoms were improving. However, her confidence and self-esteem remained extremely low, and she was still moderately depressed as well as experiencing the full range of PTSD symptoms in the form of intense anger outbursts, poor sleep, flashbacks to the postnatal incontinence, avoidance of the labor ward, and emotional numbing in addition to a degree of postnatal depression.

Lifetime prevalence of PTSD in the general population is around 5–6% for men and 10–11% for women. Women are therefore approximately two times more likely to develop PTSD than men although they are not exposed to more traumatic events than men. Thus, in any field of clinical practice, it is likely that you will encounter a few people with PTSD (1).

Approximately 6% of women have PTSD following obstetric or gynecological procedures; and recent research suggests up to 5% of men have PTSD

TABLE 13.2. PTSD in O&G

Women are two times more likely to get PTSD after a traumatic event than men
Around 6% of women will have PTSD after gynecological or obstetric events, particularly labor and delivery
Research suggests that up to 5% of men will also have PTSD after witnessing their baby's birth
Up to half of people with PTSD immediately after the event recover spontaneously without intervention in the first 3 months after the event
People who continue to have PTSD 3 or more months after the event usually require psychological intervention

---

after witnessing their partner's labor and delivery. It is not clear whether all of these cases of PTSD occur as a direct result of the obstetric or gynecological event or whether some people already had PTSD. However, at any time, 6% of postnatal women and up to 5% of their partners might have current PTSD. Many more will be distressed or have subclinical symptoms. For example, one-third of women appraise their birth experience as traumatic and approximately 10% have subclinical symptoms of PTSD. However, many people will recover spontaneously in the first weeks after birth. Up to one-half of people with PTSD symptoms recover without intervention in the first 3 months after the event, which has obvious implications for referral and treatment. Those who still have PTSD 3 months after an event are unlikely to recover without psychological intervention. In obstetrics, research suggests that between 1 and 2% of women will continue to have PTSD in the long term as a direct result of their birth experience.

Finally, PTSD is highly comorbid with other mental health problems such as depression, substance abuse, and panic. This is illustrated by the case studies in Boxes 13.1 and 13.2 where both women have concurrent symptoms of depression. PTSD and depression also have common symptoms, such as distress and sleep disturbances, which raises the issue of how to distinguish between them in clinical practice. The best indication that a woman has postnatal PTSD instead of, or as well as, depression is the re-experiencing symptoms of flashbacks, nightmares, and uncontrollable intrusive thoughts about birth. Women with postnatal PTSD also commonly have an intense fear of future pregnancy and birth (see Chapter 16) (Table 13.2).

13.2. What Causes PTSD in O&G?

Research into the causes of postnatal PTSD has identified many antenatal and delivery factors as associated with postnatal PTSD. For example, antenatal factors such as anxiety, parity, confidence to cope during labor, history of psychological problems, difficult or unplanned pregnancy, and poor social support have been variously associated with symptoms of PTSD. Delivery factors such as pain, inadequate pain relief, low control, distress, dissociation, intervention (e.g., episiotomy, induced onset), poor support, perceived inadequate care, and negative contact with staff have also been associated with symptoms of PTSD. Despite the wide array of prenatal and delivery factors associated with symptoms of PTSD, the only factors *consistently* associated with clinically significant postnatal PTSD are a history of psychological problems, mode of delivery (e.g., instrumental/surgical), and poor support during labor (4). This does not mean other factors are not implicated, only that there is not an adequate research base at present from which to draw conclusions. In addition, many factors that might be important, such as expectations, control, and a history of sexual abuse, have yet to be properly examined.

One of the difficulties that contributes to inconsistencies in research is the individual and subjective nature of postnatal PTSD. Like PTSD, after other medical events, there is not a simple dose–response relationship between the severity of obstetric complications and PTSD severity. Instead, PTSD severity is more closely associated with a woman's *perception* of the severity of the event. This is evident in Sarah's case (see Box 13.1) where her high levels of fear and panic during delivery were due to her perception of being unprepared, out of control, feeling bullied by the midwife, and believing she was going to die. Yet from a medical perspective, there is little evidence of any objective threat to Sarah's life. Emergency cesareans are another good example of different perspectives. We can compare an emergency cesarean to a dawn raid by police. In a dawn raid, a team of police officers in uniform burst into a suspect's house, shouting, and crowd into the room in a deliberate tactic to frighten and intimidate suspects. During an emergency cesarean, lots of medical personnel in uniform rush into the room, snapping commands to each other, invading the woman's space, and doing things to her that she probably does not understand. The effect can be the same on her as the police raid has on a suspect.[1]

So, it is important to remember that what is normal to us is not normal to women and their partners. In addition, as the case studies show, we cannot assume that women will only develop PTSD if they have severe obstetric complications or, alternatively, that all women with severe obstetric complications will necessarily develop PTSD. In my own practice and research, I have seen many women with postnatal PTSD following normal vaginal deliveries as well as women who suffer severe, life-threatening complications and do not develop PTSD.

Obstetric complications are therefore neither necessary nor sufficient causes of postnatal PTSD, and we need to take into account the interaction between individual vulnerability factors and the events of birth. Vulnerability can be obvious, such as a history of psychological problems or sexual abuse, or less obvious, as in Sarah's case where fear of disclosing her obstetric history led to unnaturally high levels of anxiety whenever she was in contact with obstetric personnel.

Finally, research has established that support in labor is critical, both in terms of delivery outcome (5) and in terms of postnatal PTSD. Many care factors have been associated with postnatal PTSD, such as perceived inadequate care, perceived negative staff attitudes, negative contact with staff, low

---

[1] I am indebted to Emma Cuppini for this analogy.

TABLE 13.3. Causes of postnatal PTSD and how to prevent it

What causes postnatal PTSD?
Postnatal PTSD is more likely in people with a history of psychological problems, instrumental or surgical deliveries, and poor perceived support
Perceived severity of the event is more important than objective severity
How can we prevent postnatal PTSD?
Antenatal education: recognize that women have individual needs and expectations and not imply one form of birth is "better" than another
Educate women about postnatal PTSD so that it is recognized early and they are more likely to seek help
During labor: individualize care. Remember that *what is normal to you is not normal to them*. Give women and their partners high levels of support and information and involve them in decisions
Handle emergency situations sensitively. Give women and their partners as much time and information as possible. Reassurance can greatly reduce the perception of life threat
Postnatal care should be sensitive and supportive. The issue of PTSD should be raised with women who may be at later risk of developing it
Raise awareness of PTSD in primary care so PTSD is identified early. Better liaison between midwives, health visitors, GPs, and obstetricians can help identify women at high risk and women who require help
Screen for PTSD 6 weeks after birth
If women have PTSD, screen their partners as well

support from staff or partner, not being informed of labor progress, generally feeling inadequately informed, not having views and wishes listened to by staff, not having questions answered, poor communication, and conflict with staff. The way we deal with women in O&G is therefore critical for their physical and mental health, both of which are equally important. For example, simple reassurance during obstetric complications that a woman and her baby will be alright can avoid or reduce the perception of life threat and subsequent fear.

The Birth Trauma Association (BTA) (http://www.birthtraumaassociation .org.uk) suggests postnatal PTSD can be reduced or avoided by "providing woman-centered care which includes good communication, the provision of quality information, and involving the woman in decision-making" and that women's decisions should be respected "wherever clinically possible and should not be subject to criticism." In practice the BTA proposed that this is achieved through the changes outlined in Table 13.3. These are fairly broad suggestions that are mostly basic good practice. How effective these suggestions will be is in the detail of how they are implemented. For example, if during emergency cesarean sections one person on the team is formally delegated to be with the woman and her partner, support and reassure them, and stay with them on the way to theater, it might make the difference between mental health and mental illness afterward.

13.3.   What Are the Clinical Implications of PTSD?

Postnatal PTSD has obvious implications for women and their families. Women with postnatal PTSD are more likely to report poor physical health, poor mental health, poor attachment with the baby, and strain in their marital

TABLE 13.4. How to recognize and ask about PTSD

How to recognize PTSD
Does the woman or her husband appear anxious, emotionally distanced, or flat?
If you ask her about the birth or gynecological procedure, does she show signs of distress (e.g., quiet, flushed, tearful)?
Does she not want to talk about the birth or gynecological procedure?
Are there treatments/procedures she is highly resistant to (avoidant) such as treatment that requires returning to the antenatal or postnatal clinics/ward or more contact with midwives or doctors?
Is she a repeated DNA? This is a possible indicator of strong anxiety and avoidance
Are she and/or her partner insisting on an elective cesarean for a subsequent pregnancy?
How to ask about distress
Recognise the woman's feelings: for example, "You seem to be quite upset/anxious"
Normalize: for example, "I know some women find birth difficult/have a really difficult time during birth"
Ask: for example, "is/was this the case for you?"
Validate: for example, "it's quite understandable that you feel upset/anxious"
How to clarify if it is PTSD
Normalize: for example, "when women have a difficult birth they sometimes have nightmares or flashbacks; or find that they can't stop thinking about the birth, particularly if something reminds them of it."
Ask about re-experiencing symptoms: for example, "Have you had any nightmares or flashbacks about the birth?"

relationship. If the woman has PTSD, it is also possible that her partner has PTSD, which will compound the situation further. Although we know much less about postnatal PTSD in men, a recent qualitative study interviewed six couples where the woman had postnatal PTSD and found three of their husbands also had PTSD. This has mixed repercussions with regard to health-care use. Some women and men with postnatal PTSD will avoid contact with health-care professionals if it reminds them of the traumatic event. Others will frequently attend GP practices and outpatient clinics because of these physical and mental health problems.

It is therefore important to know how to spot PTSD in clinical practice in both men and women. Table 13.4 gives guidelines on how to recognize PTSD and how to ask about it.

13.4.   What Is the Best Way to Treat PTSD in O&G?

The recommended treatment in the UK and the USA for PTSD is psychotherapy, particularly cognitive behavior therapy (CBT). For an example of how CBT was used to treat the women in the case studies, see (3). Selective serotonin reuptake inhibitors (SSRIs) can be helpful in complex cases but are not recommended for simple PTSD. Treatment by antidepressants is unlikely to be effective unless women have comorbid depression.

One of the issues in referring people for treatment is that many people recover spontaneously in the first 3 months after the event. However, it is very difficult to determine who will recover and who will not. Therefore, I believe that everyone with suspected PTSD should be referred onward to local psychotherapy services for assessment and treatment. This referral can be to adult mental health services in secondary care, community mental health teams, or primary care centers that have counseling services.

However, in a resource-strapped NHS, psychotherapy services are often sparse, and although patients are usually assessed within 6 weeks, there might be a long wait after that before treatment commences. This raises the question of what you can do in the interim to help women and their partners. Firstly, self-help information and support are available from the BTA, so you should inform women of this. Secondly, up to 94% of UK hospitals offer some form of postnatal service for women who have difficult births (6). These are usually midwife-led and offer some form of birth-debriefing service, which might be useful. It is therefore worth finding out what is available in your hospital. Research into midwife-debriefing shows that most women say it is helpful, but it has little or no effect on women's long-term mental health. There is also little evidence that debriefing is effective for PTSD in other populations, so its use is currently controversial (7). Therefore, at best, debriefing might be a useful adjunct to psychotherapy, but not a substitute. Finally, for patients who are able to fund private treatment, the British Psychological Society has a register of chartered clinical psychologists (http://www.bps.org.uk) and the British Association of Behavioural and Cognitive Psychotherapies has a register of accredited CBT therapists (http://www.babcp.org.uk).

13.5. Summary and Conclusion

In summary, up to 6% of women and 5% of men might have PTSD after labor and delivery. People who have a previous history of psychiatric problems are more vulnerable to developing PTSD, as are people who undergo instrumental or surgical deliveries and have poor support. However, the *perceived* severity of the event is more important than objective severity, so we must be aware that apparently normal procedures can be traumatizing for some men and women.

Half of people with PTSD will probably recover spontaneously in the first 3 months after the event. PTSD can also be masked by comorbid disorders, such as depression, so it is important to ask about re-experiencing symptoms, such as nightmares and flashbacks. For those who do not recover, PTSD will affect physical health, mental health, attachment with their baby, and marital relationship. It is therefore important to identify these people and refer them for psychotherapy. Self-help information and midwife-debriefing can be a useful adjunct to treatment.

In conclusion, an increased awareness of PTSD means you are more likely to pick it up in your clinical practice. In my clinical experience, cases of PTSD in O&G are often straightforward responses to a single event or procedure, such as birth. This means these cases are usually responsive to treatment if caught early enough. However, if these cases are not treated, then PTSD can become chronic and be more likely to result in other comorbid problems such as depression, panic, and drug abuse, which require more intensive treatment over a longer period of time and are less likely to be successful. Thus, identifying PTSD in clinical practice and immediately referring clients for treatment can save time, cost, and suffering in the long term.

References

1. Tedstone JE, Tarrier N. Posttraumatic stress disorder following medical illness and treatment. *Clin Psychol Rev.* 2003;23(3):409–448.
2. American Psychiatric Association. *Diagnostic and Statistical Manual for Mental Disorders.* 4th ed. Washington, DC: American Psychiatric Press Inc.; 1994.
3. Ayers S, McKenzie-McHarg K, Eagle A. Cognitive behaviour therapy for postnatal post-traumatic stress disorder: a case series. *J Psychosom Obstet Gynecol.* In press.
4. Ayers S. Delivery as a traumatic event: prevalence, risk factors and treatment for postnatal posttraumatic stress disorder. *Clin Obstet Gynecol.* 2004;47(3).
5. Hodnett ED, Gates S, Hofmeyr G, Sakala C. Continuous support for women during childbirth. *Cochrane Database Syst Rev.* 2003(3): Art no.: CD003766. DOI:10.1002/14651858.CD003766.
6. Ayers S, Claypool J, Eagle A. What happens after a difficult birth? Postnatal debriefing services. *Br J Midwifery.* 2006;14(3):157–161.
7. Wessely S, Bisson J. Brief psychological interventions ("debriefing") for trauma-related symptoms and prevention of post traumatic stress disorder. *Cochrane Library.* 2001(1).

Further Reading

Review of Postnatal PTSD

1. Ayers S. Delivery as a traumatic event: prevalence, risk factors and treatment for postnatal posttraumatic stress disorder. *Clin Obstet Gynecol.* 2004;47(3).

Role of Obstetric Events in Postnatal PTSD

1. Söderquist J, Wijma K, Wijma B. Traumatic stress after childbirth: the role of obstetric variables. *J Psychosom Obstet Gynaecol.* 2002;23:31–39.

Review of PTSD after Medical Illnesses

1. Tedstone JE, Tarrier N. Posttraumatic stress disorder following medical illness and treatment. *Clin Psychol Rev.* 2003;23(3):409–448.

14
Antenatal and Postnatal Depression

Kirstie N. McKenzie-McHarg, Jayne Cockburn, and John Cox

Whilst many obstetricians have a view that postnatal depression happens in the community at 6 weeks, there is in fact much they can do to help, prevent, and reduce the incidence antenatally. Because of the damage to babies and mortality, which is now, the second cause of maternal death in the last annual report, we urgently need to get this message across and empower obstetricians. The incidence of postnatal depression is 13%, similar to the incidence of pre-eclampsia at 10%. Like pre-eclampsia, there is a lot of mild disease, which will respond readily. However, there is severe disease, which causes serious problems. The incidence of severe depression is probably higher than eclampsia. Like eclampsia, the end result may be death of the mother and long-term damage to the child. We spend a large amount of health service resources on pre-eclampsia, for example, admission to hospital, scans, and admissions to day unit for all sorts of screening. We have practically nothing for postnatal depression. The contrast is stark yet the ability to intervene to improve outcomes for mothers and babies in depression is great. Social support has often been shown to be the key in prevention, but the obstetrician tends to think that this approach is not medical, not antenatal anyway, and therefore not in their power to influence. Nothing could be further from the truth.

Postnatal depression is probably the most widely discussed perinatal mood disorder. Defined as arising in, or persisting into, the first postnatal year, it affects around 13% of women following childbirth (1). Postnatal depression presents similarly to depression at other times. It is characterized by low mood, tearfulness, emotional lability, fatigue, excessive anxiety, attachment difficulties, and withdrawal from social events. Because of the similarity with depression arising for other reasons and at other times, there has been much debate about whether or not postnatal depression is in fact a separate diagnostic entity. There is research supporting the position that it is identical to clinical depression arising at other times (2) but also that it is a separate diagnosis (3). However, the research demonstrating the longer-term impacts on the family and children is compelling and as such it is probably unhelpful to be concerned about the precise similarity or difference of the diagnosis. It is far more important to identify and treat those women who are suffering. The NICE guidelines, published on 28th February 2007, look at treatment options for mothers. There are concerns that they do not take into account the need for early and active treatment to minimise both the short and potentially lif-long consequences for the infant. We aim to provide a comprehensive overview from why depression matters, recognising the problems, what to say in consultations as well as what treatment might be useful and when, thus empowering the clinician to be able to assess and treat each mother (and baby) depending on their individual circumstances.

14.1.   Why Does Postnatal Depression Matter?

14.1.1.   Mother

1. Psychiatric illness was the most common cause of indirect deaths and the largest cause of maternal deaths overall in the last CEMACH report (Why Mothers Die 2000–2002).
2. It is reasonable to speculate that a tremendous amount of damage was also present in families where the women did not die, but made a failed attempt at suicide.
3. Although symptoms of depression may remit spontaneously, or respond to "listening visits" or nondirective person centered counseling offered by health visitors, about one-third of women will remain depressed and need further treatment.
4. Untreated depression may contribute to the development of a chronic, refractory mood disorder in the mother, a potentially negative influence on the marital relationship with the possibility of contributing to raised rates of separation in couples. This will also have a negative impact on the infant as well as any other siblings.
5. Difficulties are often concealed. This may be due to cultural attitudes to mental health problems. Women fear the label and what they perceive as the stigma; they are afraid that they will be seen as a bad mother and the baby will be taken away. The disease process itself makes people feel isolated and not want to relate to anyone including health professionals.

14.1.2.   Impact On the Child(ren)

This is one area of research in which there is good evidence that postnatal depression, particularly if moderate or severe, can have long-lasting negative effects on any children in the family, with the new infant being particularly at risk. There appear to be both short- and long-term effects.

14.1.2.1.   Short Term

a. Infants are often reported as being of more "difficult" temperament by their mothers (although this may be because the mothers are themselves not coping well and giving poor feedback emotionally to the children, who then behave in a more difficult fashion in order to gain attention).

b. Less sensitive mother–infant interactions are seen, leading to insecure attachment patterns (4).

c. One study has even reported postnatal depression to be a risk factor for Sudden Infant Death Syndrome (SIDS), although this small study must be viewed with caution (5).

14.1.2.2. Long Term

a. A number of researchers have found adverse effects persisting for some time, and this effect appears to be more marked for boys.

b. Sinclair and Murray (6) found postnatal depression to be associated with significantly raised levels of child disturbance at the age of 5 years, particularly in boys.

c. Another group of researchers (7) has been following a cohort of 149 women recruited at 3 months postpartum. One hundred and thirty-two of their children were followed up at age 11. Children of women depressed at 3 months postnatal were found to have significantly lower IQ scores, more attention problems, and difficulties in mathematical reasoning and were more likely to have special educational needs. Boys were more severely affected than girls.

d. Finally, a meta-analysis conducted by Beck (8) concluded that "postpartum depression had a small but significant effect on children's cognitive and emotional development." For all these reasons, identification and active treatment of women experiencing perinatal depression is important.

There is much the obstetrician can do

A. In the antenatal clinic for the individual woman,

1. Picking up at risk women antenatally and raising the issue. Identification of these risk factors provides caregivers with the opportunity to observe high-risk individuals closely, provide support and preventative measures, and diagnose and treat early if the illness develops, thus minimizing morbidity for mother and baby.

2. Increasing obstetricians' awareness of how different women cope (Chapter 10) so that they can support and augment good strategies whilst helping the woman or couple to divert from less helpful ways. This is important, as doctors should not undermine the confidence of the woman—already low in depression—but can act to boost self-esteem and confidence, important in the fight against depression.

3. The obstetrician can also avoid the unintended undermining of a woman—one of those consultations that does not seem to go right despite the best of intentions.

4. Encouraging open and nonjudgmental discussion so women do not feel bad or inadequate but have confidence they will be treated well both as people and medically, should they need help.
5. Recognizing the importance of normalization of mental health to reduce the feeling of stigmatization—that is, ask the questions of everyone, be matter-of-fact, know what to do if the answers indicate problems.
6. Reassurance that the baby will not be removed and that care is aimed to help support the family unit as the best place for the infant.
7. An empathetic and supportive attitude combining social, cultural, and psychological perspectives rather than just the medical model of diagnosing abnormality which can be misinterpreted or used as "judgmental."

B. Professionally

1. Encouraging healthy attitudes to mental health problems and a nonstigmatizing culture.
2. Obstetricians are important and powerful in changing attitudes generally, in health care and society. With a problem effecting 13% of pregnancies, we need to help the argument for care and resources for this serious, but preventable and certainly treatable, problem that does so much damage.

14.1.3. Clinical Management

There are three groups to consider. "Postnatal depression" is not an amorphous subject with one management strategy and issues.

1. What to do for those currently depressed in pregnancy (also highly likely to develop postnatal depression).
2. Easy identification of high-risk groups for antenatal and postnatal depression and what to do for these women.
3. Issues of screening the general population postnatally (these are the same as for any widely implemented screening program).

In the Antenatal clinic: At the booking clinic, midwives should be able to identify mental health problems and the risk factors for postnatal depression. Special training in this area is available for midwives; this will increase their confidence in both detection and management of the "at risk" factors. Properly designed booking forms are essential. Where there is perceived to be a risk, the woman should be referred to the obstetrician for onward referral if necessary.

The current history or previous history of depression/postnatal depression should always be assessed. This can be done via two simple questions: (1) Have you ever consulted a health professional about any emotional or psychological difficulties? and (2) Has your mood been low during this pregnancy for more than 2 weeks at a time? Positive responses need follow up to elicit further details. The need to train health professionals is to ensure they acquire the ability and skills to follow up the positive answers appropriately. Whilst many health workers are instinctively sensitive communicators, this does not apply to all. Being untrained can mean this line of inquiry can be stressful, thinking up what to say, worried if the woman takes offence and how to handle that, as well as there being potential problems with transference and countertransference which they do not have the skills to unravel. Further questioning needs to discover whether the difficulty was in fact a psychotic episode (highly predictive of subsequent puerperal psychosis and which will certainly need antenatal referral to psychiatric services to coordinate the postpartum medication and possible admission to a mother and baby unit), a depressive episode (in which case, further questions can evaluate its relevance to a possible postnatal depressive problem), or some other difficulty, which whilst not directly causing depression, might indicate poor coping strategies and issues that need to be explored by counseling in respect of marital problems, bereavement, or stress (9,10). Whilst some authors feel these can be ignored, if there have been problems in previous life transitions, it does indicate there might also be difficulty coping with this very major life transition, especially as it comes at a time of sleeplessness, feeling emotional and drained as happens in the postnatal period.

Obstetricians often feel hesitant to ask about depression due to lack of experience and training. Questions to ask and to record in the notes are outlined in Tables 14.1 and 14.2 as well as the risk of recurrence. This will help get useful information as to the degree of the problem and whether to think about treatment (discussed and outlined in Tables 14.3 and 14.4).

TABLE 14.1. History taking and risk assessment where there has been previous depression

A) Questions to cover and record in notes

1 What happened?
2 How treated?
3 Any psychological input/counseling by clinic?
4 What were thought to be key factors?
5 How does the woman currently feel about these factors?
6 Any thoughts about what might happen this time?
7 Have you discussed this with your GP?

B) Interpreting the history to assess risk

Risk of recurrence	History
High	1) If only came off medication in pregnancy
	2) Reactive to key personal losses, e.g., death of first-degree relative, especially mother
Moderate	If only off medication recently
Low	1) No recent treatment
	2) Issues resolved
	3) Social situation improved
	4) Woman has insight into her own triggers, i.e., she will be able to answer the questions well

TABLE 14.2. History taking and risk assessment where there has been post natal depression

A) Questions to ask and record in notes
1 What happened?
2 When diagnosed?
3 What treatment?
4 How long to get better?
5 How long treatment for?
6 Any psychological input?
7 Any thoughts about what might happen this time?
8 Have you discussed this with your GP?

B) Interpreting the history to assess risk

Risk of recurrence if previous postnatal depression.

Low recurrence:	Improved social circumstances;
Medium risk:	Same or worse circumstances, Previous long treatment for PND
High Risk:	Continuing depression since Postnatal depression started

14.2. Antenatal Depression

This includes women who are depressed and on treatment prior to pregnancy and those who become or are diagnosed newly in pregnancy. Antenatal depression is at least as common as postnatal depression (11). It is often undiagnosed as symptoms are similar to somatic complaints of pregnancy. Women found to be experiencing antenatal depression are at an increased risk of developing postnatal depression and should be treated.

14.2.1. *Booking Already Being Treated for Depression*

With 50% of pregnancies being unplanned and up to 25% of women in child-bearing years being on antidepressant medication (12), many will fall pregnant on antidepressants and be taking them in the main period of organogenesis. The literature is small and needs to be followed, but most do not appear to cause worrying problems. The decision in this group is whether to stop or continue the medication. Avoid paroxitine in the first trimester because of the risk of fetal heart defects.

14.2.1.1. Continuing Medication

Marcus et al. (13) suggest that women in both groups—those who continue and those who cease their medication—are at an increased risk of developing depressive symptoms antenatally (which is itself a risk factor for postnatal depression). A recent article by Cohen et al. (14) additionally found that pregnancy is not "protective" of women in terms of antenatal depression. They found that of the 43% of their sample who experienced a relapse of

TABLE 14.3. Management where there has been previous depression

---

A) LOW RISK OF RECURRENCE i.e. No recent treatment, issues resolved, social situation improved. The woman has understanding and insight into her own triggers;
1) Reassure low risk of recurrence. Support a wait and see strategy with review by GP/Health Visitor.
2) Explain that having a baby causes tearfulness, tiredness, feeling emotional and up and down. This is similar to the beginning of depression, which can be scary, but does not mean they are necessarily getting depressed.
3) Discuss warning signs: If not feeling that a routine is beginning to develop at 6 weeks and still feeling low or all over the place then may be developing PND and to seek help from GP.

B) MEDIUM RISK OF RECURRENCE. i.e. If only recently off antidepressant treatment
1) Patient can "wait and see" particularly if they have good relationship with GP/Health Visitor and their ability to ask for help. They may feel better in pregnancy.
2) If the situation hasn't changed then are likely to have problems post delivery.
3) Prophylactic anti-depressants post delivery should be discussed. Start Day 1 post delivery; continue for 3 to 4 months. Come off if feeling OK in liaison with GP.

C) HIGH RISK OF PND i.e. If came off antidepressants only when pregnant or If reactive to key personal losses e.g. death of first-degree relative particularly their mother.
1) Particularly if unresolved issues psychological referral should be offered.
2) Postnatal antidepressants should be discussed, as they are likely to be needed. Start Day 1 post delivery; continue for 3 to 4 months. Come off if feeling OK in liaison with GP.

---

major depression during pregnancy, 26% were in the group who continued their antidepressants compared with 68% in the group who ceased. Although a small sample ($n = 201$), this study provides a strong indication that ceasing antidepressants during pregnancy carries a high risk of relapse of illness.

TABLE 14.4. Management where there has been previous post-natal depression

---

LOW RISK OF RECURRENCE. i.e. Improved social circumstances.
1) Support a wait and see strategy with review by GP/Health Visitor.
2) Reassure as the change plus experience of motherhood will help.

MEDIUM RISK OF RECURRENCE. i.e. Same or worse circumstances. Previous long treatment for depression.
Patient can wait and see depending on their relationship with GP/Health Visitor but should consider prophylactic anti-depressants post delivery. Start Day 1 post delivery, continue for 3-4 months. Come off if feeling OK in liaison with GP.

HIGH RISK OF RECURRENCE. i.e. Continuing depression
Recommend postnatal antidepressants, if not on them during pregnancy. Start Day 1 post delivery; continue for 3 to 4 months. Come off if feeling OK in liaison with GP. (May have antenatal depression and treatment).
5) If the woman is currently on anti-depressants:
a) Discuss history of the illness.
b) What treatment?
c) Has there been psychological input?
d) What is felt to be key factors?
e) How does the woman feel her progress has been?
The evidence to date is that it is safe to stay on anti-depressants. (Paroxetine is associated with fetal heart defects but by the time the woman is seen for booking major organogenesis will have occurred and so changing medication will not be helpful but appropriate scans should be organised). Do not make the woman feel guilty. Some women feel better in pregnancy and want to come off them but should consider going back on them postnatally or have careful surveillance with GP/Health Visitor.

14.2.2. In the Newly Diagnosed Woman

The choice of treatment is in the form of a cognitive-behavioral therapy (CBT) intervention from a trained professional (this is outlined in Section 14.3.2.1) or by prescribing antidepressants. Unfortunately, due to poor availability of psychological services and long waiting lists, prescribing may be the only option. Obstetricians should not be afraid of prescribing. The risk of antenatal depression leading onto postnatal depression should be discussed with the woman.

There is an understandable caution about using medication (particularly initiating it) in the antenatal period. The risks of medication need to be balanced against the risks of postnatal depression, the known risks for mother, and in particular, the consequences of depression for the baby's long-term health as outlined above. Obstetricians need to read the literature and keep up to date in this new area. An outline of medication risks is presented in Section 14.3.2.1. In discussing medication, many women naturally prefer not to take medication and both the risks of taking and not taking the medication should be presented. Consideration should be giving to starting medication prophylactically post-natally.

14.2.3. Untreated Depression

In terms of untreated depression during pregnancy, Bonari et al. (15) found that "untreated depression during pregnancy appears to carry substantial perinatal risks ... recent human data suggest that untreated postpartum depression, not treatment with antidepressants in pregnancy, results in adverse perinatal outcome."

14.3. Postnatal Depression

14.3.1. Factors Placing a Woman at Risk of Postnatal Depression

Those factors that are most consistently identified as predictive of postnatal depression are antenatal depression, previous clinical depression, and previous postnatal depression. In this latter case, Cooper and Murray (3) found that around two-thirds of those women entering a subsequent pregnancy were likely to experience postnatal depression again.

Other factors are reported. There are very few single factors, or clusters of factors, which have consistently been identified across many studies. Broadly speaking, the factors are divided into the following categories:

1. Perinatal factors: unplanned pregnancy; obstetric complications (these need not be particularly serious and may include multiple birth, hyperemesis, placenta praevia, fluctuating blood pressure with or without the diagnosis of pre-eclampsia, breech presentation, operative or instrumental delivery (16)).

2. Biological factors: cortisol, noradrenaline and neurotransmitter precursors such as tryptophan, estrogens, progesterone, and prolactin have all been implicated (17).
3. Individual circumstances: a poor marital relationship, a genetic predisposition, the woman's own personality characteristics (e.g., a "worrier"), poor social support, older or younger age, nulliparity or grand multiparity, concurrent life events and importantly previous psychiatric history (18).
4. Socioeconomic factors: for example, unemployment in the household.
5. Postnatal factors: include a feeling of isolation, lack of support, not breast-feeding, exhaustion, and poor physical health (19).

Protective factors may operate to prevent adverse effects in some cases.

1. Fathers good mental health (children fare worse if both parents have mental health problem)
2. Other carers' influences and support.

14.3.2. Postnatal Screening: Measurement of Risk

The most commonly used screening tool for postnatal depression is the Edinburgh Postnatal Depression Scale (EPDS). This is *not* a diagnostic tool; hence, high-risk women or women already believed to be depressed should be followed up closely and managed by midwives/health visitors with training and experience or the GP, whoever is the best placed professional.

The EPDS was designed by Cox et al. (20) and has been validated in a wide range of different languages and countries, and it has been revalidated in antenatal populations as well (21). The benefit of this tool is that it omits the somatic items commonly found in other questionnaires around items such as disturbed sleep or poor concentration, which you would normally expect to find in a postnatal population. The commonly accepted cutoffs for needing further assessment are 10 or more for minor depression, 13 or more for major depression, and 15 or more during the antenatal period. Women scoring at this level should then be assessed by a health professional with experience in making a diagnosis of postnatal depression. The questionnaire comprises only 10 items, is rapid to complete, and most women report that they do not find it invasive. In some parts of the UK, all postnatal women are now routinely screened using the EPDS. However, the National Screening Committee report found that it did not meet all the criteria for a robust stand-alone screening tool and should not be used outside the context of additional clinical experience.

Several other measures are occasionally used such as the Beck Depression Inventory (22,23)—there is a "fast screen" version of this used in medical populations, but it also omits somatic items (24). The Hospital Anxiety and Depression Scale is also used on occasion. However, the EPDS is currently the measure of choice, despite a widespread recognition of its difficulties, which include an embedded measure of anxiety (25), a sometimes poorly received question on self-harm and its lack of a diagnostic status.

14.3.2.1. Treatment

The treatment of newly diagnosed postnatal depression follows a continuum similar to that when treating depression at other times. NICE guidelines have been published 28th February 2007. We still need to emphasize the need for early intervention in order to minimize the problems for the infant.

1. The majority of postnatal depression resolves spontaneously within 6–12 months, usually either without intervention or with a simple intervention such as an increased schedule of visits from the health visitor. However, because there has already been a significant impact on the child (maximal in the first 3 months) more proactive treatment should be considered.
2. Some health visitors are trained to offer "listening visits," a form of noninterventionist person-centerd counseling.
3. Management of depression:

   a. *Mild depression*: NICE recommends structured exercise or a guided self-help program based on CBT principles. A range of psychological treatments may be of use in mild to moderate depression, including brief problem-solving or solution-focused therapy, or brief CBT interventions, provided these are administered by a trained professional. Practice nurses and GPs may have this training, in addition to any primary care based counselor. Antidepressants are not recommended for women in this category. These treatments should also be considered for women experiencing mild antenatal depression.
   b. *Moderate–severe depression*: For women experiencing moderate to severe depression either antenatally or postnatally, other interventions (medication) as well as psychological treatments may need to be considered. After a full discussion, the woman's choice for treatment must be respected and judgments must not be made, no matter how frustrating as this will only serve to alienate her rather than help health professional review and support. Respecting her choice is much more likely to initiate respect and trust and a working partnership.

4. Management and treatment in those already identified as having problems with depression in the past.

14.3.3. *The Effect of Antidepressants on Neonatal Outcome*

Research suggests that the impact of antidepressants, particularly selective serotonin reuptake inhibitors (SSRIs), is minimal in terms of major congenital anomalies, (note paroxitene is associated with fetal heart auomalies and so appropriate scans be organised). They have been associated with a risk of lower birth weight (26,27). While earlier studies found no increased risk of intrauterine death or major birth defects in women taking fluoxetine, SSRIs, or tricyclics (28), more recent studies appear to be indicating that there may be a risk of antidepressant withdrawal in neonates (29,30). In the long term, we know untreated depression gives rise to a number of problems of cognition (IQ), behavior (attention), emotionality (anxiety), and social skills at 5–11 years, as detailed at the beginning of this chapter.

Women must be properly informed of the risks and benefits of taking antidepressant medication during the perinatal period in order to make an informed decision.

14.4. Breast Feeding and Medication

It is appropriate to question the wisdom of exposing an infant to any drug during lactation, when it is possible that adverse effects will be discovered years later. However, the overall health benefits of breastfeeding to the infant and the mother are such that stopping cannot be justified on health grounds, besides which many women will refuse medication if they have to stop breast-feeding. Also there is little evidence about the long-term effects of antide-pressants in breast milk, whilst studies have shown that untreated postnatal depression often has a devastating effect on the infant. We need to keep up with the literature as evidence develops. *Despite numerous case studies, there are remarkably few reports of adverse effects in the breastfed infant.* The majority of these reports relate to the tricyclics and latterly the SSRIs. There is very little data on the newer drugs and MAOIs should be avoided.

14.4.1. *General Principles of Prescribing in the Breastfeeding Mother*

Most medications reach the breast milk in levels equivalent to 1% of the maternal oral dose and are then destroyed in the infant's gut or are poorly absorbed. Transfer of drugs to milk is greatest in the first few days of lactation. Full-term infants have low hepatic capacity for drug metabolism for the first 15 days of life, however, this increases, and by 2–3 months of age, they have a metabolic rate 2–6 times faster than adults. Premature and younger infants have less capacity to metabolize drugs, as do infants with hyperbilirubinemia, renal, hepatic, or cardiac problems.

Few drugs are "stored" in breast milk; drug levels generally reflect the maternal plasma levels. In order to minimize the infant's exposure, check the time-to-peak interval of common preparations in Tables 5 as the more predictable feeding patterns of older infants should allow the mother to plan her medication peaks away from feeds. Drugs with shorter half-lives clear from milk more quickly, so slow release preparations are best avoided.

TABLE 14.5. Brief summary of key pharmacological properties of SSRI's relevant in prescribing for breast-feeding women

Drugs	Indications main	Advice re: breastfeeding mothers	Dosing NB always aim for the lowest therapeutic dose	Time to peak plasma level (after mother's injestion)	Administration	Adverse effects reported in babies
SSRI						
Fluvoxamine	Depression	Very few reports of adverse effects or behavior have been reported in studies undertaken so far	100–300 mg/day; BD if >100 mg	4 h	Take in divided doses three times/day immediately after feeding the baby	
Fluoxetine	Depression—including that associated with anxiety	Current advice is to avoid in breastfeeding mothers due to the long half-life and adverse effects on the infant	20 mg/day (depression) 60 mg/day (bulimia)	Not known	Avoid while breastfeeding, possibility of accumulation in newborns	Excessive crying, poor sleep, colic, vomiting, and watery stools have been reported
Sertraline	Depression—including that associated with anxiety	Very few reports of adverse effects or behavior have been reported in studies undertaken so far	50–100 mg once daily, 150–200 mg/day may be used	7–10 h	Take after 1–2 h before the baby's longest sleep	One case reported withdrawal symptoms in a breastfed infant whose mother stopped Sertraline abruptly
Paroxetine	Depression—including that associated with anxiety	Very few reports of adverse effects or behavior have been reported in studies undertaken so far	20–50 mg/day (depression), 20–60 mg/day (OCD) 10–50 mg/day (panic disorder)	Not known	Take as single daily dose before baby's longest sleep. Feed the baby immediately before this dose is given	Irritability and drowsiness
Citalopram	Depression	Current advice is to use with care in breastfeeding mothers	20–60 mg once daily	Not known	Take as single daily dose before baby's longest sleep. Feed the baby immediately before this dose is given	One report of uneasy sleep in the infant of a mother who was taking 40 mg/day

Give minimum effective dose and preferably monotherapy. Further increases should be instituted under the guidance of psychiatric or psychological services. Mothers taking antidepressants should be advised to be alert for the following adverse effects in their infants:

Drowsiness
Jitteriness/hyperexcitability
Excessive crying
Allergic reaction

Always check in British National Formulary (BNF) for up to date information and prescribing data.

14.4.1.1. Psychological Intervention

In the general depressed population, there is also good evidence that a structured psychological intervention in the form of either CBT or interpersonal therapy (IPT) can be effective after approximately 16–20 sessions. CBT is generally considered the intervention of choice and is generally offered to all patients who either refuse antidepressants or are not responding to the medication. There is additionally evidence, in the general population, that a combination of CBT and antidepressants is more cost-effective than either treatment alone in the severely depressed. CBT and IPT are generally more acceptable to women than taking antidepressant medication, but the effect may take longer to become apparent and there may be long waiting lists for treatment. With the maximum effect of a depressed mother on the baby being in the first 3 months, this treatment and its availability need to be weighed up against the potential risks and benefits of immediately available antidepressant treatment.

A recent comprehensive review of antenatal and postnatal interventions of all types, other than pharmaceutical or hormonal interventions found that "strong evidence that postnatal counselling interventions...provided to women with depression or possible depression...will reduce depressive symptoms and depression substantially" (p. 140).

Antenatal interventions and universal postnatal interventions (rather than those selectively aimed at high-risk individuals) were not shown to be effective, as was the case for intrapartum and mother–infant interaction interventions (31).

14.4.2. Advice for Postnatal Support and Health for the Family

This is preferably given antenatally so plans can be made whilst not under extra stress. Look at family support, husband's support, and mothers—are they going to come and help? It is helpful to give people very detailed, structured advice. The doctor's recommendation can be very powerful in enlisting constructive family help.

14.4.2.1. Sleep

The woman needs sleep. It is reasonable to suggest that twice a week she should delegate the care of the baby overnight and have some protected sleep. This can be reciprocated for the partner so they can also get rest. She should be able to go into a quiet room far away from the baby while somebody else feeds the baby overnight. Milk can be expressed.

14.4.2.2. Household Chores

Asking friends and family to undertake definable chores and help such as washing, ironing, cooking, and cleaning at structured intervals is very useful as well as taking the baby out for an hour or two so that the mother can have a physical rest. It is easier and more useful to ask for specific structure help, advise help when no-one knows quite what to do, don't want to intrude and the women doesn't like to ask and so nothing gets done to help. Encourage the mother to have naps in the afternoon while the baby has a nap, leaving the housework.

14.5. Conclusion

Much can be done by obstetricians to help, support, and diagnose women struggling with depression in pregnancy and postpartum. We hope this chapter has provided some useful ideas for the trainee to use.

References

1. O'Hara MW, Swain AM. Rates and risk of postpartum depression—a meta-analysis. *Int Rev Psychiatry.* 1996;8:37–54.
2. Whiffen VE. Is postpartum depression a distinct diagnosis? *Clin Psychol Rev.* 1992;12:485–508.
3. Cooper PJ, Murray L. Course and recurrence of postnatal depression: evidence for the specificity of the diagnostic concept. *Br J Psychiatry.* 1995;166:191–195.
4. Murray L, Cooper PJ, Wilson A, Romaniuk H. Controlled trial of the short- and long-term effect of psychological treatment of post-partum depression: 2. Impact on the mother–child relationship and child outcome. *Br J Psychiatry.* 2003;182:420–427.
5. Mitchell EA, Thompson JMD, Stewart AW, Webster ML, Taylor BJ, Hassall IB, et al. Postnatal depression and SIDS: a prospective study. *J Paediatr Child Health.* 1992;28(Suppl 1):S13–S16.
6. Murray L, Sinclair D, Cooper P, Ducouranau P, Turner P and Stein A. The Socioemotional development of 5 year old children of postnatally depressed mothers Journal of Child Psychology and Psychiatry and Aelied Disciplines. 1998;40(8):1259–71
7. Hay DE, Pawlby S, Sharp D, Asten P, Mills A, Kumar R. Intellectual problems shown by 11-year-old children whose mothers had postnatal depression. *J Child Psychol Psychiatry.* 2001;42(7):871–889.

8. Beck CT. The effects of postpartum depression on child development: a meta-analysis. *Arch Psychiatric Nursing.* 1998;12(1):12–20.

9. Seguin L, Potvin L, St Denis M, Lioselle J. Chronic stressors, social support and depression during pregnancy. *Obstet Gynaecol.* 1995;85:583—589.

10. Kitamura T, Shirmura S, Sugawara M, Toda MA. Clinical and psychosocial correlates of antenatal depression: a review. *Psychother Psychosom.* 1996;65:117—123.

11. Kumar R, Robson KM. A prospective study of emotional disorders in childbearing women. *Br J Psychiatry.* 1984;144:35–47.

12. Yonkers K, Little B, eds. *Management of Psychiatric Disorders in Pregnancy.* Paris: Arnold; 2001.

13. Marcus SM, Flynn HA, Blow F, Barry K. A screening study of antidepressant treatment rates and mood symptoms in pregnancy. *Arch Women's Mental Health.* 2005;8:25–27.

14. Cohen LS, Altshuler LL, Harlow B, Nonacs R, Newport DJ, Viguera AC, et al. Relapse of major depression during pregnancy in women who maintain or discontinue antidepressant treatment. *JAMA.* 2006;295(5):499–507.

15. Bonari L, Pinto N, Ahn E, Einarson A, Steiner M, Koren G, et al. Perinatal risks of untreated depression during pregnancy. *Can J Psychiatry.* 2004;49(11):726–735.

16. Patel RR, Murphy DJ, Peters TJ for ALSPAC. Operative delivery and postnatal depression: a cohort study. *BMJ.* 2005; doi: 10.1136/bmj.38376.603426.D3 (published 25 February 2005).

17. O'Hara MW, Zekoski EM. Postpartum depression: a comprehensive review. In: Kumar K, Brockington, eds. *Motherhood and Mental Illness.* New York: Academic Press; 1989.

18. Kearns RA, Neuwelt PM, Hitchman B, Lennan M. Social support and psychological distress before and after childbirth. *Health Social Care Community.* 1997;5(5):296–308.

19. Small R, Brown S, Lumley J, Astbury J. Missing voices: what women say and do about depression after childbirth. *J Reprod Infant Psychol.* 1994;12:89–103.

20. Cox JL, Holden JM, Sagovsky R. Detection of postnatal depression: development of the 10-item Edinburgh Postnatal Depression Scale. *Br J Psychiatry.* 1987;150:782–786.

21. Eberhard-Gran M, Eskil A, Tambs K, Opjordsmoen S, Samuelsen SO. Review of validation studies of the Edinburgh Postnatal Depression Scale. *Acta Psychiatr Scand.* 2001;104:243–249.

22. Beck AT, Ward CH, Mendelson M, Mock J, Erbaugh J. An inventory for measuring depression. *Arch Gen Psychiatry.* 1961;4:561–571.

23. Groth-Marnat G. *The Handbook of Psychological Assessment.* 2nd ed. New York: Wiley; 1990.

24. Beck AT, Steer RA, Brown GK. *Manual for the Beck Depression Inventory—Fast Screen for Medical Patients.* San Antonio, TX: Psychological Corporation; 2000.

25. Jomeen J, Martin CR. Confirmation of an occluded anxiety component within the Edinburgh Postnatal Depression Scale (EPDS) during early pregnancy. *J Reprod Infant Psychol.* 2005;23(2):143–154.

26. Simon GE, Cunningham ML, Davis RL. Outcomes of prenatal antidepressant exposure. *Am J Psychiatry.* 2002;159(12):2055–2061.

27. Hendrick V, Smith LM, Suri R, Hwang S, Haynes D, Altshuler L. Birth outcomes after prenatal exposure to antidepressant medication. *Am J Obstetr Gynecol.* 2003;188(3):812–815.

28. Wisner KL, Gelenberg AJ, Leonard H, Zarin D, Frank E. Pharmacologic treatment of depression during pregnancy. *JAMA*. 1999;282(13):1264—1269.
29. Koren G, Matsui D, Einarson A, Knoppert D, Steiner M Is maternal use of selective serotonin reuptake inhibitors in the third trimester of pregnancy harmful to neonates? *Can Med Assoc, J.* 2005;172(11):1457–1459.
30. Maciag D, Simpson KL, Coppinger D, Lu Y Wang Y, Lin-R, Paul I, et al. Neonatal antidepressant exposure has lasting effects on behavior and serotonin circuitry. *Neuropsychopharmacology.* 2006;31(1):47–57.
31. Lumley J, Austin M-P, Mitchell C. Intervening to reduce depression after birth: a systematic review of the randomized trials. *Internatal J Technol Assess Health Care.* 2004;20(2):128–144.

15
Maternal Suicide

Carol Henshaw

'Why Mothers Die 2000—2002' (1) the report on Confidential Enquires into Maternal Deaths in the United Kingdom has, like the two triennial reports before it, highlighted suicide as a major cause of maternal death and like the 1997–1999 report, found suicide to be the leading cause of indirect or late indirect deaths for the year following delivery.

There is significant psychiatric morbidity associated with childbirth. Nonpsychotic postnatal depression follows 13% of deliveries (2) and a similar number of women are depressed during pregnancy. One-third to one-half of these women will have moderate to severe illnesses. At least 2 per 1000 new mothers develop a psychotic illness (3), usually a mood disorder. Approximately two-thirds of them will experience a depressive psychosis and one-third a manic episode. In addition, women suffering a wide range of other mental disorders from chronic schizophrenia, eating, and anxiety disorders to substance misuse, learning disability, and personality disorder become pregnant. These disorders may make women vulnerable to suicide or self-harm through psychosis, alcohol or drug consumption, or poor impulse control, which is a feature of some personality disorders. Substance misuse may coexist with other mental disorders. The mental health problems of minority women, particularly refugees and asylum seekers, are likely to coexist with serious physical health problems, severe adversity, trauma and difficulties in communicating with and understanding an unfamiliar culture.

A recent review assessed 27 studies that reported rates of suicidal ideation, intention, attempts, and completed suicide in pregnant and postpartum women (4). Suicidal thoughts (assessed by endorsement of item 10 on the Edinburgh Postnatal Depression Scale, "The thought of harming myself has occurred to me") occurred in up to 14% of pregnant women. The review found lower rates of suicide during pregnancy than that in the general population but when it did occur, violent methods were used. Particular groups at risk are teenagers and women from cultures where being unmarried and pregnant is stigmatized. Women with past histories of abuse are more likely to commit suicide.

15.1. Deliberate Self-Harm (DSH) in Pregnancy

Earlier reviews estimated that 5–12% of women attempting suicide are pregnant. Around half of the attempts by pregnant women occur during the first or second trimester and the drug taken is commonly an over-the-counter analgesic, iron, or a vitamin. Studies in Sweden and the USA have found that issues relating to pregnancy and interpersonal difficulties are often cited as the main provoking factorsfor DSH in pregnant women. These may include prior loss of children (through death, termination, or adoption), desire for a termination, or the potential loss of a partner as reasons for their act.Women who have experienced abuse may be more likely to harm themselves.

15.2. Pregnancy Loss

The standardized mortality ratio for women who have experienced a stillbirth is 1.05, six times higher than that for all postnatal women and closer to that of women in the general population. If women who experience a stillbirth have no other children they can be considered as being without the protective effect of a child. Such women may leave hospital quickly and may be reluctant to remain in contact with health professionals. The low rates of stillbirth may lead to a sense of isolation, with women not knowing anyone else who has experienced this. There are active voluntary organizations but they may be more acceptable to or more easily accessed by middle-class women leaving other groups with less support.

15.3. Methods

Postnatal suicides tend to use violent methods, a reversal of the usual trend of women using nonviolent methods such as overdose. Self-incineration, jumping from bridges, high buildings, or in front of trains, intentional road traffic accidents, hanging, drowning, or throat cutting have all been methods used by postpartum women. The timing and choice of method strongly suggests that many of these postnatal suicides were psychotic at the time of death.

Women who kill themselves tend to be older, from comfortable backgrounds, in stable relationships, well educated, and with professional qualifications at the time of suicide. Very few were from ethnic minority groups. As many of these women were well during pregnancy, well supported, and some time had elapsed since their last illness, there appeared to be little suspicion that they would be at high risk of a serious mental disorder after delivery.

15.4. Chronic Mental Illness

Two of the cases described in the CEMD had histories of chronic mental illness, one a recurrent depressive disorder and the other bipolar disorder (manic depressive illness). The second woman had had her prophylactic medication discontinued prior to conceiving. Bipolar patients are at considerable risk of relapse, especially of mania, on discontinuation of lithium, or other maintenance therapy (5). The risk can be reduced somewhat by a gradual rather than rapid discontinuation. These women are at substantial risk of recurrence (one in two or three) following delivery (6). This will occur at the same time after each delivery, with a similar presentation and degree of severity. Relapse of a psychotic illness may involve considerable risk to the woman, her fetus or infant, and/or others before she can be treated. Treatment may involve admission (perhaps under the Mental Health Act) and require considerable amounts of medication.

Such patients require careful evaluation of the risks of relapse versus any potential risk to the fetus of continuing with medication. The risk of fetal exposure to lithium is now known to be less than previously believed (7) but each case requires careful individual evaluation by a psychiatrist aware of all the issues at stake. Certainly prophylaxis immediately following delivery should be offered. This could involve restarting lithium or, if the woman wishes to breastfeed, an alternative medication such as an antipsychotic. Women with prior nonpsychotic postpartum depressions or recurrent depressive disorder may benefit from antidepressant prophylaxis (8). Hence a psychiatrist should assess any pregnant woman with a history of serious mental illness so that a management plan to prevent recurrence can be agreed, communicated to all, and placed in the patient's handheld record.

15.5. Problems in Identification and Risk Assessment

The CEMD cites lack of information relating to past psychiatric history or current involvement with mental health services from the GP referrer, poor recognition of mental disorder during pregnancy and the risks involved, together with poor liaison between obstetric and psychiatric professionals and lack of management plans for recurrence after delivery, as being important factors which increase the likelihood of suicide. One-third of the psychiatric deaths in the last enquiry were due to physical illness. In half of these, physical symptoms or behavioral disturbance were attributed wrongly to psychiatric illness when there was, in fact, a serious physical disorder present, which ultimately led to death.

15.6. Practice Recommendations

15.6.1. Antenatal Booking

The first recommendation relates to the antenatal booking interview. The midwife should systematically enquire and take details about current or past maternal psychiatric disorder, substance abuse, social problems, and self-harm. Such sensitive and stigmatized topics require careful appraisal and a sufficiently private environment in order to encourage disclosure. In recent years, partners and other relatives have been encouraged to attend antenatal appointments and to participate in the process. Many appointments take place in the woman's own home. Under these circumstances it may be difficult to ensure the privacy which is required in order to undertake a full assessment of these areas. Women may be fearful that disclosing mental illness, substance abuse, or physical abuse will result in their children being taken into care.

15.6.2. Screening Questions

The midwife carrying out the booking interview should at an appropriate point in assessing significant past history ask if the woman has ever had a serious mental health problem after previous births or at any other time. The terms used should be appropriate to the locality, culture, and educational level of the woman. This might be the most useful point at which to enquire about family history. Questions such as "Has anyone in your family ever had a serious mental health problem?" and "Did your mother/sisters/aunts have any problems after their babies were born?" are appropriate. If the answers to these questions are negative, then the midwife can move on to other areas of the assessment. If, however, there is a history of problems, then the nature and severity of the problem requires exploring.

Questions such as "What was it like?," "How was it treated?," and "How long did it last" help to assess this. If the illness required psychiatric treatment or hospitalization or was treated with lithium, divalproex semisodium, or antipsychotics, it is likely to have been severe. A problem that was entirely managed within primary care is likely to have been much less severe.

Those women with a history of serious mental illness will often be well during pregnancy and hence this provides an ideal opportunity to get to know her and agree a management plan. This assessment should be carried out by specialist psychiatric services if the woman has a current or past history of schizophrenia, bipolar disorder or schizoaffective disorder, or severe unipolar depression. Those with lesser mental health problems, stressors, or adversity would benefit from more attention from their GP, health visitor, or community midwife, perhaps with increased social support. They should be monitored and if problems do occur, intervention by the primary health-care team is usually sufficient. Those with moderate to severe mental health problems might be managed by primary care but if there is comorbidity, learning disability, multiple stressors, or major physical health problems then referral to psychiatric services should be considered. Midwives may need to seek advice from mental health professionals if they are in doubt and may need to clarify the woman's account of her problems by seeking more information from her GP. The obstetrician should ensure that a clear management plan for those at high risk of recurrence after delivery is obtained from the psychiatric assessor and that this is communicated to all involved in the care of the woman and placed in her handheld record.

Clearly, responsibility does not end at booking. Those caring for pregnant or postpartum women need to be aware of the implications of suicidal ideation and threats and what action to take. Many of the CEMD patients who committed suicide had made threats prior to killing themselves but this was often not taken seriously and acted upon.

Midwives undertaking postnatal care need to be aware of the early symptoms of mental illness arising in the puerperium as not all women who develop a psychotic illness will have had a past history. Early symptoms are often nonspecific, for example, sleep disturbance, irritability, and agitation, but may be the precursor of florid psychotic symptoms. Particular attention should be paid to these symptoms in a woman with a past history. Almost 50% of maternal suicides occur within the 3 months before or after birth.

Many midwives have little experience of psychiatry during their preregistration training and few have undergone training since registration. This may be true for obstetricians too. The majority of midwives surveyed in two adjacent health districts (9) indicated that while they agreed that they had a role to play in managing perinatal mental disorder, they lacked the skills and confidence to do so. Very few had had any formal training. The CEMD refers to "techniques being piloted" but does not elaborate. Clearly should these interventions prove successful, there are organizational and resource implications in ensuring all midwives undertaking perinatal mental care receive appropriate training. Obstetricians should ensure that those undertaking booking interviews in their unit have been adequately trained, supervision is available, and there are clear referral pathways for women identified as being at high risk and requiring further assessment.

15.6.3.   Liaison

Midwives and obstetricians should also ensure that they are familiar with statutory and voluntary services for the mentally ill and how to access them locally. They may be managed by a different trust and/or on a different site from maternity services. This will become more likely with the move toward specialist mental health trusts and may make liaison work more difficult. Community midwives may find that they can meet with, for example, community psychiatric nurses, also working in primary care settings. Women with severe mental disorders will have their care coordinated via the Care Programme Approach with regular review meetings involving all the relevant professionals, the patient, and carers. This provides a forum whereby maternity staff can link up with all concerned. Such women might be best managed in specialist antenatal clinics with regular obstetric review like women with other medical disorders, such as diabetes or epilepsy, who are pregnant.

Most of these measures are to be incorporated into auditable standards for midwifery care in the near future but clearly each service has to develop a training strategy for its staff, and obstetricians could take a lead in this.

15.6.4. Specialist Services

The CEMD proposes the identification of a clinician in each district who should manage a perinatal mental health service on a sessional basis. Shortages of psychiatrists and other mental health professionals make this unlikely to be achievable in the short term even if sufficient resources can be identified. Perinatal psychiatry is not an identified subspecialty of psychiatry leading to a CCST, and training posts do not exist on all higher training rotations. There are, however, a growing number of psychiatrists who have gained relevant experience and a number of societies including the Marcé Society and the British Society for Psychosomatic Obstetrics and Gynecology which seek to educate and research this area as well as pressing for improved services.

Current specialist services are patchy. Mother and baby inpatient units exist in some centers and can act as a focus for services linked in to obstetric, primary care, and generic mental health services. They could have a training and consultation/liaison role. However, they are not universal and many women who require admission still face the choice between admission without their baby to a general psychiatric setting or transfer to a mother and baby unit at some considerable distance. Some trusts feel they have addressed the issue by the provision of a small number of beds attached to a general psychiatric ward. Such units are usually without specialist psychiatric cover, designated and skilled nursing staff or nursery nurses. Infants in this setting may be particularly vulnerable.

Some areas have developed health visitor screening and counseling intervention for nonpsychotic postnatal depression. However, in places this has been implemented without considering links with or the implications for secondary mental health services. This approach clearly does not meet the needs of the more severely ill mother nor of those women with disorders other than depression and may not screen pregnant women.

15.6.5. Psychological Autopsy

Obstetricians and pediatricians have led the field for years with multidisciplinary detailed audit of perinatal morbidity and mortality. Psychiatrists have been slow to follow and only in recent years has the National Confidential Enquiry into Suicides been instituted. Psychiatric services are beginning to hold "Postincident Reviews," which are multidisciplinary reviews of suicides or "near misses." These could provide a valuable means of learning and reshaping services. Where such incidents involve pregnant or postpartum women there is a clear case for joint review with maternity services.

15.7. Summary

In summary, the greater focus on psychiatric causes of maternal mortality in the CEMD should be welcomed by all who care for pregnant and recently delivered women and their infants. It remains for the recommendations to be taken seriously by all and resourced adequately. Only then might we see a reduction in these often-preventable deaths.

Key Points

The Profile of Women Who Commit Suicide Due to Perinatal Mental Illness

She is likely to be an older white woman, married, and in comfortable circumstances. This will be her second or subsequent pregnancy and she will have a past history of mental illness, will be in contact with psychiatric services, and may be in treatment currently. Her baby is likely to be under 3 months old and she is likely to die violently. This profile is very different from other women and men.

Risk of Recurrence

Women with a past history of severe mental illness after delivery have a one in two or three chances of recurrence.

Guidelines

Guidelines for the care of women who are at risk of recurrence or relapse of serious mental disorder following childbirth should be in place in every maternity unit.

Antenatal Booking

A systematic enquiry should be made about past or current mental disorder, its severity, treatment, and presentation. The term "postnatal depression" or "PND'" should not be used as a generic term for all types of mental disorder.

Sharing of Information

General practitioners, obstetricians, midwives, and psychiatrists must share information and management plans.

References

1. Lewis G, Drife J. Why Mothers Die 2000–2002: The Sixth Report of the Confidential Enquiries into Maternal Deaths in the United Kingdom. London: CEMACH; 2004.
2. O'Hara MW, Swain AM. Rates and risks of postpartum depression: a meta-analysis. *Int Rev Psychiatry.* 1996;8:37–54.
3. Kendell RE, Chalmers J, Platz C. The epidemiology of puerperal psychosis. *Br J Psychiatry.* 1987;150:662–673.
4. Lindahl V, Pearson JL, Colpe L. Prevalence of suicidality during pregnancy and the postpartum. *Arch Womens Ment Health.* 2005;8:77—87.
5. Suppes T, Baldessarini RJ, Faedda GL et al. Risk of recurrence following discontinuation of lithium treatment in bipolar disorder. *Arch Gen Psychiatry.* 1991;48:1082–1088.
6. Cohen LS, Sichel DA, Robertson LM et al.Postpartum prophylaxis for women with bipolar disorder. *Am J Psychiatry.* 1995;152:1641–1645.
7. Cohen LS, Friedman JM, Jefferson JM et al. A reevaluation of risk of in utero exposure to lithium. *J Am Med Assoc.* 1994;271:146–150.
8. Wisner KL, Perel JM, Peindl KS et al. Prevention of postpartum depression: a pilot randomized clinical trial. *Am J Psychiatry.* 2004;161:1290–1292.
9. Stewart C, Henshaw C. Midwives and perinatal mental health. *Br J Midwifery.* 2002;10:117–121.

Further Reading

1. Yonkers KA, Wisner KL, Stowe Z et al. Management of bipolar disorder during pregnancy and the postpartum period. *Am J Psychiatry.* 2004;161:608–620.
2. Akdeniz FS, Vahip S, Pirildar S et al. Risk factors associated with childbearing-related episodes in women with bipolar disorder. *Psychopathology.* 2003;36:234–238.
3. Llewellyn A, Stowe ZN, Strader Jr. JR.The use of lithium and management of women with bipolar disorder during pregnancy and lactation. *J Clin Psychiatry.* 1999;59:57s–65s.
4. Viguera AC, Cohen LS, Baldessarini RJ et al. Managing bipolar disorder during pregnancy: weighing the risks and benefits. *Can J Psychiatry.* 2002;47:426–436.
5. Yonkers K, Little B, eds. *Management of Psychiatric Disorders in Pregnancy.* London: Arnold; 2001.

16
Tokophobia: A Profound Dread and Avoidance of Childbirth (When Pathological Fear Effects the Consultation)

Kristina Hofberg and Mark Ward

16.1. Introduction

Fear of childbirth is not pathological. On the contrary, it is well known that pregnancy can be a time of considerable but appropriate anxiety. Symptoms of anxiety and fear increase in the third trimester, especially if the woman is expecting her first child. However, for some women, there is no reassurance in the fact that obstetric services have developed and risks related to childbirth have reduced. For them the danger of parturition feels real and the fear of death believed to be a genuine and terrifying risk.

Tokophobia was described in 2000 (1) but is certainly not a modern day phenomenon. Fear of parturition was described by Marcé (2), a French psychiatrist, in 1858. He said of women, "If they are primiparous, the expectation of unknown pain preoccupies them beyond all measure, and throws them into a state of inexpressible anxiety. If they are already mothers, they are terrified of the memory of the past and the prospect of the future."

When significant anxiety and fear of death during parturition precedes pregnancy and is so intense, *tokos* ("childbirth") is avoided whenever possible, this is a phobic state called tokophobia.

16.2. Psychosocial Considerations When Women Fear Childbirth

16.2.1. Tokophobia: An Anxiety Disorder

A phobia is an avoidance response. This may be learned through frightening experiences, vicariously by seeing the fearful responses of others or through instruction. It has been recognized that a pregnant woman's expectations of the delivery are relevant to how she experiences the delivery and behaves throughout. In addition her appraisal of the last delivery will include the anxiety associated with it and will indicate the level of fear for a future delivery (3). Fear of childbirth has been associated with anxiety proneness in general and can be classified as an anxiety disorder.

16.2.2.   Social Culture

Women can accurately recall details of childbirth 20 years later (4). Fear of childbirth may be transmitted over generations and represents a second generation effect of a mother's own unresolved frightening experience. Interestingly there is evidence to suggest that women's reproductive adaptations resemble their mothers'. Dread of childbirth may be further highlighted for girls when their parents have a negative attitude towards sexuality.

16.2.3.   Childhood Sexual Abuse (CSA)

Significant numbers of women describe being sexually abused before the age of 16. It is known that the psychological morbidity secondary to CSA is both immense and diverse. As adults these women suffer increased rates of sexual dysfunction, anorexia, and posttraumatic stress disorder (PTSD). A history of CSA is sometimes associated with an aversion to gynecological examinations, including routine smears and obstetric care. The trauma of vaginal delivery or even the contemplation of it may cause a resurgence of distressing memories. This can lead to anxiety, then dread and avoidance of childbirth, even when a woman wants a baby.

16.3.   Treatment Studies for Fear of Childbirth

Treatment studies are problematic because of the developments and changing expectations in obstetric care. Today a woman is more likely to request or demand a delivery of choice in the UK than a generation ago. Nevertheless, studies that aim to reduce fear of childbirth date back to the 1920s. Psychoprophylaxis was investigated in the 1950s and again in the 1980s. Psychoprophylactic preparation courses were offered to women, who were afraid of childbirth, in the 1980s. They made no significant difference to obstetric outcome. Psychological outcomes were not investigated. The benefits of hypnosis were investigated in the 1990s.

Much good work has come from Sweden where women have been, for many years, able to make choices about vaginal versus surgical delivery. Ryding (5), a Swedish obstetrician and psychotherapist, offered either counseling or short-term psychotherapy to pregnant women demanding a cesarean section (CS) the obstetrician thought was unnecessary. At term, half the women chose vaginal delivery.

Sjögren (6), another Swedish obstetrician, investigated 72 women with severe anxiety about childbirth. They were offered psychotherapy or extra obstetric support. Subsequently, some women chose a vaginal delivery. These women experienced the delivery as positively as a reference group.

Saisto et al. (7) in Finland randomized women, referred to an antenatal clinic for fear of childbirth, to receive either psychotherapy or usual care. There was no difference in the proportion of women who chose to deliver by CS between the two groups. However, there were differences for the women in the intervention group who had vaginal births. Fewer reported fear of pain in labor and they were noted to have shorter labors.

Tokophobic women who strongly desired a surgical delivery and were refused suffered greater psychological morbidity than those granted their chosen delivery method. The number of women demanding elective CS in the UK because of tokophobia is not known.

16.4. Classification of Tokophobia

Tokophobia can be classified as follows:

1. Secondary: previous traumatic obstetric experience
2. Primary: nulliparous
3. Secondary to depressive illness in pregnancy.

16.4.1. Tokophobia Secondary to Childbirth

Mothers and doctors alike will challenge the idea that tokophobia secondary to childbirth is indeed a phobia. Both may suggest that the fears could be reasonable and therefore not a phobic state. However, the psychological manifestation remains one of extreme anxiety and avoidance.

So some women develop a dread and avoidance of childbirth after a delivery. Most typically this is a traumatic delivery. It could also occur after an obstetrically normal delivery, a miscarriage, a stillbirth, or a termination of pregnancy (TOP). The fear may be manifested either as a wish to have a CS or to avoid the current pregnancy and childbirth. Research has suggested that women requesting an elective CS due to fear of childbirth were more likely to have experienced a spontaneous miscarriage, a longer time between pregnancies, a longer duration of second stage of labor, and a previous assisted vaginal birth or emergency CS. Some women feel so traumatized that they avoid a further pregnancy altogether even when they want a baby.

Secondary tokophobia has a close relationship with PTSD (8). PTSD is increasingly recognized as a consequence of childbirth and is associated with a pathological dread and avoidance of further childbirth experiences. Bydlowski and Raoul-Duval (9) documented the "nightmare of childbirth." They stated "Parturition—especially the first—can, by its obligatory violence and confrontation with an imminent and lonely death, put the mother under extreme stress." They suggested that subsequent pregnancies intensified the aftermath of previous pregnancy trauma. Some of these women avoided further childbirth because of the trauma experience. Some suffered terrifying nightmares and were afraid to even go to sleep. PTSD may even follow deliveries that were not abnormal from the clinician's perspective. Some traumatized women terminate pregnancies because—untreated and unrecognised—they cannot face any method of delivery.

16.4.2. Primary Tokophobia

When dread of childbirth predates the first conception, this is primary tokophobia. The dread of childbirth may start in adolescence or early adulthood. Although sexual relations may be normal, contraceptive use is often scrupulous. Pregnancy is avoided to prevent parturition. Some women will actively seek out an obstetrician who will perform an elective CS before becoming pregnant for the first time. Some women never overcome their fear of childbirth and remain childless or adopt. Many feel shame at their perceived inadequacy. Some women enter menopause having never delivered a much-desired baby and grieve this loss into old age.

16.4.3. Tokophobia as a Symptom of Depression

Less commonly, prenatal depression may present as tokophobia. The morbid dread of childbirth is in stark contrast to the woman's prepregnancy and euthymic beliefs. The woman may present with recurrent intrusive beliefs that she cannot deliver her baby and if she is made to she will die.

16.5. The Obstetric Consultation

Women with fear of childbirth may present to the obstetrician in the first instance. Medical presentation is multifaceted. What these women will have in common is extreme anxiety about the pregnancy with the recurrent intrusive beliefs that they are unable to deliver their babies, and either they or the baby will die if they are forced to proceed with the delivery.

A nulliparous woman may present before she conceives for the first time. A parous woman may present in the aftermath of delivery. A pregnant woman may present at any time during the pregnancy. Some women believe that private obstetrics can ensure the delivery of choice. Often a woman with tokophobia is anxious, fearful, and concerned she will be dismissed. A tokophobic woman would have been told already that her fears are "normal." She knows they are not "normal" but they are extreme and dominate her thinking and her pregnancy.

The obstetrician may be faced with a woman who appears angry and demanding and is insisting on a specific method of delivery without discussion of medical risk or benefit. It is easy for the obstetrician to feel defensive and dismissive. To be challenged about a professional decision—perhaps before adequate discussion—requires the obstetrician to be sensitive. The easy option would be to believe the woman has a "neurotic personality." What may seem to the obstetrician and other professionals working with the woman as a problem based entirely "in the mind" merely alienates the problem. Time needs to be taken to

- Consider her reasons for the request
- Consider one's own emotional response to the challenge.

16.6. How the Obstetrician Recognizes Tokophobia

16.6.1. The Pregnant Woman with Tokophobia

When a woman presents during pregnancy with a profound fear of delivery, this needs to be addressed as soon as it is recognized. Ironically, the woman will know that her fears are overwhelming but the team looking after her may not recognize the situation as such. The obstetrician may just see an angry and distressed woman making what seems an unreasonable request.

It is recognized that some women with fear of childbirth also have fears of other medical interventions. The woman may be terrified of needles, hospitals, and medical and nursing staff. With the substantial publicity on MRSA and other hospital-borne infections she may be excessively fearful of even entering a hospital. This woman may well request a home delivery even for her first baby.

The other extreme case is the woman who just "wants the baby out." She requests the maximum intervention and minimum responsibility. She wants the doctors to deliver the baby, even requesting general anesthetic in some cases.

16.6.2. The Pregnant Woman with Tokophobia Requesting a Termination of Pregnancy

This woman will have an unplanned pregnancy. In fact she may well want to have a baby and be in a social and financial position to accommodate this decision. However, she is terrified of delivering a baby. She does not believe anyone will take her fears seriously. She can find no obvious solution other than terminating the pregnancy. She may present distressed or angry and defensive—terrified that her request for TOP will be refused. A proportion of TOPs may be requested from women who suffer from tokophobia and want a baby but cannot understand their own strong aversion to parturition. In the absence of an empathic professional listener or relevant medical literature, their only choice may be to terminate the pregnancy.

16.6.3. The Pregnant Woman with Tokophobia and Hyperemesis Gravidarum

Women with tokophobia may present with *hyperemesis gravidarum*. A psychological component to *hyperemesis gravidarum* has been postulated. This may be relevant to tokophobia when rejection of pregnancy, failure to bond with the fetus, attempts to obtain a TOP and terror of an impending delivery may occur.

16.6.4. The Pregnant Woman with Depression

It is increasingly recognized that women develop depression during pregnancy at a similar rate to postnatally. Occasionally the pregnant woman can develop psychological symptoms associated with the depression which include tokophobic ideas. However, these women do have other significant symptoms of the depressive illness, both biological and psychological. If feelings of low mood are considered to be a concern a specialist psychiatric opinion would be appropriate and helpful. In such situations the tokophobic ideas resolve with the treatment of the illness.

16.6.5. The Woman with Secondary Tokophobia

Some women present with a change in attitude towards future delivery following their previous experience of childbirth. A previous childbirth experience may be obstetrically normal with a healthy child or may have been more obviously traumatic. However, the woman experiences the process as a significant trauma and is terrified of facing a repeat even though she may desperately want another baby. She may present not pregnant but wanting guarantees about a future pregnancy and delivery.

When a woman has experienced childbirth as a traumatic event she is vulnerable to developing a number of mental health problems. Postnatal depression is a well-recognized condition that can occur spontaneously. It can also affect women who have been psychologically traumatized through childbirth. In addition, symptoms of posttraumatic stress disorder following delivery have been described. Both these are described in significant detail in two other chapters of this book. The profound dread of childbirth may be just one of several psychopathologies consequent on childbirth.

16.6.6.   The Nulliparous Woman

This woman may present before she has conceived. She may be sexually active. She may use several contraceptive methods simultaneously. She may have wanted a baby for several years and be in a stable relationship.

This woman wants assurance from the obstetrician that when she becomes pregnant her chosen delivery method can be guaranteed. This may be an elective CS for no obvious medical reason. Her proposed birth plan may include the promise of a general anesthetic. The woman may appear resistant to discussion or negotiation. This can produce a deadlock between the woman and the obstetrician. The obstetrician may see this as a consumer-driven mentality that is "too posh to push" rather than an overwhelming phobic state.

When a woman presents before a pregnancy with either primary or secondary tokophobia, there is time and opportunity to consider a satisfactory and humane approach to the obstetric care.

16.6.7.   Tokophobia and Request for Permanent Contraception

The proportion of women with tokophobia and their partners are overrepresented in couples seeking permanent contraceptive methods. Ekblad (10) addressed the issue of "fear of pregnancy" as a reason for requesting sterilization. Some childless women presenting for sterilization may be tokophobic and respond to a psychological approach to dealing with the phobia.

16.6.8.   The Pregnant Woman with Psychosis

Occasionally a woman with a severe and enduring mental illness can present whilst pregnant. If her illness is poorly controlled she may have somatic hallucinations and/or delusions, often religious, relating to the fetus and delivery process. This situation will require joint working with her Community Mental Health Team and perhaps the reinstatement of psychotropic medication if this has been discontinued through pregnancy. If a clinical situation involves psychotic symptoms this is not the phobic state of tokophobia.

16.7.   Managing the Consultation

The most important aspect of the consultation is to recognize the psychpathology. This then allows the obstetrician to engage in discussion on aspects of the woman's personal and obstetric history and consider her management. Some work may be usefully approached through psychological services. Certainly a woman with depression, PTSD, or severe anxiety may benefit from specialist treatment through mental health services and perhaps work psychologically or respond to pharmacological treatments. It is important that such women are recognized and treated.

16.8.   Conclusion

The prevalence of tokophobia is unknown. We can only speculate at the etiology. There are no clinical trials that allow precise replication in clinical practice. However, the problem is real for the women who suffer.

Tokophobia is in fact managed by many women by avoiding childbirth altogether. One could speculate that the most severe cases are indeed the ones that are never witnessed or addressed.

The role of the obstetrician is to recognize the distress and acknowledge the seriousness of this. With an empathic approach the obstetrician and the woman can work with psychiatric and psychological services as appropriate to diagnose and treat mental health problems that exacerbate the situation.

References

1. Hofberg K, Brockington I. Tokophobia: an unreasoning dread of childbirth. A series of 26 cases. *Br J Psychiatry*. 2000;176:83–85.
2. Marcé LV. *Traité de la Folie des Femmes Enceintes, des Nouvelles Accouchées et des Nourrices*. Paris: Baillière; 1958.
3. Lazarus RS. *Emotion and Adaptation*. New York: Oxford University Press; 1991.
4. Simpin P. Just another day in a woman's life? Part II: Nature and consistence of women's long term memories of their first birth experiences. *Birth* 1992;2:64–81.
5. Ryding EL. Investigation of 33 women who demanded a caesarean section for personal reasons. *Acta Obstet Gynecol Scand*. 1993;72:280–285.
6. Sjögren B. Fear of childbirth and psychosomatic support—a follow up of 72 women. *Acta Obstet Gynecol Scand*. 1998;77:819–825.
7. Saisto T, Ylikorkala O, Halmesmäki E. Factors associated with fear of delivery in second pregnancies. *Obstet Gynecol*. 1999;94:679–682.
8. Ballard C, Stanley AK, Brockington IF. Post-traumatic stress disorder (PTSD) after childbirth. *Br J Psychiatry*. 1995;166:525–528.
9. Bydlowski M, Raoul-Duval A. Un avatar psychique méconnu de la puerpueralité: la névrose traumatique post obstetricale. *Perspect Psychiatriques* 1978;68:321–328.
10. Ekblad M. The prognosis after sterilization on social–psychiatric grounds. A follow-up study on 225 women. *Acta Psychiatr Scand*. 37(Suppl. 161):9–162.

General Reading

1. *Motherhood and Mental Health*. Oxford: Oxford University Press; 1996.

17
Psychological Aspects of Stillbirth

Jayne Cockburn

17.1. Introduction

Obstetrics is a joyful job, a job welcoming new life. Therefore it is much harder when all goes wrong. Loss in the form of stillbirth touches on everyone's core identity, personal dreams, and life construct and is more painful to bear in comparison to losses in other areas of medicine where death is expected. We all hate failure, and it asks a lot more of us to provide quality care in such adverse circumstances. The staff, as well as the patients, need support, time, and space. In the original plan for this book we wanted to write about management of pregnancy subsequent to stillbirth, as much of the management of stillbirth itself is covered by guidelines written and endorsed by the RCOG, as well as all the other relevant organizations. However, so much in the subsequent ongoing pregnancy is determined by the experience in the pregnancy resulting in stillbirth, neonatal loss, or termination for abnormality that we felt it essential to provide an outline of key issues in the management of the stillbirth process. The death will affect all the family and possibly attitudes and feelings in the next generation. The more we can do to give insight and understanding to the family about their experience and its effects, the more it appears to help them with the process of childbearing and rearing in subsequent years and generations, reducing the negative emotional effects.

The experience for the individual doctor in managing and discussing stillbirth may not be great because of (a) relatively small numbers, (b) respect for the couple's privacy, which excludes "training observers" from the process (particularly medical staff), (c) a tendency to admit "non-urgent" losses at weekends when the unit is quieter and there are less people around. Yet O&G trainees find themselves in senior positions and are expected somehow to know what to do. This chapter is to help guide professionals through what little evidence there is and to provide some guidance as to what might be helpful to say. Hopefully this chapter can provide some useful generalities, which provide a framework for clinical work and consultation. By knowing the outlines and basic concepts, it is hoped that trainees will have more confidence when approaching stillbirth in the clinical situation.

The keys to managing any loss are twofold:

1. Understanding the basic processes of grief and breaking bad news
2. Listening to the individual and adapting to her needs whilst addressing basic issues for the good management/care of the woman

17.2. Key Concepts

17.2.1. Stages of Grief

The stages of grief described by Kubler-Ross (1969) when patients receive a catastrophic diagnosis are useful as they are short and easy to remember:

1. Denial: "This can't be happening to me."
2. Anger: "Why me?"
3. Bargaining: "I'll be a better person if only…"
4. Depression: Overwhelming feelings of hopelessness, frustration, bitterness, self-pity, loss of hopes, and dreams for the future.
5. Mourning: Acceptance of the reality of the loss, experiencing the pain of the loss, readjustment to reality—life without the lost "object," finding the good out of the pain, good memories, and the establishment of a new life.

Progress along the emotional framework is not linear. Grief is complex and individual. People do not have to go through it in any one order, or just experience a stage once.

Expanding from the Kubler-Ross's five stages, Ramsay and de Groot (1977) give a more detailed insight into what is going on:

1. Shock: "Feelings are turned off."
2. Disorganization: Unable to do the simplest thing (especially take that complicated regime of tablets drive home).
3. Denial: (Seeking a second opinion, "if he/she was only moving this morning)
4. Depression: Desolate pining, a feeling of emptiness (especially in pregnancy when the mother is literally emptied of the baby, thereby creating a physical void to correlate with her emotional emptiness).
5. Guilt: "Was it something I have done? Mothers so often blame themselves, even in circumstances where clearly they had no part in the problem. Repeated reassurance will need to given, especially as in subsequent pregnancies we know women are prone to take on a great personal responsibility for the welfare of their fetus/baby, which is unjustified and can

cause huge anxieties and start off mental health problems, for example, obsessional compulsive disorder.

6. Anxiety: Of losing control of one's feelings or more general apprehension of what the future now holds for them.
7. Aggression: This can be against anyone, family friends, god, fate, and of course doctors and nurses. (Outbursts should be understood in this context and communication skills used to calm the situation down if at all possible, rather than punish people by calling security.)
8. Resolution: Taking leave of the dead and accepting life must go on and that there will be good things again.
9. Reintegration: The practical acceptance of resolution, with building a new life (sometimes literally after stillbirth). At times regression will occur, for example, anniversaries—doubly difficult, if the woman is pregnant again, for her to have both happy feelings for the future as well as feel overwhelmed with sadness for the past baby and dreams of the family she should already have. This will occur both on the date of death/birth and when the baby was actually due.

This helps us to recognize the stages and what bit of the emotional process the patient is grappling with. Thus we can communicate appropriately for that stage and can monitor her progress as she feeds back her feelings as she talks.

If you are not getting any feedback and so are unsure of what is happening emotionally, if a patient is quiet and withdrawn after delivery, do not be afraid to ask how she is actually feeling. By doing this you can give permission to feel and can ask without being directive or making assumptions. By quoting how other women have talked and felt, you look informed but stay talking about generalities. By asking if she feels the same, you are both giving permission to feel "normal difficult feelings" but also asking what she as an individual is feeling. She may have returned to "shock" as the experience is so far from expectations. If this is the case then you know it is too early to proceed with giving lots of detailed instructions.

17.3. Cultural Differences

All health professionals need to remember that there are cultural differences, with different beliefs and cultural and religious constructs for behavior and thoughts about loss. If you are not sure, be sensitive and open. Ask what their preferences and needs are. Equally, there is likely to be an effect of Westernization and so we need to be doubly sensitive to what is needed. Do not rush in with assumptions. Follow the standard "breaking bad news" practice. Allow time and open-ended questions to give the woman/couple/family chance to say what they need or for you to have confidence that you have a good relationship to ask about differing culture needs. If we do not rush talking to cover our own discomfort, the patient will usually tell us very clearly what they need.

17.4.   High Risk for Difficulties

There are some who are at a particularly high risk of difficulty in coping with stillbirth. These include women who have a history of recurrent miscarriage, infertility, termination, and multiple pregnancy. Also women who have become "stuck" in grieving for other losses or who have had recent (and therefore probably unresolved) losses are all very vulnerable. Your clinical antennae need to be alert to monitor these couples to enable you to offer help quickly if necessary.

17.5.   Breaking Bad News

Key elements of this skill adapted from Chapter 1 are as follows:

- Preparation for the encounter (Quiet setting, enough time, is all the information needed available? Is the patient alone or accompanied by a family member or friend? What is the emotional situation of the physician?).
- Introduction (a brief summary of the previous events and the objective of the consultation)
- Announcement ("Unfortunately I have to give you bad news").
- Statement (Give the diagnosis in simple words).
- Waiting for the individual reaction of the patient (Stunned, paralyzed, confused, shocked, desperate, crying, stoic, denying, etc.).
- Response to the reaction (Emotion handling, reflecting, summarizing).
- Encouraging questions and giving further information in small pieces.
- Structure the near future (What is the patient going to do next—define the next steps to be taken and give details).

17.6.   Stillbirth

Prior to the 1970s the attitude to stillbirth had been to hide and remove the baby immediately after birth and to encourage the mother to "forget about it." The hospital usually disposed of the baby for the couple. This was well meaning. However, greater understanding of the grief process, together with reports by Emanuel Lewis and others in 1969 of depression and anxiety up to 50 years after a stillbirth, brought about a societal change in attitudes. A much more open, compassionate, and sensitive approach was adopted. Patient support organizations such as the Stillbirth and Neo-Natal Death Society (SANDS) and Support After Termination For Abnormality (now ARC) grew up. SANDS have drawn up guidelines for professionals endorsed by many Royal colleges and other involved organizations. (Newly revised guidelines are being published 12th June 2007.) Many labor wards have these guidelines available or have incorporated them into the unit policies and procedures.

All doctors and health professionals should refer to their unit's guidelines. SANDS and ARC can also provide support if the woman or couple wants to contact them. It is very likely that the unit will have leaflets for the women and provide support numbers to ring if they want to.

The comprehensive guidelines are helpful to the health-care team in providing emotionally aware care for the couple and also for the staff looking after them. They do concur with the professional wish for sensitivity, but give little guidance as to how to actually manage the tragedy of stillbirth. Much of the advice is based more on intuition than our factual evidence. Intuition may be wrong and it is important that we acquire and integrate more research-based evidence. Perinatal loss is relatively common and has a huge impact on parenting, attachment, and bonding, vital parts of healthy functioning in society, and these effects also transfer to subsequent generations.

The SANDS guidelines are for all staff. We discuss the process for the doctors as they have a key role of breaking the news. They also have the responsibility for all subsequent care. The doctor is responsible for key elements of management, delivering and investigating afterwards, and imparting all the information to the distressed couple in a way that is sensitive and understood, but allows them to feel some control. The doctor has to give difficult and painful medical advice about delivery and investigation including postmortem. Not doing this is to fail the patient. The doctor is often juggling work, caring for many patients at a time, and also can feel very isolated, with little support that is obvious. Being sensitive to the patient's distress is not the same as avoiding giving correct and good medical advice to prevent causing distress.

17.7.   Breaking the Diagnosis of Death

The doctor is called in as soon as the death of a baby is suspected. The woman/couple are already worried and anxious. The doctor's job is to confirm the death and to break the news. Many doctors find themselves on the frontline, with the aspiration to be sensitive and kind, but with no training in what to say and how to say it.

Introduce yourself simply and explain who you are. The couple will not want prevaricating small talk. They already suspect the worst. Small talk makes the doctor look uncertain as to what to do, not very confidence inspiring when the couple will need to be able to trust the medical staff to listen and help them emotionally and physically at a very stressful time. In order to give them some control, let them know what is happening at all times and the expected timeframe. If this is not working out, say why. A quick simple explanation of what is going to happen next will do, for example, you are going to get the scanner and do a scan yourself or that it does not look very hopeful, but you are going to organize a scan to come up to the room. Show you are aware of their worry, and tell them it is coming, for example, the scanner is coming immediately and will be here in 10 minutes. The shorter the time to official confirmation the better. Horror stories of a woman having to wait till 9.00 next morning when the scanning staff came on duty are hard to listen to. The midwife should stay and support the couple and help with all the rhetorical questions that may follow. The midwife must not be called to deliver another baby. Her job must now be to stay with this woman/couple and help them bear the uncertainty and loss. The doctor should confirm that they will return once the scanner has arrived. If bleeps go off and have to be attended to, say "I have to answer this, I am sorry," and be as quick as possible, not "I have to go to an emergency"—"What can be more of an emergency than them?" they will feel.

The natural feeling for staff is to want to do something, make it better, try and pretend it is not as bad, make a cup of tea. It is important to stay. Many of the questions asked around the time of stillbirth are rhetorical. You do not need to answer these questions; in fact you probably should not, except to generally acknowledge that it is normal to search for answers and to reassure the couple that nothing they could have done would have helped and that they did their best. Note down any specific questions for later.

Once the diagnosis is confirmed a simple statement such as "I am sorry. I cannot find the baby's heartbeat. I'm afraid your baby has died" is enough. Then stop to allow the couple to take this in and react. Wait for subsequent statements and questions to guide through what they want to know about the death and what is the next step. Again there is likely to be a lot of rhetorical questions. Keep the language brief and simple. There will be lots of time for explanations. *Do not* be drawn into reasons or blame. So many times a clear-cut case has changed after a postmortem. But the harm of blame has already been done. Reassure all complaints or questions will be looked into thoroughly—write them down in the notes at the time so they are being taken seriously, but do not be drawn, for example, "Yes, that sounds worrying, and yes, we will investigate that, have a full enquiry." Be open without being critical, no matter how big the temptation. We will all be feeling emotional and so there is potential for us to want to judge and apportion blame. Do not do this, no matter how clear cut it may look. Bad communication is remembered more clearly at times of stress and can affect the whole management.

If they are angry, remember that it is not likely to be with you as a person, but with their loss, that anger being projected around, and at people, which is entirely natural. Sit down close to the patient (less adversarial than standing over them). Giving straightforward replies to angry comments, for example, "it's very understandable and normal to feel angry, you have lost a baby, it's a big loss," without being patronizing can validate the anger whilst stopping it from attaching to anyone. Providing anger is accepted, listened to and reacted to calmly, in a problem solving way or just listened to (again note down any complaints which can be investigated at any later stage after dealing with the current situation "I am keeping a record of these questions and we will investigate them and try to answer them"); this angry phase too will pass and the patient can refocus on what has to happen next. The parents of course may be angry with themselves and will need reassurance such as "I am sure that lifting the shopping did not kill the baby." Parents commonly ask "Was it my fault?" They are looking for reasons and apportion blame widely, including themselves. Consistently parents look at the actions leading up to stillbirth and accuse themselves bitterly of doing things wrong.

17.8.   Staff Reactions: Sadness, Guilt

17.8.1.   Sadness

It is natural to be sad. No patient was ever upset because the doctor looked upset, but if the doctor appears rushed or uncaring that does get remembered. However, if the loss touches upon deaths or losses of your own, be clear that these are your feelings being reawakened. It is all right to say you are sorry for the loss, and it is important to acknowledge this when meeting an affected couple for the first time.

17.8.2.   Guilt

Looking at the way everyone checks in the notes of an undiagnosed breech to make sure it was not them who "missed it" makes me feel that everyone feels guilty about a stillbirth. For example, "Could I have noticed something earlier?". This is a natural reaction but again is not always helpful. Even where we may have a reason to feel guilty, it is important not to rush in or apportion blame. The whole point of a process and investigation is to come up with a systematic view and I have seen huge differences in causes of the death, particularly after a good postmortem. So talk with your consultant or the consultant responsible in this case about your thoughts and worries.

It is, however, important that we reflect on our feelings and ensure that we have given good care.

17.9.   Delivery

Once the death has been confirmed and the couple have had time with the doctor, with staff, and with themselves, the question of "what next?" will naturally come up. The doctor is responsible for assessing and planning the delivery.

It is likely that delivery will be via induction. This usually brings up the question why not a cesarean section? Get it all over and done with? These questions need to be answered patiently and time given for them to be taken in and understood. A cesarean is not the quick fix. It leaves a lasting scar, increases the risk of infection and complications both now and for the future. And there is no quick fix for the loss of a baby. The doctor should sit with the couple during this discussion, through the anger and frustration that it cannot "just be solved," as they come to grips with the reality of facing the death and its implications.

Induction where there is an intrauterine death can be particularly difficult. We do not rupture the membranes because of the risk of infection. The primigravida with an unripe cervix may have a very drawn out induction experience, with repeated prostin and repeated change of staff. A poorly managed induction is very damaging with a high risk of PTSD. This in turn will affect subsequent pregnancies and deliveries, attachment, bonding and mental health of subsequent children, as well as the mental health of the mother in the here and now, making it harder for her to get over the stillbirth. Units need to have policies and plans and clear guidance as to which consultant should be informed and be responsible.

The doctor has the difficult job of helping the woman/couple learn about the labor and delivery. They are in shock, with emotions rising high; this is something they have never thought about before and it is not a situation that they have prepared for or expected. It is important that the doctor explore a few different scenarios and how the picture might look in several days time, depending on which choices they make or which options they choose, thus helping the couple understand the process and the potential problems. For example, anticipate that there might be difficulty in ripening the cervix, then if it does prove difficult the patient does not feel she has failed again.

Modern prostaglandin analogs (mifegyne) can be very useful in making it an effective labor and delivery. They just need to be taken beforehand and then induction with prostaglandin delayed for 48 h. Couples desperate to start delivery still benefit from taking them in my experience; even if prostaglandin is started straight away for induction and if the initial induction fails, then they are in the system for the second try. So it is a win–win situation. With a good explanation, couples usually welcome the chance to draw breath between the emotion of the diagnosis and the energy needed to face the delivery. They should be asked whether they want to go home or stay in the hospital in the specially designated room. Some prefer to be in familiar surroundings, but some prefer the support of the sympathetic unit before facing the world and the telephone or people who will not know what to say. Some researches, however, have shown that delays of greater than 24 h are risk factors for increased psychological sequelae. It is unclear as to whether this is because it meant a long drawn-out labor which is bad for you or because of the delay itself. More research is needed to help us to accurately advise the best course of action and anticipate problems depending on the individual choices.

It is important that the care team speak with one voice to instill a sense of confidence at this confusing time (i.e., the voice of a well-prepared unit). The team must be open to questions at all times and they must communicate well within the team.

17.10.   Analgesia

Epidural is particularly useful as it reduces the stress hormones—already at a peak—and prevents further exhaustion for the mother who will still need reserves to cope after delivery. It also allows good doses of Syntocinon for effective contractions. You do not have to wait for labor to put it in. Get a good experienced anesthetist wherever possible, as it may need to be there for several days. Work with the woman with whatever she chooses. If an epidural is not wanted, remember larger doses of pethidine and morphine or infusions can be used, as sadly there is no worry about respiratory depression.

17.11.   Postdelivery

In the cases described by Emmanuel Lewis in 1969, the women were not allowed to see their stillborn babies. Their longing, sadness, and continued questions led to the establishment of a much more open process. Now the convention has become to see, and hold and cuddle the baby, somehow saying hello in order to say goodbye. Whilst being advised to respect the wishes of those who do not want to see or hold the baby, the prevailing wisdom has been that if in doubt it is better to see the stillborn infant, with guidance for those unsure being "No one has reported regret for seeing their baby".

Evidence looking at the problems in the next pregnancy, however, has shown that seeing and/or holding the baby may not be a neutral intervention. Earlier studies did not find any worsening of outcome, but these were not controlled studies and did not look at the next pregnancy. A case-controlled study of primigravid women suffering a stillbirth confirmed that though there was less anxiety and depression at one year for the mothers who had seen and handled the baby, confirming previous findings, this was not the case when looking at the next pregnancy. Very worryingly there are significant problems for mothers and quite dramatic differences for babies. Anxiety and depression and PTSD in the subsequent pregnancy were worse for those who saw the baby (21%) compared to (6%) for those who never saw the stillborn infant. The incidence was even higher for those who held the child (39%). Most importantly nearly half the babies (42%) in women who had seen or held the baby had disordered attachment compared to 8% in those who had done neither. No effect was seen for keeping mementoes or having funerals. As secure attachment is a fundamental need for good mental health in later life, these data need to be taken into consideration when advising women.

The pendulum does not need to swing back to not seeing the stillborn infant. We need to keep the sympathetic, open culture. We need to keep the respect for women who are sure what is right for them. However, we need to advise them well, to be aware of the implications on the next pregnancy of what they have chosen, and to look out for problems well into the year postdelivery. In this way we may ameliorate the effects of the death by reducing poor mental

health, and hopefully improving the outcome for future babies. We also have
to be circumspect in what we advise those who are not sure what to. Do not
hurry them. Remember these women and their partners are still in the shock
stage of grief and so good decision-making for them is difficult. Thus the
professionals have a bigger burden to give user friendly, unbiased information
and try and help the couple decide what is consistent with their usual coping
strategies. Not rushing into anything is certainly good advice for the couple.
Not suggesting anything is good advice for the doctor. It is probably easiest
and correct to say that some studies are concerned that if you do not see
the baby that you may have increased anxiety and depression; however, other
studies do not show this. Whilst people who have opted to see the baby have
not been reported to have regretted it, some studies are concerned that it can
affect how you feel in the next pregnancy, leading to anxiety and depression
and posttraumatic disorder then, and that the relationship you have with that
infant afterwards may be more difficult. Doctors can empathize with couples
on what is the right information as it is not straightforward and how difficult
it can be to work out what is the right thing to do. There are no studies of the
effect of wanting one thing and having to do the other!! That is, if you want to
see the baby and you do not, is that protective or if you do not really want to
see the baby but think it is the right thing to do, is that more traumatizing? So
research is certainly needed to try and work out what is the best advice. It is
also worth saying that 14% of people in recent studies did not see their baby,
giving them permission for this option. Remind them that photographs and
so on will be taken and kept on file if they change their mind about seeing
the baby.

All couples are different and need to come to their best answer depending
on what seems right for them. Some people feel they do want to see their baby,
some definitely do not, some need to think longer about what they think is
right for them.

Using research examples and underlining how conflicting it is at least gives
information and permission for the couple to relate to and means information
is less likely to be biased.

There is clearly a need for much more research to be done in this area
particularly because of the profound impact on the health of subsequent
generations.

17.12.   Postmortems

The doctor and midwife on the active delivery suite have the difficult task of
explaining about the postmortem. The couple are still in shock and distressed,
so they do not want to think about it. Health professionals can also have
difficult feelings about the postmortem process and the excuse of not wanting
to cause more distress allows us to hide our own feelings. Yet often the
professionals on the front line, the busy difficult delivery suite, do not see

the therapeutic benefits of a postmortem, regardless of answers, at the 6-week visit, or the sadness and regret—"Why didn't they explain how important it was at the time?" when this one-off opportunity has not been taken and there are no answers and no choice or ability left to look for them. Whilst not riding roughshod over people's feelings, the doctor must give the message of the need for, and the approval of, postmortems. They must have no doubt that it can be very beneficial and useful. We are not doing our medical duty if we fail to give good accurate advice: if we do not advise of the importance of the postmortem in truly looking for underlying causes and how they might feel later if they have not explored all possible avenues to find some answers.

In the case of recurrent genetic disorders the postmortem is vital to alert us to this and it may not be discovered any other way. Where there is a medico-legal concern it is also vital for both parties to have accurate information.. Distress soon changes and grief and regret in not having a postmortem is often expressed at the 6-week visit when no answers are available. I have never met anyone who regrets having a postmortem, but I have met many people at the 6-week visit who regret not having one. The mixture of shock, distress, and not wanting to think about it all conspire to not wanting one at the time.

The difficulties are understandable. The thought of babies undergoing a postmortem involving being cut up is like a nightmare. There is a belief that often answers are not found and so the distress is not worth it. This is not true. There have been huge inroads into finding a reason, particularly before 36 weeks, where nearly always extra useful information is found. The findings can contradict previous suspicions as to the cause. This can change the whole management and outcome in subsequent pregnancies. The modern perinatal pathology service is very sensitive, showing great respect for the stillborn infant. The pathologists want to ensure that the maximum amount of information is obtained at this one-off opportunity. They know they are performing a delicate task and are doing the utmost to get information that will give some answers. They know that this information is vital for the parents' own questions, as well as their future plans, and indeed for the next generation who will need to know for their own pregnancies what the effect might be.

It is important that the medical staff take the lead and responsibility. They are responsible for investigation and providing answers. Doctors are not distant observers in this decision, but the key in providing accurate information and explanations at every stage. Their job is also to explain to other professionals involved why it is important, so they can also respond accurately to the couples' questions.

The possibility of a postmortem should be brought up early, as the couple start their questions and search for an answer as to why this has happened.

After the delivery of the stillborn infant, doctors must choose their time sensitively and have time to sit with the couple. They must metaphorically hold the couple's hands as they work through this important issue, recognizing how awful a decision it might be to make, yet so important, so there are no regrets either way in the future.

The doctor should ensure the forms are given and the process explained to help consent. Since the Alder Hey enquiry, there should be specific consent forms to help professionals take the couple through the process of what they are consenting to, which have usually been designed by an expert committee. These help a lot by breaking the process down into manageable bits and by providing good information as to exactly what will happen. Some couples may just want to sign without hearing too much of the detail, for others it is important to take time so they can feel in control.

Most services can fit in with religious needs of speed if they are telephoned and made aware. There is also the option of at least a limited postmortem if the parents do not want a full postmortem. Whilst not a good substitute, some disorders can be ruled out by this, giving some reassurance.

All the forms need to be filled in with great accuracy and the pathologist needs as much information and detail as possible. Sometimes this part of the process is overlooked. The couple can then be let down at the last minute.

The couple should have as long as they need to be in hospital and see the baby. Some go home and are supervised by their community midwife in coming back for a final visit. The postmortem should not affect this time of visiting.

It is helpful to have a designated worker (some units have a dedicated midwife for the service to parents of a stillborn infant) to track where the infant is in the process so that the couple can have accurate information for the undertaker and funeral preparations. A designated worker should be available to coordinate after care and to answer any questions. A follow-up visit should be organized before discharge or the couple should know who is sending it to them. Whilst a 6-week visit has always been the standard, the actual timing can depend on many things, including the postmortem results. There is little point in attending for results when they are taking longer. So the guidelines for aftercare need to take into account individual variations. The couple should be given the outline of what will happen and when. Whilst it is the hospitals responsibility at all times to contact the couple, a designated worker or secretary's number is useful for the couple for if they need to ask anything.

17.13. Communication

This can often be poor, partly due to the distress and partly due to the fact that many other things are going on and it may not be clear who is responsible for notifying other carers. Not knowing about a stillbirth is very upsetting for the community carers and they can easily feel at a great disadvantage if not informed.

The GP and community midwife should have been informed personally of the stillbirth by phone and in writing, so they can take steps to visit and provide the immediate after care upon discharge. It is also vital to inform all agencies providing care, for example, the antenatal clinic and scan clinic so that "DNA" letters are not sent. Each unit should have accurate and specific guidelines about this communication need for their setup. Also contact the partner's GP if that is different as he may well be visiting for sick notes or other support.

17.14. Discharge Advice

17.14.1. *Factual Information for the Next Stage*

We know from studying our grief stages that there is still likely to be some elements of shock. All information should also be backed up by written booklets. Write down instructions, for example, for antibiotics and milk suppression. Write down when next to expect a visit. Ensure all relevant booklets have been given and contact telephone numbers.

17.14.2. *Emotional Support for the Next Stage*

It is useful to rehearse with them some of the likely "life scenarios" to give them some confidence when going home and help them think about the next stage so that problems do not just hit them, and they have some defenses and healthy coping strategies ready.

a) *The effect on the other children in the family.* The other children will know of the loss even if they are at a preverbal development stage. They are likely to think that if one baby can go, so can them, and so they play up to get lots of contact and reassurance. It is worth warning the parents that they are not going to get a quiet time. Early and factual discussion with existing children, whatever the stage, followed by frequent reassurance, is encouraged to limit their acting out and will be rewarded usually by good behaviour. It is all right to cry, though both parents helpless with overwhelming grief at the same time can feel like no one is looking after that child, and may mean they need to get someone in to look after them all at this critical phase. You can reassure them that usually the grief comes and goes, and so couples find that they can cope and share this with the family. Rehearse what they might say to the child, and what questions they think the child will ask. How will they be able to respond to the child's emotions and questions?

b) *What to say to their parents* if they have not told them yet, again rehearse how they will be told, and what their reaction might be.

c) *Friends, family, and work*: What will they say to sympathetic phone calls? Do they want to see people? Do they want a few days on their own? Who is going to come and support them? Always ensure that the man is also asked. Too often the man is expected to be strong and supportive to his partner, but is never asked about what he is doing to cope and his experience with work, friends, and family. Give him permission to have time off work—advise him to see his GP and get a note for time off work, whilst also being aware that many cope by just getting on with things.

d) *What to say to people you meet in the street.* Many people do not know what to say or do and can easily say the wrong thing without meaning to. You might want to help them with some ideas on what to say to them, to comments like "How are you?" It is likely that they will come up with their own answers but suggestions could be "It has all been very sad but we are coping. We are getting a follow-up appointment at the hospital and hopefully we will get some answers then" or "The midwife is coming in regularly to support us and we are coping thanks." They do not have to prolong the conversation if they are feeling overwhelmed but can politely move on.

e) *Angry feelings* will naturally surface and the couple may want to work out how they are going to deal with that, rather than lash out at someone.

f) *Other people are pregnant.* It is inevitable that others will get pregnant and be pregnant. Especially if this was a second child it is likely that a lot of antenatal friends from before are pregnant or planning to be. The couple may want to think about that and how they want to respond. It is sad that they have lost their baby but they can still be pleased for their friends or family. Remember these people will be feeling awkward and guilty and also worried about their own pregnancy. Encourage them to tell their own midwives and obstetrician that this has happened, so they can discuss their anxiety with the appropriate person.

17.15.   The Follow-Up "6-week" Visit

This visit is critical both to help towards resolution of the loss of the stillborn infant, and to give accurate and helpful advice about subsequent pregnancies. As ever the distress surrounding the loss may distract the couple from retaining information. It is important then that we have clear communication and strategies to help this.

A recent study of the knowledge of mothers about their previous loss, was striking, showed often women have a poor or confused knowledge of events surrounding the death. For example, mothers of stillborn infants were significantly less likely to know the birth weight. Only 29% were satisfied with the information they had received; 40% did not take the advice of doctors about their next pregnancy.

17.16.   Preparation for the Poststillbirth Appointment

Where? We traditionally see the patient back at the hospital. Some find this traumatic, to visit the place where it happened, though a well-managed stillbirth, despite leaving sad memories, should also leave memories of good caring staff and an expectation of sensitive care at this appointment. Avoidance of long waits in the waiting room surrounded by pregnant women should be organized.

This visit should normally take 30–60 minutes depending on the complexity and the questions of the couple; 10 minutes in a gynecology clinic is not sufficient and ought to be separate. It is important that they are separate and specific times and this should be encouraged as a health policy.

I personally limit all of these consultations to 1–1.5 h and do not go over. After 1 h you are drained if you have been listening hard and the quality of work you are doing will go down. The couple will also be drained. When you are both tired your communication quality will go down and misunderstandings are more likely to occur, sabotaging all your previous good work.

Check the notes for all the results the day before. Read the notes. Always be accompanied by a midwife or other appropriate professional. They can help the couple feel supported and also provide comfort if needed so you can concentrate on your role of explaining and listening, being sensitive to their pace and feelings and responses as you progress through the consultation. It is also useful to have a member of the hospital team with you to help clarify, understand, and also be a witness. People tend to behave better if there are others around and this will minimize difficulties you may experience with anger.

We need to be open and honest. Covering up, not giving details or explanations do not help the couple come to terms with their loss. Good mental health is best served by an open approach. Feeling they have no alternative but go to litigation means they have not felt heard and feel something has not been told to them. Women undergoing litigation have a much higher incidence of PTSD, not good for the mother or for the rest of the family.

17.17.   Conduct of the Appointment

Briefly check how they are and how they are feeling coming back to the hospital. This needs to be done but should not be used as an excuse to prevaricate as the parents are there for some answers and the postmortem results.

After this brief enquiry, outline the framework for the consultation and what you are going to talk about,

1. The postmortem.
2. What are the implications?
3. How do they feel after hearing the results?
4. What advice might be there for the future retiming of pregnancy and what extra care will be needed and choices to help with anxiety?

Ask them if they have brought a list of their questions or anything they specifically wanted to talk about that they have been thinking about over the last 6 weeks, to ensure that these are covered during the discussion. You may well have records noting their questions from when they were admitted and can revise that before starting.

This reassures them that they will be heard. Take a copy of the list, so that you can refer to it in the consultation and later when writing the letter of summary/follow-up letter.

Outline that the consultation will be for an hour, so they can be reassured they will have time to cover the points. Reassure them that if more time is needed another appointment can be arranged. Sometimes you will go over the hour a little way. It is rare to actually need another appointment.

Keep notes of the discussion. Warn them you will be taking notes in order to have a record and that this final report will be sent to them, as it is well known not everything is remembered.

17.17.1. *Giving the Results*

Give the postmortem findings first. Give them a copy of the summary to take home and read later. The postmortem is usually the key report working towards a diagnosis. The rest of the results, for example, blood tests follow. Discussion of what happened naturally follows after that. If necessary the report is supplemented by some basic interpretation. Keep statements brief and to the point. After discussing the postmortem there should be time to take it in. The couple may want 5 minutes on their own to think about it.

The main postmortem report is very medical, for example, weight of organs and does not contain any extra helpful information. If the couple want this too, read a piece out to make sure they understand that it is very basic and medical, so that they do not get shocked when they come to look at it in the future.

If the questioning around the results has not led on to a review of the pregnancy as a whole then this can now be done by going through the notes, picking up their questions, and generally completing the picture. It is specifically useful to listen to the couple and woman. Her feelings about the problem may not be the same as the facts. They are, however, real and pertinent. Feeling listened to is important. Recording and summarizing the feelings in the final report is useful in making people feel that they have been heard and heard accurately.

Sometimes they feel that this is the biggest battle–getting heard clearly and it is reassuring that you are going to deal with them openly and honestly. For many, however, it will be a time of trying to come to terms with the loss.

This can then lead on to a discussion about whether something was missed or whether it should have been picked up and something done at an earlier stage if appropriate. Where there is cause for complaint it is useful if this can be documented, and if necessary arrange to meet them at a later date if further investigations or information needs to be gathered.

Where no cause for the stillbirth is found, it is important to empathize with just how inadequate this feels, no answer to explain their hurt and loss. The only advantage is that it tends to give a more positive result for the next pregnancy, should they want one in the future.

At the end, return to how they are feeling now that they have heard the results. Silently check where the couple is on the grief pathway. (See above.) Find out how they are coping—help them to adjust to reality.

17.18.   Implications for Future Pregnancy

For implications for the management of the next pregnancy and when to go ahead and try for another child, you can say to the patient, "We do need to talk about the next pregnancy, it may be far from your mind but it is important to give you some guidance". It is quite natural not to be thinking about it at this time but it is also natural for people to wonder whether it would happen again as they begin to recover whether or not they decide to go ahead with a further pregnancy.

The advice for the management of the next pregnancy will depend on the diagnosis of the stillbirth. If there is a specific diagnosis then the options for diagnosis, management and monitoring need to be outlined e.g. genetic abnormality then the options for prenatal diagnosis and possible termination, or if there was pre-eclampsia, the role of Doppler ultrasound and aspirin can be mentioned. Also discuss the emotional aspects, particularly the anxiety and how this might be helped by extra checks, that is, extra scans. Not everyone will want them, having a check reminds them things can go wrong and can cause anxiety rather than reassurance. No one knows yet exactly how they will feel in the next pregnancy; however, knowing what options there are gives them some control and help. Other psychological aspects as outlined in the chapter on pregnancy after stillbirth need to be mentioned.

When to start the next pregnancy. Whilst physically there is no problem in starting straight away, many women feel they have hardly stopped being pregnant for 2 years by the end, which is exhausting in itself. There are concerns that the mother needs some time for mourning and if there is not enough time for that process then the issues of unresolved mourning can affect the attachment and mental health of a subsequent child. There are some worries about whether with a short gap this will be seen as a replacement child and not a child in their own right. This can lead to confusion for the next child. There is also idealization of the lost child "The first child would have been a good feeder and not kept me up all night." At least if this is explained then the mother can be aware of the thought processes and not get caught up in this harmful line of thinking. The problem of going through anniversary dates of the death and when the baby was actually due can be more difficult if pregnant. This also affects the anxiety in the next pregnancy.

Do not be didactic. Women do not like to be told when to have their next baby. About 50% of women become pregnant within the first year despite medical advice. If a woman feels strongly that she wants to get pregnant quickly, then it is likely to be the right thing for her and depression may ensue with enforced waiting. However, all things being equal it is probably best to wait for a year. Some women, for example, older mothers and those that had difficulty conceiving, may feel they do not have the luxury of waiting. Advise them that support and help can be given if they do run into sequelae in the next pregnancy. At least we can be forewarned to watch out and so work towards a good outcome.

At the end of the meeting: Summarize what has been said. Repeat that the report will be on its way. (I would dictate this immediately and minimize delays in sending it off). If another appointment is to be made, make it there and then. Leave at least 2 weeks before the next appointment. (It will take 3–5 days for your letter to arrive and allows some time for reflection) If further information is needed, indicate when that will be ready and who will contact them.

Follow-up letter: This is a useful transcription of your notes into legible writing. Use the original appointment outline. Go through their questions and ensure they are answered or outline what is still outstanding for the next appointment. Add in any extra points that need looking up. Also include the list of suggestions for the management of the next pregnancy. This can be kept in the notes for when she represents. Also the couple have it if they go to another hospital to help the next obstetrician.

If there are unresolved issues: There are mechanisms for complaints or second opinions to which your patient is entitled. These can be given calmly and readily when you feel you have exhausted the help, support, and information you can give. It is also worth reflecting about the dissatisfaction. Is this the anger of loss displaced on to you? Do you feel helpless to solve it? Perhaps so do they. They want you to feel it and feel unhappy too. If the anger or frustration is open, there may be benefits for them to talk to a professional unrelated to the stillbirth, such as a psychologist. Other options are to liase with their GP.

Remind them that questions may come up in the future and that they should be free to phone your secretary at any time to see you or write in and that this is an open ended invitation at any time.

Bibliography

1. Kohner N. Pregnancy Loss and the Death of a Baby. Guidelines for Professionals: Revised edition. London: SANDS (Stillbirth and Neonatal Death Society); 1995.
2. Kohner N, Henley A. *When a Baby Dies: The Experience of Late Miscarriage and Neonatal Death*. Revised edition. London: Routledge; 2001.
3. Don A. *Fathers Feel Too*. Bosun Publishing on behalf of SANDS 2005.
4. Hughes P. Psychological effects of stillbirth and neonatal loss. In: Clement S, ed. *Psychological Perspectives on Pregnancy and Childbirth*. London: Churchill Livingstone; 1998:145–166.

5. Hughes P, Riches S. Psychological aspects of perinatal loss. *Curr Opin Obstet Gynaecol.* 2003;15(2):107–111.
6. Hughes P, Turton P, Hopper E, Evans CD. Assessment of guidelines for good practice in psychosocial care of mothers after stillbirth: a cohort study. *Lancet.* 2002;360:114–118.
7. Bowlby J. *Attachment and Loss: Loss: Sadness and Depression.* London: Hogarth Press; 1980.
8. Chambers HM, Chan FY. Support for women/families after perinatal death. *Cochrane Database Syst Rev.* 2000;(2) CD000452.
9. Defey D. Helping health care staff deal with perinatal loss. *Infant Ment Health J.* 1995;16:102–111.
10. Lewis E. Mourning by the family after a stillbirth or neo-natal death. *Arch Dis Child.* 1979;54:303–306.
    Grief stages:
11. Kubler-Ross E. *On Death and Dying.* New York: Macmillan; 1970.
12. Ramsay RW, de Groot W. 9 Components of Grief. A Further Look at Bereavement paper presented at EATI Conference Uppsala sited in PE Hodgkinson 1980 Treating Abnormal Grief in the Bereaved Nursing Times 17 January; 1977:126–128.
13. Murray L. The impact of post-natal depression on infant development. *J Child Psychol Psychiatry.* 1992;33:543–562.
    Post-natal visit:
14. Crother ME. Communication and following a stillbirth or neonatal death, room for improvement. *Br J Obstet Gynaecol.* 1995;102(12):952–956.
15. **Davis DL, Stewart M, Harmon RJ.** Postponing pregnancy after perinatal death: perspectives on doctor advice. *J Am Child Adolesc Psychol.* 1989;28,4:481–487.

18
The Next Pregnancy After Stillbirth

Patricia Hughes and Jayne Cockburn

Whilst much is written about SB, little guidance is given in respect of managing either the physical or psychological hurdles in the next pregnancy. The experience of stillbirth is a significant trauma and the next pregnancy may be a time of high anxiety and sadness for both mothers and fathers, with around 20% of parents suffering from Post Traumatic Stress Disorder (PTSD) related to the stillbirth experience and triggered by the new pregnancy. If the mother remains unresolved in her mourning for the dead infant, the next born may show disorganization of infant–mother attachment. Early infant–mother problems may lead to long-term developmental and behavioral problems. Other members of the family are also vulnerable when there has been a stillbirth and there is a tendency, notable in the literature, for failing to recognize that fathers too have suffered a loss and may find the subsequent pregnancy difficult. Current children have been reported to be vulnerable to psychological problems, possibly related to maternal anxiety.

18.1.   What Are the Physical Problems of Pregnancy After Stillbirth?

There is evidence from a number of studies of physical problems that arise in the pregnancy after stillbirth (Table 18.1).

Though the actual percentages may vary between studies, the problems identified in different studies are similar. The increase in "fetal distress," and operative deliveries, forceps, and emergency caesarean section, is independent of the extra risk of induction of labor. Postpartum hemorrhage is more common. There was an observable but not statistically significant increase in obstetric intervention for unclear medical reasons. The studies were too small to be able to detect this, as there was already a high intervention rate, but may well reflect obstetrician anxiety (1).

TABLE 18.1. Maternal physical complications in the pregnancy after stillbirth

Antenatal	Post SB (%)	Control (%)
Abnormal GTT/gestational diabetes (36)	7.9	1.9
Placental abruption (37)	5.4	0.7
Medical complication (38)	58	30
Admission to hospital (38)	46	26
Delivery		
C section (37)	30	13.4
Induction of labor (37)	20.6	10.7
Elective C section (36)	21.2	21.5
Fetal distress (36)	18.3	8.3
PPH (36)	7.2	3.4
Forceps (IIL)	7.9	3.9
Instrumental deliveries (36)	9.8	5.3
Emergency c section (36) (IIL)	13.6	7.1

IIL, independent of induction of labor.

18.2.   Complication for the Baby In Pregnancy After Stillbirth

With the extra care given, it might be expected that complications be reduced. However, studies of outcomes after stillbirth compared to control populations show that this is not the case.

Small studies show no increase in mortality compared to controls. Larger epidemiological studies are needed to confirm this.

Evidence is beginning to suggest that there is a psychosomatic contribution related to some of these complications. Maternal anxiety in pregnancy is associated with earlier births, lower birthweights (2,3), and impairment of fetal brain development (4). Mediating mechanisms may include abnormal uterine blood flow (Teiweira et al 2002) and increased cortical transfer from mother to fetus (5). Maternal anxiety is natural. It is the obstetrician's job to help the mother cope and minimize it. Antenatal depression is associated with poor clinic attendance and poor self care (6) likely to lead to small babies.

TABLE 18.2.

	Post SB (%)	Control (%)
Preterm birth (36) (IIL) <37 weeks	10.4	4.8
Preterm birth (36) (ILL) <32 weeks	2.5	0.8
Complications (38)	28	20.4
Low birth weight (36)	6.3	3.7
Very LBW <1.5 kg (36)	2.2	0.9
Intubation (38)	11	5
SCBU admission (38)	13	7
Delivered preterm (38) because of complications	6.7	1.6

18.3.   Mental Health Problems in Next Pregnancy After Stillbirth

There is a significant morbidity for parents, and the parents' state of mind may affect the development of the next born infant.

18.4.   Women's Mental Health Problems

There is increased anxiety, depression, and PTSD in the pregnancy following stillbirth, and the symptoms often occur together (7–9). These are maximal in the third trimester and if symptoms have not been present before, they should be asked about again. The pregnancy itself is a potential reactivating factor for PTSD. For nearly all women, PTSD symptoms remit by 1 year postpartum. However, as a small proportion of women continue to suffer chronic symptoms, the possibility of this diagnosis should be recognized.

These symptoms are distressing for the woman herself, and may have implications for the family and the next born child if symptoms persist after the birth, as maternal psychiatric disorders of all kinds increase the risk of disturbance in child development (10).

18.5.   Risk Factors for Psychological Problems

Not all mothers develop severe psychological problems, though understanding of the emotional journey provides the opportunity to intervene, provide appropriate support for all, whilst identifying and following closely those at risk (11–13).

TABLE 18.3. Outcome measures in women who had had a stillbirth and in controls

	Stillbirth n = 60	Control N = 60	p	95% CI difference
Third trimester depression (EPDS >12) (mean)*	10.8	8.2	0.004	0.91–4.7
Third trimester depression (EPDS >14)	28%	8%	0.004	8–34%
Third trimester anxiety (SSA) (mean)*	39.8	32.5	0.001	3.0–11.6
Third trimester PTSD	21%	0%	< 0.001	11–32%
1 year after birth				
Depression (BDI) (mean)*	6.0	5.1	0.39	-1.2–3.0
Depression (BDI >10)	10(18%)	4.0(8%)	0.18	-5–20%
Anxiety (SSA) (mean)*	32.9	32.4	0.36	-2.5–6.7
PTSD	2 (4%)	1 (2%)	1	-4–7%
Disorganized attachment	19 (36%)	8 (13%)	0.03	7–36%
Overall poor outcome	39 (65%)	23 (38%)	0.007	8–42%

*Analyses by paired t-test, other analyses by McNemar test with exact p value
EPDS, Edinburgh Postnatal Depression Scale
SSA, Spielberger State Anxiety Scale

TABLE 18.4. Risk factors for psychological problems

Problem	Risk factor
Active/increased grief	High self criticism, Later gestational age of loss
Unresolved grief	Conception within 1 year
Difficulty coping despair	Longer between loss and conception
PTSD 20%	Felt lack of social support at time of loss. Holding the dead infant. Conception within 12 months.
Depression 20%	High self criticism, conception in first 12 months
Specific anxiety	Belief that their behavior directly affects fetal health—a lot of personal responsibility, which needs to be reduced.
Unresolved grief	Holding the dead infant

Fifty percent of women conceive within the first year, and this is of concern as early conception is associated with increase in psychological symptoms.

18.6.   Fathers' Mental Health Problems

Although, research on perinatally bereaved fathers is limited compared to that on mothers, it is similar in its methodological quality and findings. However, there are some important differences. In addition to grief, qualitative studies emphasize fathering and supportive roles; that is, the experience of becoming a father and the perceived need to provide emotional support to the mother (14,15). Most quantitative studies comparing fathers to mothers have found lower levels of grief (16–18) and lower levels of anxiety and depression in fathers than in mothers (19,20). A study of fathers in the pregnancy following stillbirth, found significant anxiety which resolved with time, and case-level PTSD in 20%. As with mothers, these symptoms were associated with holding the dead infant, but symptom levels fell after the next infant's birth (21). Vulnerability factors are similar to those in mothers (16,21).

18.7.   The Baby's Psychological Development

Mental health disturbances of all kinds in the mother of a young child increase the risk of difficulties arising in the child's psychological and emotional development (10,22). A range of problems for the baby has been described: -

1. "Vulnerable child syndrome" where the child is treated with particular anxiety (23).
2. "Replacement child" where the child's needs are idealized, or denigrated as less than the lost child's would have been (24,25) and the "Replacement child maneuver" where child is treated as special and yet is neglected because of the mother's continuing ambivalence (26).
3. Single case studies have been reported where another child in the family develops somatic symptoms such as abdominal pain assumed to be related to maternal anxiety (27).

4. One study reported that two out of seven mothers felt unable to respond to their children's needs due to negative feelings about them (28).
5. "Disorganized attachment" in 36% of infants compared to 8% in a nonbereaved control group (29) mediated by continuing maternal preoccupation with the lost child. This is a predictor of poor socio-emotional development in later childhood and adolescence (Main, Kaplan, & Cassidy 1985; Lewis & Feiring 1989; Wartner, Grossman, Bremmer-Bombik & Suess wartner1994, 30).
6. Anxiety disorder in adolescents has been found to be associated with maternal experience of stillbirth (31).

18.8. Clinical Outline of Management

Women in the pregnancy after perinatal loss feel that they have to invest in the pregnancy by doing all that they can to ensure that the baby will be healthy. At the same time, irrespective of their gestational age or loss history, some women seek self-protection by holding back emotionally, and not believing too strongly in a positive outcome in case the worst happens.

18.9. Women's Coping Strategies in Pregnancies After Stillbirth

Most people do find a way to cope with the strain of the next pregnancy, and for many people these strategies are helpful to get through a difficult time. Two references catalogue coping strategies. In "One Foot In, One Foot Out. Weathering the storm of Pregnancy after Perinatal Loss," women were able to navigate the pregnancy through 7 activities or themes:

1. Setting the stage.
2. Weathering the storm.
3. Gauging where I am.
4. Honoring each baby.
5. Expecting the worst.
6. Supporting me where I am, and
7. Realizing how I have changed (Loss of innocence/less naive).

Another description of coping (32) includes:

a. Developing emotional armor.
b. Limiting disclosure of the previous and present pregnancy.
c. Delaying attachment to the baby.
d. And forming a strong attachment to healthcare professionals and other people with similar experiences.

It is important for clinicians to be aware of what means women have found to cope so that they can support and augment healthy, useful mechanisms, and be aware of their needs.

18.10. General Principles of Care

i. Continuity of care should be provided by a consultant/clinician with experience in managing the pregnancy after stillbirth wherever possible.
ii. Women should be seen in a high risk clinic by a clinical team well versed in counseling (listening) and support, comfortable in discussing reality for the couples both physically and emotionally in an open and honest way, and ideally with ready access to psychological services if needed.
iii. Midwifery teams or day-assessment units should offer a variety of well qualified and confident staff that will provide a feeling of safety and allows parents to ask questions they may not ask of the "busy" consultant. Midwifery models have been used in other countries and we may be able to learn from those (33).
iv. It is helpful to see both parents, if possible regularly, to build a relationship for later times in the pregnancy when there may be increased stresses.
v. If the usual obstetrician is not going to be in the clinic the next visit, the couple should ideally be introduced to the person who will see them, and who ensure that he/she is familiar with the history so they don't have to go through it again, something many couples find irritating and distressing.
vi. Try to ensure parents are seen quickly: lengthy time hanging around the waiting room increases anxiety.
vii. Demonstrate a problem solving approach to problems—emotionally neutral and factual. Do not let parents feelings of distress, anxiety or even panic become yours. Try not to speak down to parents, who may feel patronized, and ensure that they are involved in getting information and in making choices.
viii. Interpret whatever scientific evidence that there is, and try to do so in the context of the individual couple's values and experience.
ix. Use technology appropriately, knowing why we are using it but also being aware of its limitations.
x. When ordering a test discuss the implications, what the results might be and what might happen. This can help keep anxiety in proportion, and allows the parents to feel some degree of control and reduce anxiety. It also helps establish a trusting relationship so that parents will feel more confident about telling you other worries that they may fear are irrational.

Routine testing may not be found as reassuring as we professionals expect, but may actually increase anxiety—"there might be something wrong and I have to face it every time I have a scan." So check this out with the mother and ask what would be helpful for her.

18.11. Emotional Care

At appointments, check how the mother is feeling. This is not a social question. Chatting about her daily life and worries allows you to get a measure of how she and the couple are functioning. Ask about sleep, work, and other members of the family. Mentioning anxiety may help normalize the mother's anxiety and signal that it is natural to worry. Watch for depression—again, you can reassure the mother that feeling sad or having some experience of low mood is normal when the last pregnancy ended with a loss. Remember that antenatal depression is the biggest predictor of postnatal depression, which may require psychological intervention.

With fathers, remember that the father of this pregnancy may not be the father of the stillborn child, and adapt your approach accordingly. For those fathers who did suffer a stillbirth, regardless of the timing of the loss or the investment in the previous pregnancy, the father is liable to feel anxiety about the outcome of a subsequent pregnancy, with a heightened sense of risk and a need for increased vigilance (34). It is easy for the father to be excluded or to exclude himself with the result that all the support is given to the mother. If the father attends with the mother, give attention to him, both in recognizing his own possible upset and his own need for support, as well as mentioning your appreciation of the support that he is giving his wife.

18.12. At Booking

This is a key visit to establish the relationship and make an outline plan.

18.12.1. Establish That You Listen

Hear the parents' story of what happened last time and their worries for this pregnancy. Ask what they were told last time about the causes as well as how they felt. Ask if there was any course of action for a subsequent pregnancy recommended after the loss. It is likely they will expect these questions from you. Try to incorporate these recommended actions if at all possible, or if you feel they are not helpful then explain clearly why you want to do something differently. If you do not do so, then you may undermine your good working relationship with the parents.

18.12.2. Establish a Clear Outline Plan for the Pregnancy

Rehearse the key issues

a) What is needed for any physical problems that arose last time, both in terms of prevention and what action will be taken if they recur.
b) Record the anniversary times of death, delivery, funeral and previous EDD. As 50% of women are pregnant within a year, these important first

anniversaries will occur in this pregnancy, and commonly are associated with increase in stress.

c) Discuss the emotional issues:

i. There is an increase in incidence of antenatal depression and PTSD, and you should be aware of this. This acknowledgment may implicitly give the mother permission to ask for help. In many women a degree of low mood is entirely normal and not something to worry about. If you are seriously concerned (for example, if the woman cannot manage her usual responsibilities, or seems severely depressed), then you may consider referring to a psychiatrist/psychologist for a consultation.

ii. Discuss the emotional armor needed to cope with fears and "expecting the worst" which can contribute to becoming overanxious. Do not criticize, it is very natural for the parents to be anxious, and professionals need to help the mother behave as " normally" as possible, and to expect that the symptoms will get better.

18.13.   The First 13 Weeks; Fear and Risk of Miscarriage

18.13.1.   Anxiety

a. There is an increased anxiety about miscarriage compared to the general population. Parents may expect the worst to happen—it did before. Offer reassurance, and ask what would be helpful. A midwife can listen to the fetal heart either at home or at the surgery. It is a further loss for the parents to suffer such anxiety that they cannot enjoy being pregnant and cannot welcome the congratulations and pleasure of family and friends.

b. If a miscarriage does occur, this may trigger serious distress. The woman may feel that she will never get it right, will never be a success and always be a failure. This group may need more support from professional staff both after the loss and in planning a subsequent pregnancy.

18.14.   Previous Mid-Trimester Loss and Cervical Cerclage

If there was a mid-trimester loss and a cervical cerclage is needed this should be arranged in line with unit guidelines. The term "weak cervix" is preferable to incompetent cervix, which may be experienced as dismissive of the woman's body.

You should have a plan for gestation at the time of removal. Parents must be warned that the mother may go into labor when the stitch comes out. Have a management plan both for that, and for the mother not immediately going into labor so that parents are prepared for either and are not made unnecessarily anxious.

18.15.   After the First 13 Weeks

A "honeymoon period" may develop where the pregnancy is going well and loss is less likely. Not all women experience this, and it may be ended when the gestation of the previous loss approaches. This can be a good time to establish a trusting and collaborative doctor–parent relationship which will stand you in good stead for dealing with future stresses, and where you can signpost psychological issues for the mother.

18.16.   Physical Issues

Be clear and business like. Stay focused on the planned tasks for the pregnancy.

18.17.   Monitoring

Organize appropriate monitoring, which will depend on the cause of the previous loss, but remembering that the parents' personality will affect how they experience monitoring as reassuring or anxiety-provoking, raising questions about whether the baby is healthy. The role of a scan is dubious: there is unlikely to be benefit in scanning more often than monthly for reassurance, so more frequent scans should be for physical concerns such as suspected IUGR. Where possible, the same person should do the scans, as there is significant inter-observer error. Iatrogenic error can only increase anxiety and will not help to reach a secure diagnosis of IUGR.

Reassurance is often helpful, for example, by saying, "you are doing everything right" and to acknowledge to the couple that they are trying hard.

It may not be so helpful to say "only 100 days to go," which can seem an eternity of worry and sleepless nights. Better to offer "so far, things are going well" which is true but recognizes that we cannot predict the future.

18.18.   Maternal Behavior Toward the Unborn Baby

Talk about attachment issues with the mothers. Reassure them that it is not uncommon after a pregnancy loss for a woman to hold herself back from becoming too attached to her unborn baby, but that for the vast majority this feeling disappears when the baby is actually born. Remind them that the loss may leave them with some sadness and regret for years afterward, but that it is important for the new baby that he or she has the mother's full attention. It is appropriate to remember the lost baby, but not to make it the focus of the parent's lives, especially when a new baby needs their care. When the baby is born, reassure parents that this is a healthy child who is as fit as any other in terms of his or her physical well being and he or she will need the same care, stimulation, and freedom to explore as any other. Point out that some parents do find it rather difficult to believe that their baby is as vigorous as others, but reassure them that with time, they can be as confident as any other parents.

18.19.   Coming up Toward the Indexed Time of Loss

1. Increase the antenatal visits to weekly to check mood, provide support and discuss how parents are coping with thoughts and remembrances from the last pregnancy. Reassure them that it is normal to feel rather "down" at an anniversary and that it will pass.
2. Ask parents what they are doing. They are most likely happy to tell you whether they want to put it out of their minds, or whether they want to visit the grave, taking the rest of the family with them, to have a quiet time at home, or find some other way to note the anniversary. People use different ways to deal with the pain of loss: their strategy may not be yours, but may work for them. In general it is best not to criticize.
3. Review the initial plans in terms of on-going support, and check that this is still what suits parents and helps most with anxiety. If they are well, then parents may choose what they feel most comfortable with, varying from nothing additional, to day unit review. You may observe that an intensely anxious woman may feel she needs the reassurance of being admitted to hospital. If you have medical concerns then you should recommend the clinically appropriate intervention in the usual way.

   Once that day has passed and certainly after that week of gestation, it is usual to see an increase in parents' confidence and a gradual realization that a baby will actually arrive. Now it is time to talk about the delivery and postdelivery feelings.

18.20.   Delivery

18.20.1.   Feelings About Having a Baby After a Stillbirth

Coming up to delivery is the next potential peak of anxiety. Remembrances of last time are likely to be in the parents' minds alongside wanting to be excited for this baby. A common concern is whether this baby will look like the last one and remind parents even more. The mixed emotions of sadness and excitement can be hard. Ask parents whether memories of the last delivery are troubling them. Parents are usually pleased that this is recognized, and happy to tell you. They can also be reassured that such mixed feelings are normal after stillbirth.

Women may also benefit from discussion about their thoughts on the reality of having a baby, and what preparations they and the family have put in place. Remember that some may be so anxious that they don't "want to tempt fate" by making plans. Psychologically the mothers have not fully integrated the fact of the coming baby and therefore cannot plan for potential problems afterward. This is the parents' emotional armor, and if it is necessary for their psychological survival then it should be respected. We can, however, help by organizing good postnatal support where we can check that all is going well or establish whether additional support or treatment is required.

18.20.2. Mode of Delivery

There is no indication for Caesarean section other than the usual ones (including tokophobia and PTSD due to bad induction the first time). Vaginal delivery, if appropriate, should be encouraged to reduce medicalization, and to encourage the mother to feel confident in her abilities again. Normal delivery of a live baby can reaffirm to the mother that her body does work normally after all.

18.20.3. Timing of Delivery

Early delivery may seem harmless, gives the parents a live baby sooner, treats the obstetrician's anxiety and usually results in grateful parents. However, it is not to be advocated because of the associated medical problems that may result. However anxious parents or staff become, unless there is a good medical reason for an early delivery, we should aim to manage anxiety in the parents and the staff, rather than cause iatrogenic problems.

Reassure parents that anxiety about this child is because of the mother's previous experience rather than because of the problems of this pregnancy. Your excellent care has ensured a healthy baby. Admitting a baby to SCBU because of unwarranted early intervention only serves to "prove" that the anxiety was appropriate rather than due to the previous stillbirth, and may encourage parents to regard this baby as less than healthy. This is very unhelpful and increases the risk of maternal anxiety about this child, with potential fear that she may lose another child. Although there is no firm research evidence that prematurity and admission to SCBU has an adverse effect on parent–infant attachment, it is unlikely that a separation with the infant in a high tech unit will improve a comfortable early attachment. Feeding problems from iatrogenic prematurity reduce the mother's confidence and increase her anxiety.

This can be a hard time for obstetricians as well as the parents. Support from colleagues can be helpful to reassure you that the decision making is appropriate and offer back up in holding out for a normal delivery time

It may be useful to offer a planned delivery. If this is the decision, then the consultant should follow the unit guidelines for "high concerns" pregnancies. This is likely to be induction at 38 weeks or caesarean section at 39 weeks. Some mothers want to wait to term for natural labor, but will not tolerate the anxiety of going overdue. System factors such as availability of the requested midwife and doctor may also affect the timing of delivery. This can be agreed in discussion with the parents. Confidence in staff, and therefore having an environment which is supportive, is helpful in producing a good outcome. Unless unavoidable, delivery dates should aim to avoid anniversary dates—the death of previous baby and the estimated date of that baby's delivery.

18.21.   Other Issues

18.21.1.   Sexing of Baby

Many units now do this routinely. It can be a sensitive issue for parents: while some will not have strong feelings about the baby's sex, others may react emotionally to finding that it is the same or the other sex from the stillborn infant. Some parents may be relieved to have a same sex baby as the lost one, but this may raise the possible hazard that the child could be more likely to be seen as a replacement child, rather than a new person in his or her own right. Some parents may feel better if the child is the other sex, and may have a rather superstitious sense that having the other sex reduces the likelihood of loss happening again. In this context, note the belief that some women can never carry boys.

18.21.2.   Work

Traditionally advice has been for lots of rest in high-risk pregnancies. Bed rest has been shown to increase placental flow as measured by Doppler studies. Some women find that their worries mean they find it difficult to concentrate and cope with the extra of work. However, there is no evidence that not working helps emotionally, and it could work in the opposite direction. There is a well-established association between not working and depression, and this is especially likely to be the case if the woman is isolated at home and apprehensive about the forthcoming birth. Some women find that work and company helps, keeping them distracted from their fears, and on balance, unless there is a good medical reason to advise giving up work, then work that the woman enjoys, and that is not too tiring, is likely to be more of a help than a problem.

18.22.   Postnatal

If possible, parents need the following:

1. A single room, to help them have own physical space to adjust emotionally
2. Extra help and midwifery support if the mother wants to breast-feed.
3. Calm support to reduce anxiety handling the baby, and to reassure that attachment will happen naturally with time

4. A visit from the consultant who cared for the mother antenatally. The consultant may be the most familiar person involved in the care and the one most trusted to listen to the mix of emotions. In general this may include:

  i. Calm listening, rather than advice.
 ii. Admiration for the baby, like any other. This baby deserves it. You may want to say "he/she is a lovely baby, but I realize it is not always easy, when you had such a bad experience last time."
iii. Asking about other family members, asking, "What does your husband/partner think?" "What did the grandparents say?"
 iv. Talking through the family's coping strategies as they go back to the outside world, e.g. people saying that "they are lucky" (when they have had to cope with a lot to get to this stage) or "Is this your first baby" (when it is the second baby not first). You can ask the parents how they might cope with these comments, to plan for dealing with this sort of remark when they go home.
  v. Reassurance about the normal range of feelings that come with having a new baby. However, much the baby is wanted, it is normal for parents to feel tired, frustrated, and even angry, for example, when the baby needs attention in the middle of the night and cannot be calmed, despite the parents' best efforts. A useful suggestion is to give relatives and friends, who want to help, structured tasks such as help with housework and shopping, and explaining to them that the mother is very tired.

18.23. Postnatal Adjustment Problems/Differences in Women in Next Delivery After Loss

Anecdotally, midwives have reported that women with a previous pregnancy may have more worries about their new child, and about handling the baby. Research has confirmed this observation. Women having a subsequent child after having lost a baby because of congenital abnormality, were compared with women who had not suffered a pregnancy loss. The bereaved women said that their healthy baby experienced more problems with sleeping, crying, eating and acquiring a regular pattern of this behavior than the average baby. They also perceived their baby as being less ideal than the women without a previous pregnancy loss. These problems were particularly apparent four weeks postpartum and were positively correlated to trait anxiety (35). This suggests that those such as GPs and Health Visitors who routinely see mothers in the community after the birth should be aware of possible anxieties for the mother in her confidence and in her handling of the baby particularly in anxious women.

18.24. Six-Week Visit

Postnatal visits have gone out of fashion. However, the extra care that the parents needed in this pregnancy, and stress that the consultant has dealt with, may have established a strong bond between the obstetrician and parents. It may be important for the parents to have opportunity to say good-bye to the obstetrician and other team members when they have recovered from the birth and are feeling more confident in their ability as parents. It is also useful to check about any continuing psychological problems including rational or irrational anxiety about the baby. If parents are having problems at this stage a psychological referral may be helpful to discuss the real anxieties and how to cope with them.

18.25. Subsequent Pregnancies (For Example, A Third Pregnancy, That Is, the Second Pregnancy After Stillbirth)

We should always be cautious about assuming that problems are all over now the mother has one live child. However, in a subsequent pregnancy the mother is likely to be less anxious, and may be more able to think calmly about the loss and experience of the stillbirth, with more questions and sadness. Normal openness, with support is usually all that is needed.

18.26. So What is Success?

The aim is to have a couple leave with a live baby, accepting that the new birth does not wipe out the loss, and that this has been a pregnancy where there have been ups and downs, and much anxiety. This is a celebration that is tinged with sadness. The parents will know, better than we do, that the memory of the loss will not disappear, but our hope is that it has its place in the past, and will not interfere with their pleasure in their new child. This may leave you as well as the parents with a feeling of poignancy rather than great rejoicing, but that is appropriate. It is tempting to go home thinking how well we have done getting them a live baby, but that in itself is only one part of success with these parents.

References

1. El-Bastawissi AY, Sorensen TK, Akafomo CK, Frederick Io, Xiao R, Williams MA. History of fetal loss and other adverse pregnancy outcomes in relation to subsequent risk of preterm delivery. *Mater Child Health J.* 2003:7(1):53–58.
2. Wadwa PD, Sandman CA, Porto M, Dunkel-schetter C, Garite U. The association between prenatal stress and infant birth weight and gestational age at birth: a prospective investigation. *Am J Obstet Gynaecol.* 1993;69:858–865.

3. Cooper RL, Goldenberg RL, Das A, Swain M, Norma G et al. The pre-term prediction study: maternal stress is associated with spontaneous preterm birth at less than 35 weeks gestation. *Am J Obstet Gynecol.* 1996;175:1286.

4. Lou HC, Hansen D, Nordentoft, Pryds O, Jensen F, Nim J et al. Prenatal stressors of human life affect brain development. *Dev Med Child Neurol.* 1994:36:826–832.

5. Gitau R, Cameron A, Fisk NM, Glover V. Fetal exposure to maternal cortisol. *Lancet.* 1998;352:707–708.

6. Zuckerman B, Amaro A, Bauchner H, Cabral H. Depressive symptoms during pregnancy: relationship to poor health behaviours. *Am J Obstet Gynaecol.* 1989;160:1107–1111.

7. Hughes PM, Turton P, Evans CDH. Stillbirth as a risk factor for depression and anxiety during pregnancy and the postpartum year in the pregnancy after stillbirth; to assess relevance of time since loss. *BMJ.* 1999;318(7200):1721–1724.

8. Turton P, Hughes P, Evans CDH et al. The incidence and significance of post traumatic stress disorder in the pregnancy after stillbirth. *Br J Psychiatry.* 2001;178:556–560.

9. Sierles FS, Chen J-J. Concurrent psychiatric illness in non-Hispanic outpatients diagnosed as having post traumatic stress disorder. *J Nerv Ment Dis.* 1986;174:171–173.

10. Rutter, M. Pathways from childhood to adult life. *J Child Psychol Psychiatry & Allied Disciplines.* 1989:30(1):23–51,

11. Hughes P, Turton P, Hopper E, Evans CDH. Assessment of guidelines for good practice in psychosocial care of mothers after stillbirth. *Lancet.* 2002;360:114–118.

12. Franche RL. Psychological and obstetric predictors of couples grief during pregnancy after miscarriage or perinatal death. *Obstet Gynaecol.* 1997;(4):597–602, 2001.

13. Franche R L and Mikail S F. Impact of perinatal loss on adjustment to subsequent pregnancy, *Soc Sci Med.* 1999;48(11):1613–1623.

14. Samuelsson M, Radestad I, Segesten K. A waste of life: fathers' experience of losing a child before birth. *Birth.* 2001;28(2):124–130.

15. O'Leary J, Thorwick C. Fathers' perspectives during pregnancy, postperinatal loss. *J Obstet Gynecol Neonatal Nurs.* 2006;35(1):78–86.

16. Zeanah CH, Danis B, Hirshberg L *et al.* Initial adaptation in mothers and fathers following perinatal loss. *Infant Ment Health J.* 1995; 16:80–93.

17. Theut SK, Pederson FA, Zaslow MJ, Cain RL *et al.* Perinatal loss and parental bereavement. *Am J Psychiatry.* 1989;146(5):635–639.

18. Helmrath T, Steinitz EM. Death of an infant: parental grieving and the failure of social support. *J Fam Pract.* 1978;6(4):785–790.

19. Vance JC, Najman JM, Thearle MJ, Embelton G *et al.* Psychological changes in parents eight months after the loss of an infant from stillbirth, neonatal death, or sudden infant death syndrome—a longitudinal study. *Pediatrics.* 1995;96(5):933–938.

20. Dyregrov A, Matthiesen SB. Anxiety and vulnerability in parents following the death of an infant. *Scand J Psychol.* 1987;28(1):16–25.

21. Turton P, Badenhorst W, Hughes P, Ward J et al. The psychological impact of stillbirth on fathers in the subsequent pregnancy and puerperium. *Br J Psychiatry.* 2006;188:165–172.

22. Murray L. The impact of postnatal depression on infant development. *J Child Psychol Psychiatry.* 1992;33:543–562.

23. Green MG, Solnit AJ. Reactions to the threatened loss of a child: A vulnerable child syndrome. *Pediatrics.* 1964;29:58–65.

24. Cain AC, Cain BS. On replacing a child. *J Am Acad Child Psychiatry.* 1964;3:443–445.

25. Pozanski EO. The "replacement child": a saga of unresolved parental grief. *J Pediatr.* 1972;81:1190–1193.

26. Akhtar S, Thomson JA. Overview: narcissistic personality disorder. *Am J Psychiatry.* 1982;139:12–20

27. Jolly H. Family reactions to child bereavement, current children have been reported to be vulnerable to psychological problems, possibly related to maternal anxiety. *Proc R Soc Med.* 1976;69:835–837.

28. Forrest GC, Standish E, Baum JD. Support after perinatal death: a study of support and counselling after perinatal bereavement. *BMJ.* 1982;285:1475–1479.

29. Hughes P, Turton P, Hopper E, McGauley G, Fongay P. Disorganised attachment behaviour among infants born subsequent to stillbirth *J Child Psychol Psychiatry.* 2001;42:791–801.

30. Carlson EA. A c prospective longitudinal study of attachment disorganization/disorientation. *Child Dev.* 1998; 4(69):1107–1128

31. Allen NB, Lewinsohn PM, Seeley JR. Prenatal and perinatal influences on risk for psychopathology in childhood and adolescence. *Dev Psychopathol.* 1998;10:513–529.

32. Rillstone P, Hutchinson SA. Managing the re-emergence of anguish: pregnancy after a loss due to anomalies. *J Obstet Gynaecol Neonat Nurs.* 2001;30(3):291–298.

33. Caelli K, Downier J, Letendre. A parents experiences of midwife-managed care following the loss of a baby in a previous pregnancy. *J Adv Nurs.* 2002;39(2):127–136.

34. Strong DR. Exploring fathers experiences of pregnancy after a prior perinatal loss, *Am J Maternl Child Nurs.* 2001;26(3):147–53.

35. Hunfeld JA, Taslaaer-Kloosak, Agterberg G, Wladimiroff JW, Passchier J. Postpartum adjustment anxiety, negative emotions and the Mother's adaptation to an infant born subsequent to late pregnancy loss: case control study. *Prenat Diagn.* 1997;17(9):843–851.

36. Robson S, Chan A, Kean ERJ, Luke CG. Subsequent birth outcomes after an unexplained stillbirth: preliminary population base but prospective cohort study, *ANZ J Surg.* 2001;4(1):29–35.

37. Heinonen S, Kirkinen P. Pregnancy outcome after the previous stillbirth resulting from causes other than maternal conditions and foetal abnormalities. *Birth.* 2000;27(1):33–37.

38. Crowther ME, Obstetrical and neonatal outcome in subsequent pregnancies *J R Army Med Corps.* 1995;141(2):92–97.

39. Cote-Arsenaultd, Marshall R. One foot in, one foot out. weathering the storm of pregnancy after perinatal loss. *Res Nurs Health.* 2000;23(6):473–85

40. Lewis E. Mourning by the family after a stillbirth or neonatal death. *Arch Dis Child.* 1979;54:303–306.

41. Lyons-Ruth K, Easterbrooks MA, Cibelli CD. Infant attachment strategies, infant mental lag and maternal depressive symptoms: predictors of internalising and externalising problems at age 7. *Dev Psychol.* 1997;33(4):681–692.

42. Sroufe LA. Infant care-giver attachment and patterns of adaptation in preschool: The roots of maladaptation and competence. In: Perimetter M (ed.). Minnesota Symposium in Child Psychology. Vol. 6. Hillsdale, NJ, Eribaum. 1983:41–81.

43. Teixeira JM, Fisk NM, Glover V. Association between maternal anxiety in pregnancy and increased uterine artery resistance index: cohort based study. *BMJ.* 1999;318(7177):153–157.

Part Three
Gynecology

19
Health Care and Young People: A Challenge

Mary Pillai

Currently there are 7 million 10- to 19-year-olds in the UK population. A wide range of problems that may result in referral to a gynecology clinic is listed in Table 19.1, yet traditionally gynecologists have received little or no training in this area of practice. As a result management has often been less than optimal and at worst has caused or exacerbated problems (Vignette 4). The Royal College of Paediatrics and Child Health recognize "There is presently no formal clinical training in any area of adolescent health in the UK outside mental health."[1] In contrast to all other age groups mortality in this age group did not fall significantly in the second half of the twentieth century, the main causes being accidents and self-harm. The risky behavior underlying mortality also attracts considerable morbidity for sexual and reproductive health. Adolescents are very vulnerable to falling under adverse influences leading to conduct problems, substance misuse, pregnancy, sexually transmitted infections, and accidents (e.g., failure to use seat belts). In regard to sexual behavior serial monogamy may explain the extraordinarily high rate of chlamydia in teenagers. Children, and especially adolescents, who are stressed by social and emotional problems may present with a complex picture of physical and psychological problems which are challenging and require multidisciplinary management.

Case Vignette 1

Jennie, age 15, was admitted for the third time with abdominal pain. On the first occasion all investigations were normal, apart from an abdominal X-ray showing fecal loading. This responded to regular laxatives, however within days of going home her GP requested readmission following repeated requests by her mother for home visits. On this occasion she underwent removal of a normal appendix. Her third admission coincided with a heavy painful period. Her mother said she was prone to cyclical mood swings and the family were now

---

[1] Bridging the gaps: healthcare for adolescents: the intercollegiate adolescent working party report. *Royal College of Paediatrics and Child Health*, June 2003. Also available at www.rcpch.ac.uk/publications/recent_publications/bridging_the_gaps.pdf.

TABLE 19.1. Problems referred to gynecology (or obstetrics) in order of frequency

Menstrual problems
Dysmenorrhea/menorrhagia/polymenorrhea
Oligomenorrhea/secondary amenorrhea
Abdominal pain
Pelvic pain (sometimes associated with school refusal)
Teenage pregnancy
Hirsutism/acne
Hymen problems (unable to use tampons)
Discharge
Vulval itching/vulval pain
Puberty
Primary amenorrhea
Primary/premature ovarian failure
Sexual health issue
Genital warts, chlamydia, or other STI
Body image
Breast or labia dissatisfaction
Genital injury
Accidental
Forensic: child sex abuse/sexual assault
Urinary incontinence
Cancer treatment
Reproductive concern

unable to cope with her temper. She had been violent toward her younger sister and had recently been excluded from school for a week following an assault on a fellow pupil. Her mother was convinced her hormones were to blame.

On the children's ward it was difficult to find somewhere to talk to Jennie alone. She was a very unhappy young person. Her father walked out 2 years earlier and her grandmother, who she had always been close to, had suddenly died. She suffered with quite severe acne and was being bullied at school. Addressing these issues in a multidisciplinary team was productive in controlling her pain and integrating her back into school. During six sessions with a clinical psychologist she explored her feelings and learned anger management. This progressed to three family sessions, which further reduced tension in the house. The school nurse talked to her in confidence every fortnight about any problems within school, and the school enhanced enforcement of the bullying policy. The gynecologist established that Jennie would be happy to have more control over her periods and particularly that the pill would also help her acne.

For some the easiest path is to believe their symptom has a purely physical cause. For women hormones are often blamed. The seriousness of the psychosocial problem may often be insoluble for the health professional. This case was gratifying in that, largely owing to her age, the multidisciplinary team approach was more effective than for many cases. Were she an adult the availability of psychology support would not have been a possibility.

Children with a chronic diagnosis will sooner or later need to make the transition to adult services, and for some gynecology will be a key service. Examples include girls with Turner's syndrome and androgen insensitivity. Although there is much expertise between the specialties, it is not structured or coordinated into a service that maximizes on knowledge between pediatric and adult services. So it is especially difficult for adolescents to access this expertise. Factors to be addressed at the time of transition to adult services include the following:

- Evaluation of knowledge/understanding of their diagnosis. This may have been limited in a long-term pediatric doctor–patient relationship.
- What are their concerns, especially in relation to sexual and reproductive function?
- What are their continuing medical needs?—Continuing services are often not well defined and in some cases not funded at all. For example egg donation for young women with ovarian failure.

There may still be young adults who have been brought up in a conspiracy of silence, although hopefully this is now rare as attitudes have changed in the last 15–20 years. Today respect for autonomy would outweigh any concern to protect a child or young person from upsetting information about their diagnosis. This raises challenging issues of how and when to tell the diagnosis, and how to avoid or minimize disruption to family relationships.

The age of menarche has fallen to a mean of 12.8 years, compared with around 16.5 years according to records from the mid-nineteenth century. Problems associated with sexual and reproductive function, including pregnancy, have therefore increased among young people who have not attained intellectual maturity and are still minors in law. Sexual relationships are an accepted and expected dimension of adult life. In making the transition to adulthood young people need the skills to make healthy decisions about their sexual and reproductive lives. These skills and knowledge do not come naturally. Unfortunately there is a strong focus on negative aspects of young people's sexual and reproductive health and a tendency for societies to view adolescents as problems.

19.1. Considerations of Adolescence

Early adolescence is defined by the pubertal transition, a period in which young people undergo intense physical growth and often feel self-conscious about their changing bodies (1). We form opinions about ourselves based on the reactions we elicit from those around us. In this way negative self-appraisal and self-rejection result when the individual perceives negative attitudes from the wider social group. Young people react to the real or perceived stigma of their physical appearance by attempting to change their appearance, often creating more anxiety in the process.

Most young people become sexually active between the ages of 12 and 19, but many will do so without the knowledge and skill to negotiate safe sex. Often they are viewed as risk takers and blamed for negative outcomes, seen as rebellious, irresponsible, and antisocial. In contradictory ways they are also seen as dependent, innocent, and in need of protection.

Teenagers are more likely than adults to engage in high-risk sexual behavior, making them vulnerable to repeat pregnancies and sexually transmitted infections. Sixteen- to nineteen-year-old women have the highest rate of chlamydia of any age group.[2] Thus opportunistic care should include explaining the value of using condoms in addition to any other method of contraception and screening for chlamydia.

When adolescent girls choose to have sexual intercourse, it is important for them to have the knowledge, resources, and communication skills necessary to avoid unintended pregnancies. There are many barriers to contraceptive use that are specific to adolescents. Addressing these barriers requires increasing knowledge and access to contraceptive services and enlisting support from significant others, such as parents and educators. This is part of the health-care provider's role when engaging parents and young people in the process of fostering consistent contraceptive use. Parents influence adolescent contraceptive use through many factors, including the quality of their relationship and the communication of sexual values and beliefs (2,3). It is clear from research that young people who have open discussion with their parents about sex and relationships become sexually active at a later age and are more likely to use contraception (4,5). Adolescents with greater family connectedness are significantly less at risk of all forms of adverse sexual outcome, including unintended pregnancy (6,7).

When the opportunities arise health-care providers should discuss contraception with adolescent males and females directly. These discussions with young men can help them view contraceptive decision-making as mutual and collaborative and as extending beyond condom use. Even though contraceptive discussions with males are important, most of the research has focused on condom use and has described unilateral approaches, such as no condom/no sex. The unilateral approach may not be the best strategy to help young people gain additional skills in order to have mutually intimate relationships.

As part of these discussions with males and females the health-care provider should assess the adolescent's comfort with talking about sexuality and their skills to negotiate with partners. For example the adolescent may appear uncomfortable (e.g., move around more in the chair, avert eye contact, blushing, providing fewer words in their responses) when the topic of sexuality is addressed. For some the discomfort with these discussions also may exist with their partners. If this is the case then they may need additional opportunities to enhance their communication and relationship skills.

---

[2] Data source: KC60 statutory returns and ISD(D)5 data, HPA Centre for Infections, 29/6/2005, available at www. hpa.org.uk/ infections/ topics_az/hiv_and_sti/ sti-chlamydia/epidemiology/epidemiology.htm.

While strategies for supporting parent and partner involvement in contraceptive behavior are ideal, some adolescent–parent relationships do not provide the young person with the guidance and support they need, and not all adolescents are in healthy and safe relationships.

Case Vignette 2

Leanne, age 18, presented with a request for emergency contraception during a Thursday evening clinic, having had unprotected intercourse in the early hours the previous Monday. The doctor explained that she was outside the 72 h window, and that it had been noted this was the second time she had come this month for emergency contraception. The doctor's immediate reaction was a feeling of annoyance at this irresponsible request; however she managed to resist the temptation to let her irritation show through a disapproving tone or comment. As she explained the relative risk of pregnancy the doctor remarked that she wondered what it was that had delayed Leanne coming to the clinic on this occasion and also why she did not get her boyfriend to use a condom. Leanne began to cry. The doctor handed her some tissues and said nothing for a moment. Then she asked if there was a problem with her boyfriend. Leanne revealed he would become angry if she asked him to use a condom or tried to talk him out of sex. His demands for sex were unpredictable, and he also told her she was not to take the pill. He did not like her seeing doctors and became violent when he found out about her last visit to the clinic, even though she had assured him there were only female doctors at the clinic. For this reason she had to wait until she knew he was out before she could seek emergency contraception.

Some young women fear aggression from partners if they request condom use and need sensitive awareness of their need for alternative methods of contraception. They also need help to recognize their relationship is abusive and to address their risk for and avoidance of sexual violence, together with knowledge of local resources to tackle domestic violence.

19.2. Sexual Assault

Young women, especially those under 16 years of age, are at great risk of predatory behavior by adult men (Vignette 5). Teenage girls are many times more likely to be assaulted or raped than the rest of the population.[3] Most incidents occur during high-risk behavior, and most involve considerable quantities of alcohol. Risk taking is common, but at the same time young teenagers are less likely to have acquired the social skills to recognize or disengage themselves from situations of danger. A wide range of conditions, including peer group pressure, conflict with authority figures, and also the

---

[3] Crime in England and Wales 2004/5. *Home Office Statistical Bulletin*. July 2005, also at www.homeoffice.gov.uk/rds.

coexistence of psychiatric morbidity may all contribute to impair the mechanisms that keep young people safe when they take risks. Risky behavior and omnipotence of the peer group may lead young teenagers to believe they should have sex but with no expectation of how they will be treated. Physical violence is relatively common in teen dating, and young teenagers tend to romanticize jealousy. This perpetuates a culture of disrespect, particularly for women. A study of young people in New Zealand found that only 0.2% of young men but 7% of women reported being forced to have intercourse on the first occasion (8). For women there were increasing rates of coercion with younger age at first intercourse. Most women regretted having sexual intercourse under the age of 16.

Sexual health concerns bring young people into contact with services, and this provides an opportunity to screen for abuse. It is a considerable challenge to know how best to engage young people in keep safe work. For example one can inquire if sex was enjoyed and wanted, whether they have any concerns, whether their boyfriend is ever violent or jealous, and whether they have felt pressured to have sex. If one is perceived judgmental, they will not use your service again. However if provided with an opportunity to talk about their experience in a safe, unpressured environment, a significant number of young girls seeking emergency contraception do reveal that the episode was not only unprotected but was unwanted and unenjoyed. This provides the best opportunity for discussing preventive strategies. In many cases of this nature a formal complaint to the police is never an issue and would not be helpful.

Vulnerability may be by age, learning disability, or it may be due to family factors such as abusive relationships or young people with inappropriate and inconsistent boundaries, for example young teenagers out clubbing late at night. Children in care are especially at a high risk. Running away is common and carries high vulnerability to exploitation. Within relationships teenage girls are also at relatively high risk of abuse. Low self-esteem with lack of expectation about how they will be treated is more common than among older women. Domestic violence frequently includes sexual violence, lack of family support, and social isolation.

19.3.   Pitfalls of Adolescent Medicine

Gynecologists often forget a developmental history and growth, while pediatricians may forget to take a sexual history or consider the possibility of pregnancy and sexually acquired infections. Gynecologists are often unskilled at managing third-party consultations, ensuring any intrusion of mother does not compromise the best interests of the patient. The purpose of parental rights is to benefit the child, *not* to further the interests of parents. Most gynecologists are familiar with the Gillick/Fraser ruling[4] but may not have

---

[4] Gillick versus West Norfolk and Wisbech HA and the Department of Health. [1985] 3 All ER 402.

thought through the assessment of competence and its importance to medical practice with those considered in law to be minors. Moving onto an adult patient–doctor relationship is not merely age dependent. In particular those individuals with special needs are often not well addressed.

Case Vignette 3

Nicola, age 14, started her periods at 11. They are heavy and painful, resulting in absence from school. Mother answers all questions and her response to the pill as a proposed therapy is absolutely not.

It is important to explore Nicola's views on her problem, as well as establishing whether she has yet been sexually active. Neither can be done with the mother present.

It is equally important to explore the basis to the mother's objection. Not uncommonly there is a perception that "the pill" is dangerous and that fertility will be impaired in the longer term, and also that it encourages sexual activity. This provides an opportunity for clarification that in *reality* induced oligomenorrhea may have significant advantages for young women including

- effective control of menstrual distress
- improved quality of life—resolution to disturbance to school and other activities, especially important at key exam times
- improved self-esteem and self-confidence
- more self-confidence may equate with less susceptibility to peer pressure to engage sexual activity and *later* onset of sexual activity
- there is no evidence that making contraception more available encourages underage sex
- there is no evidence that making contraceptive services less available will alter the likelihood of young people engaging in risky sexual activity.

It is important to balance advocacy with not antagonizing the parental relationship with both the doctor and the patient. "[A]dvocacy is not about saying what is best for a child/young person but about enabling the child/young person to come to informed decisions about matters affecting their lives."

Case Law in the UK has determined that young people may consent to treatment provided they are

1. adequately informed
2. doing so voluntarily (no external coercion and understanding they have a choice)
3. competent.

In the Gillick ruling, overturning the decision by the Court of Appeal that a child under 16 could not give valid consent, the House of Lords determined that the test to be applied was whether or not the child had sufficient understanding to enable him or her to understand fully what is proposed. This test of maturity must be assessed in respect of the individual and is the responsibility of the doctor offering treatment. Quinn has expressed reservations as to whether legal or clinical definitions of maturity can ever really be given to courts (9). There is however evidence that the majority of adolescents are well able to understand the issues of consent to treatment. A series of vignettes describing various treatment dilemmas were assessed among groups of subjects aged 9, 14, 18, and 21. The 14-year-olds demonstrated a level of competence identical to that of the two older groups (10).

Competence is function specific, not determined by age. The ability of children to make valid decisions is frequently underestimated and will be facilitated by

- a supportive parental relationship
- trust and confidence in the doctor
- adequate information presented in an appropriate way
- freedom from pressure, panic, pain, "temporary factors" that impair judgment.

The Fraser Ruling (also known as "Gillick competence") confers on children the right to consent to treatment. However cases of enforced treatment of minors subsequent to the ruling have demonstrated flaws in the notion of Gillick competence applied to minors. Gillick competence does not confer upon a child the power of veto over treatment. The judiciary and doctors are uncomfortable with children's rights where this may result in serious harm or death of the child. Courts will force very ill adolescents to undergo life-saving treatments against their will.[5] [6] [7] This is contained in the Family Law Reform Act.[8] It concludes that children over 16 can consent as if they were of full age but preserves the common law powers of parental consent up to age 18. Thus, unlike adults, children may be forced to take account of their own best interests. This remains a contentious area, particularly in light of the Human Rights Act, which may have implications for young person's refusal of treatment.[9] Since enactment (October 2000) this legislation "obligates doctors, in all decision making, to have regard to whether their actions involve a person's human rights, and if so whether those rights can legitimately be interfered with." It seems likely this may be used to challenge enforced treatment of a competent child.

Case Vignette 4
Kate, age 15, presents to the clinic with a request for the emergency pill. She is concerned that a neighbor may have seen her in the waiting room and will tell her mother she was seeing the doctor. She wants the doctor's assurance that her mother will not be told. The doctor explains her right to confidentiality

---

[5] Re R (*a minor*) [1992] 1 FLR 190.
[6] Re W (*a minor*) [1993] 1 FLR 1 and 4 All ER 627.
[7] Re M [1999] 2 FLR 1097.
[8] Family Law Reform Act 1969, Section 1.
[9] Human Rights Act, 1998.

and that this will be respected. The doctor asks when she had unprotected intercourse and also how long she has been sexually active. She has had sex with her boyfriend several times during the past three months. Kate expects and wants the relationship to continue. They usually used a condom but on this occasion they took a risk. Besides prescribing Levonelle the doctor discusses with Kate using more reliable contraception in addition to condoms.

The Fraser guidelines currently state that under-16s can be prescribed contraception provided

- they are competent to understand the advice
- the doctor cannot persuade them to tell their parents or allow the doctor to tell the parents that they are seeking contraceptive advice
- the young person is likely to begin or continue having sex without protection
- that as a result of this, the young person's physical and/or mental health is likely to suffer
- that the young person's best interests require the doctor to give contraceptive advice/treatment without parental consent.

This requires that the doctor discusses with young people the advantages of involving a parent in their sexually related decisions and encourages them to do so. Their response should be documented as this is actually a legal requirement of treatment for those under 16. From a practical point of view the following points are key to effective use of contraceptive pills by young teenagers:

- encourage knowledge of mother
- a visual reminder that they cannot miss a day
- emphasize what to do if pills are forgotten and ask them to repeat this advice back to you before concluding the consultation
- encourage charting for first three cycles
- suggest the option of tricycle or continuous regime to improve efficacy
- explain there is *no need to have breaks*, unless they prefer to
- explain the length of the break and hence pills taken just after any break are critical to avoiding the risk of a pill failure
- emphasize condom use with the pill to protect against STIs

It is important to consider the relative merits of an injectable or implant in those with a chaotic lifestyle or learning disability.

The doctor discussed pill taking with Kate, particularly how she was going to remember it every day. Kate acknowledged this was going to be extremely difficult with the additional pressure of trying to keep the pills and her pill taking a secret at home. The doctor inquired further about Kate's relationship and established it was with a boy of 15 and she was happily consenting to this activity. Kate was particularly afraid of her father finding out as he was a policeman and she thought he might try to prosecute her boyfriend. The doctor asked more about her relationship with her mother. Kate thought her mother would be cross if she found out, but pleased they were trying to be responsible about protection. Kate acknowledged that there might be some advantages in her mother knowing, particularly that her mother reminding her about her pill every day would help. The doctor suggests she could see Kate together with her mother if Kate decides to tell her mother and would like support when doing so.

Unlike analytic philosophers who are trained to work deductively from general principles, doctors are trained to work in the opposite direction, beginning with the case and then seeking the principles that might apply. The doctor used a narrative approach to explore with Kate the hypothetical scenario of confiding in her mother. Sometimes clarifying the situation in this way may change the perspective on the scope of confidentiality to be maintained. From a legal stand point it is crucial that some record is made of this conversation to show that the doctor has fully considered Kate's best interests and made every effort to act in accordance with guidelines.

19.4.   Problems for Adolescents Using Medical Services

Kate's case highlights some of the problems adolescents experience with medical services:

- concern about confidentiality
- ignorance of rights and services available
- concern about who they might see (*or who may see them*)
- fear of what might happen, *especially genital examination*
- fear of disapproval.

To begin to address these doctors must have a strategy for confidentiality:

- How will you obtain a social history from the girl alone?
- How will you talk about STIs and pregnancy risks?
- How will you judge needs for those with learning disability as distinct from those of their carers/family?

19.5.   The Consultation

The definition of adolescence is from the onset of puberty to adulthood. In practice this will mostly include the age range 12-17 years. The two biggest concerns to this group are *confidentiality* and *body image*. Understanding these concerns is crucial if any professional encounter is to engage them successfully.

Where the teenager has come about a general medical problem, they will rarely enter the consultation alone. Inclusion of the mother (usually) necessitates skill and understanding of three way consultations and the pitfalls. Asking questions inappropriately within hearing of an authority figure may significantly compromise the welfare of young people.

Case Vignette 5
Libby, age 14 years 10 months, was referred with abdominal pains. The GP
had taken blood tests and had organized a pelvic ultrasound scan. These were
normal. Her mother requested a private referral to a gynecologist.
Although the gynecologist directed questions to Libby, generally her mother
gave the answers. The consultant then suggested Libby might prefer to be seen
alone, explaining this was usual practice with adolescents. Her mother turned
to Libby and asked if she wanted this. The girl looked uncomfortable and
shrugged her shoulders. The mother made no move to leave, so the consultant
continued taking the history. Libby had been feeling tired and nauseated with
the pain and had noticed increased urinary frequency. Her periods were always
irregular, and she could not remember when she last had one.
Before examining Libby the consultant explained the needed to check Libby's
height and weight and took her to another room to do this. Once alone the
doctor asked about sexual activity, explaining this was in confidence. Libby
said she had been sexually active for 8 months and had gone to the local
family planning clinic a couple of times for Depo-Provera. She thought her last
injection had been about 5 months ago. She was worried the injections were
making her fat so she did not go when the last one was due. She had meant
to ask for something else but had not got round to it. Under no circumstances
did she wish her mother to know she was sexually active.

It is imperative that adolescents are seen in confidence for at least part
of the consultation. There are many ways of facilitating this. For example
saying openly at an opportune moment that it is usual good practice to see
adolescents for part of any consultation on their own and ask the parent to
leave or take the young person to another room. If the examination room is
separate from the consulting room this also affords an opportunity to talk in
private.

The consultant felt increasingly compromised at the situation unfolding. The
most immediate diagnosis that needed consideration was pregnancy. First in
the circumstance that Libby had presented with pain, it was a priority to exclude
ectopic pregnancy. Secondly she needed screening for sexually transmitted
infection, especially chlamydia. However proceeding with a pelvic examination
and relevant investigations would compromise an adolescent who was not
supposed to be sexually active. Her mother had not indicated any willingness
to leave the consulting room. To ask her to do so now would certainly arouse
suspicion. Thirdly her mother was also paying for the consultation. Any bills
arising from testing would go directly from the private hospital to her mother
and would itemize the tests. This precluded doing the most relevant and urgent
tests in the setting in which the referral and consultation had been made.
The consultant acknowledged Libby's wish to keep this information confidential
and suggested that they ask her GP to do the tests. Libby was adamant the GP
should not be informed, saying the GP was also her mother's GP and a family
friend. They lived in a small village where everyone used the local practice,
so she also feared whether someone would see her and tell her mother she

had been there. The consultant then suggested the family planning clinic could ensure complete confidentiality.

They rejoined her mother in the consulting room. The consultant examined Libby's abdomen and then explained to her mother that they needed to exclude a urinary tract infection. While Libby went to pass urine her mother asked the consultant what she thought was wrong and what tests she was going to do. The GP had suggested that a laparoscopy might be necessary. The consultant replied that it was very reassuring that the scan was normal, so a laparoscopy would not really be appropriate at the present time. She explained that often no explanation can be found for abdominal pains and commented how much pressure young people were under with exams and peer expectations.

Libby attended the family planning clinic the following evening. Fortunately her pregnancy test was negative and contraceptive care was resumed.

The three-way consultation is one of the biggest pitfalls in adolescent medicine. The mother showed concern for Libby and wished to be there throughout the consultation. However the dynamics that unfolded led the doctor to feel this was inappropriate. The doctor had to calculate the right action to be taken. GMC guidance on good clinical care outlines duties which includes[10]

- You must make adequate assessment of the patient's condition
- Because the doctor–patient relationship is based on trust you have a special responsibility to make the relationship with your patients work.

Confidentiality is a duty of any doctor–patient relationship. The deontological (or Kantian) approach is concerned with duties and so tends to consider the intentions rather than consequences of actions. The strict Kantian views lie as an act that cannot be universalized as normative conduct and hence the doctor's behavior toward the mother was improper. This theory faces an impossible conflict of obligations between truthfulness and confidentiality, leaving the doctor stuck between a rock and a hard place. In this circumstance the doctor picked the least bad option of not telling the mother the whole truth, in order to respect Libby's request for strict confidentiality.

19.5.1. Probity

Libby had been referred on a private basis, and her mother had attended the consultation and paid for it. This meant there was a contract between the mother and the doctor. The doctor was unsure what duty of care was therefore owed to the mother. In this circumstance the doctor should seek advice from their professional indemnity organization and is not breaching confidence by doing so. The doctor arranged an alternative appointment within the NHS to perform the necessary investigations. There was no intention to abuse the

---

[10] *Good Medical Practice.* General Medical Council, May 2001.

NHS/private system to save the patient money. Libby was entitled to use the NHS, and there was no other means of carrying out necessary investigations while safeguarding confidentiality. In these unusual circumstances this action was morally justified.

19.6.   Obtaining a History from Young People

Young people must never be asked a sexual history while a parent or authority figure is within hearing. It is imperative that they receive reassurance that any disclosure will be kept in strict confidence. Equally any inquiry about smoking or use of recreational drugs must be in confidence. Confidentiality is a duty of any doctor–patient relationship, and this includes a duty to avoid landing the patient in a position from which she has to choose between lying or compromising her own position. Young people will be compromised by inappropriate questions in the presence of those with whom they do not wish to share their personal information. When a parent then directly asks for confidential information (for example asking what is wrong when the girl may be pregnant), the doctor must explain the young person's rights mean they cannot discuss this information. The only exception to this rule is where a doctor has reason to suspect a child is being abused.[11]

Conversely when young people engage services to address a sexual health need, they will most often come alone or with a friend or boyfriend but strictly in secret from family members. Fear of being seen may be a significant deterrent to young people needing to access services.

Case Vignette 6

Victoria, age 14, has come to see you because she suspects she may be pregnant. She requests a termination and is adamant that her parents must not find out. As she goes back to the waiting room you notice she is accompanied by a man who looks at least 30.

19.7.   Child Protection

The relative ages involved raised the specter of sexual abuse, and in this circumstance the doctor's obligation to protect Victoria may override the duty of confidentiality. The doctor is therefore obliged to explore this concern, not because Victoria was having sex at an age not permitted in law, but because the age difference increased the risk her autonomy might be impaired. This impairment could range from frank coercion to persuasion or manipulation by false information. The young person should be questioned to elicit whether sexual activity is

---

[11] Responsibilities of doctors in child protection cases with regard to confidentiality,. 2004. Royal College of Paediatrics and Child Health, also available at www.rcpch.ac.uk/publications/recent_publications/confidentiality.pdf.

voluntary. Young women presenting for emergency contraception often describe having been pressured. Obviously if the partner is present it is important this question is posed when they are not within hearing. A difficult issue emerging for the profession concerns "what is the boundary between acceptable behavior and rape?" In this particular case it was appropriate that the doctor called Victoria back to the consulting room and established that this man was the partner. It was then important to establish what she had told him about her age and to discuss with her the doctor's obligation to contact child protection agencies. Each Trust has a named senior doctor for child protection, and this person would be the first point of contact for the doctor in this case.[12]

19.8. Young Age and Pregnancy

The teenage pregnancy rate in the UK is the highest in Western Europe and one of the highest worldwide (11). There were 42.1 conceptions per 1000 15- to 18-year-old girls and 9.3 conceptions per 1000 13- to 15-year-old girls in 2003. Once a young woman conceives friends and others in her social networks can exert verbal or other pressure on her to terminate or continue the pregnancy (12). Friends who have experienced birth might constitute role models in the eyes of the pregnant young woman (13). The visibility of other young women who are pregnant or parenting and their acceptance, or otherwise within the community, sends out a strong signal about local attitudes to early motherhood. It is not difficult to envisage how a normative environment where friends and neighbors begin childbearing in their teens might help create local cultures of early fertility.

In general society has a negative attitude to teenage pregnancy, and this is understandable when viewed in the context of the risks associated with pregnancy at this age. The infant mortality rate among babies of mothers under 20 years in England and Wales in 2000 was 53% higher than rates for babies born to women of all ages.[13] Teenage mothers must interrupt their education, rely more on state benefits and have fewer employment opportunities, leading to lower income, poorer housing, and poorer health. A high proportion book late, with over 20% booking after 20 weeks.[14] The Confidential Enquiries into Maternal and Child Health (CEMACH) reports have found that late booking and poor attendance are risk factors for maternal death.[15] The majority of under-18s are single mothers and as a group, single mothers are three times

---

[12] What to do if you're worried a child is being abused. Department of Health. London: Department 2003. Avaiable at www.doh.gov.uk.
[13] Infant and perinatal mortality by social and biological factors, 2000. Office of National Statistics. Health Stat Q 2001;12.
[14] Gloucestershire local statistics for 2004/5.
[15] Why Mothers Die 2000–2002: Confidential Enquiries into Maternal Deaths in the United Kingdom. RCOG Press. CEMACH 2004.

more likely to die than those in stable relationships. An important consideration often overlooked is that teenagers who are pregnant are at high risk of partner violence. Smoking rates in pregnant women are an important risk factor for low-birth-weight and are highest among teenagers. National surveys have consistently demonstrated lower breast-feeding rates among teenage mothers, and there is a considerable literature supporting the view that young parents may lack effective parenting skills. The risk of family instability or breakdown is high, leading to a poorer environment for teenage parenting.

Most studies on adolescent pregnancy have focused on the female, with their male partners largely escaping scrutiny; however, it is the male who may have the decisive role in initiating the sexual encounter. Teenage pregnancy prevention programs need to target male behavior and also consider the apparent desire to father a child, which is a factor in some cases (14). Compared to partners of older women, males involved in teenage pregnancy have typically achieved a lower level of education, have higher rates of unemployment with lower socioeconomic status, and have more behavioral problems such as smoking, drinking, and illicit drug use. They also have more simultaneous sexual partners and sexually transmitted infections, engage in more aggressive behavior, and adopt poorer attitudes toward their partner's pregnancy by being less involved in the postpartum care of the mother and infant (15). These negative associations have great potential to aggravate the problems of teenage mothering.

Case Vignette 7

Tracey is a 15-year-old primigravida. She has not attended school for over a year and admits to multiple substance misuse, including alcohol, cannabis, benzodiazepines, amphetamines, ecstasy, and street heroin (anything she can obtain). On three occasions she has been hospitalized for overdoses. Tracey's mother was 16 when she had Tracey, and they have a poor relationship. Her mother also has two younger children (3 and 5 years) from a new relationship. Tracey was taken into care by the local authority following four cautions for shoplifting in the past 2 years. She has repeatedly run away from the children's home and has been living in a squat with several drug addicts. Her pregnancy was diagnosed when she was admitted to hospital with dehydration due to vomiting and diarrhea. She is unsure who the father is and from her evasive responses it seems likely the pregnancy is the result of prostitution to feed her addiction. A scan shows that Tracey is already 19–20 weeks.

Tracey is an extreme example but she presents the whole range of problems that are more common in teenagers who are pregnant. She lives in poverty, she has no family support and no partner, and only a long history of chaotic and dysfunctional family and interpersonal relationships. The only means by which she can address her own physical needs and her addiction is crime. She has no aspirations for her future and trusts no one. Building a relationship with Tracey will be challenging for all professionals with whom she comes into contact.

Tracey expresses negative feelings about her mother. A little probing reveals she feels shunted aside by her mother's "new family." Tracey's risk for early childbearing has been increased by what she admits is looking for "someone to love who will love me." Unfortunately this often equates, in the adolescent psyche, with a baby. She responds affirmatively when asked, "During the past month, have you been bothered by feeling down, depressed, or hopeless?"

Depressed adolescents often engage in high-risk behaviors, such as unprotected sex, binge drinking, dropping out of school, smoking, and become victims of physical or sexual assaults (16). Clinical experience has shown that depression is a frequent pre-existing condition among adolescents who become pregnant. The risks to her child if she continues the pregnancy are enormous. Yet at almost 20 weeks time is extremely short to help her come to an informed choice about the pregnancy. The procedure of termination, even if she did come to this decision in time, would be daunting for an unsupported 15-year old. Unsurprisingly Tracey does not come to any decision and continues her pregnancy by default more than choice.

Standard antenatal care does not address Tracey's complex needs. Her immediate need is for a place of safety, housing, and social support. She needs assessment and treatment for her depression and testing for the whole range of sexually transmitted infections. The result most likely to be positive is chlamydia, but if positive there is a high likelihood she will not comply with a 2-week course of erythromycin. She declines hepatitis and HIV testing as if wanting to deny the reality of her risky lifestyle.

In terms of supporting Tracey, careful thought needs to accompany pre- and post-birth child protection assessments and encourage her participation and understanding of the processes involved. A positive presentation of the importance of assessment with a focus on support for her and the child is crucial. Linked to this is the need for an independent advocate or neutral source of support for all young parents involved in child protection procedures. A midwife trained in substance misuse and child protection procedures can be extremely useful working with young people in Tracey's situation. The pregnancy may occasionally provide a means to motivate a change in behavior and new aspirations for a different future, but also there must be careful recording of factual information to help guide any decisions affecting the prospective child's future.

Half of under 16-year olds and two-thirds of 16- to -19-year olds who conceive continue with their pregnancies, necessitating strategies for the support of teenage parents as well as preventing pregnancy in the first place. The relatively high infant mortality rate among children born to teenage mothers highlights the focus needed in postnatal care:

1. to prevent serious illness, including accidental or non-accidental death to the infant
2. to provide adequate nutrition and child care while mothers are working or in school
3. to monitor the young person's care of their children.

Good antenatal care is associated with improved outcomes amongst teenagers, and this is most likely to be accessed where specially designed programs are targeted at teenagers by midwives and health visitors, working in liaison with other professionals. Accordingly the national teenage pregnancy network was founded in the UK in 2001 (http://www.dfes.gov.uk/teenagepregnancy/dsp_ content.cfm?pageid=240). Its principle aim is to increase support for midwives working specifically with young parents and also to enable midwives to share good practice and innovative work ideas. At a local level establishing a midwife with a special remit for under 18 pregnancies to establish a specific service to address their needs. Examples include an antenatal drop-in session with joint support from health and social care agencies such as Connexions, Sure Start, state benefits, housing, smoking cessation, and a nutritionist. Midwives who have run flexible and friendly sessions have been encouraged by the numbers who attend drop-ins, and at least anecdotal evidence suggests that young pregnant teenagers want this service.

The Social Exclusion Unit (SEU) report on Teenage Pregnancy published in June 1999 set out a 10-year national strategy to halve the rate of conceptions among under-18s by 2010 and to increase the participation of teenage parents in education and work to reduce their risk of long-term social exclusion.[16] The 2003 data shows that under-18 conception rates have fallen by 9.8% since the strategy began, but this is nowhere near the rate needed to meet a target of halving under-18 conceptions by 2010 (http://www.dfes.gov.uk/teenagepregnancy/dsp_showDoc.cfm?FileName= Government% 20 Response% 2Epdf).

An important consideration for after the pregnancy is that Tracey is unlikely to effectively use birth control unless her mental health and dysfunctional relationship issues respond dramatically to therapy. Her motivation to avoid a pregnancy is questionable, which reduces her chances of remembering to take a pill every day or to change a patch every week. She might be persuaded to accept the Depo-Provera (DMPA) injection every 12 weeks, but a more long-term method such as Implanon will probably serve her needs best.

19.9.   Examining Young People

Adolescence is equated with feeling intensely self-conscious about body changes. In contradiction to increasing social acceptance of nudity and sexual behavior, young people need considerable sensitivity to their body fears and their need to be covered up. It is therefore imperative to use a drape sensitively during any examination to minimize vulnerability. So, if for example Tanner staging is necessary, only uncover one part at a time, having carefully explained what you are looking for and let him or her know your findings.

---

[16] *Teenage Pregnancy*. Report by the Social Exclusion Unit, June 1999. The Stationary Office.

Body fears are common among young people and it is very important to know he or she is like other people and not abnormal. Thus the findings must be carefully explained within the context of sensitive inquiry into what concerns the young person has. The appropriateness or otherwise of a pelvic examination requires careful consideration. In general a pelvic examination is contraindicated if the girl has not yet been sexually active. It is indicated for those who are sexually active with discharge, pelvic pain, or intermenstrual bleeding in order to assess for any infection, pelvic mass or tenderness. For other problems, especially amenorrhea or dysmenorrhea, better information will be obtained from a pelvic ultrasound scan. The transvaginal route may not be appropriate in those who have never been sexually active, although the author has found that with careful explanation and sensitivity this route may be acceptable to girls who are tampon users.

General rules to observe when conducting any examination are the following

- discuss what you want to do and why
- do not do anything that he/she is unhappy with
- give her any instrument you wish to use and explain it
- communicate the findings, assuming complete ignorance of anatomy
- ensure a chaperon and a locked door
- do not encourage mother's presence
- remember teenagers need to be covered up.

Unfortunately a small but significant number of women feel they have been "abused" by a doctor conducting a pelvic examination. Often the context was an adolescent examination.

Case Vignette 8 – A Deep Dark Secret

The referral letter for Joanne, age 39, stated she would need an anesthetic in order to have a smear test. The GP had been unable to examine her and Joanne explained it was just not possible for her. The gynecologist wondered if she actually needed screening at all but also wondered whether sexual assault or abuse might underlie the problem with examination. She explored this by explaining "only women who have had a sexual experience, either consensual or due to abuse, need screening. I am therefore wondering if you do need screening?" Joanne started to cry, and the doctor acknowledged that this was something very upsetting for her. Joanne replied that when she was 17 she had been referred to a gynecologist because of period pains. He seemed very dismissive, saying that it was "just something she would grow out of, especially when she started having babies." She was taken to a cubicle by a nurse and told to undress. She was very embarrassed, especially when the doctor entered the cubicle and announced loudly that she was supposed to take her pants off as well. He told her to bend her knees up and proceeded to insert his fingers into her vagina. She cried out in pain and was told "relax, this will only take a moment." She was so traumatized that she could not remember the rest of the consultation but only that she went home and washed many times. She did not go for her follow up, and when her GP asked why she told him her periods were OK now. She was so embarrassed that she told no one and suffered her periods rather than seek further help. When she started being called for smears she always ignored the letters. Then in her early 30s she had a relationship but every attempt at intercourse failed so the relationship ended. The man had told her that his previous partner had suffered with genital warts and her GP had said that the attempts at a relationship meant she should have screening. The consultant acknowledged how poor her initial experience of gynecology services had been, and she could now better understand why she had been unable to tolerate a pelvic examination. She remarked that "hopefully doctors are better trained now." She suggested to Joanne that it might be helpful to have a look at her on a couch but stressed that she would be in complete control. Joanne was given privacy to undress and encouraged to cover herself with the drape. The consultant asked her understanding of her genital anatomy. She was not a tampon user and assumed that she must be abnormal and too small since it had hurt so much when the first gynecologist examined her and when she had tried to have intercourse. The consultant used this opportunity to explain how vaginal muscles control the size of the vagina and sometimes can close off the vagina, making penetration impossible. Attempts to do so would be extremely painful and might even cause tearing. She encouraged Joanne then to squeeze her pelvic floor as tightly as possible. When she relaxed she suggested Joanne might try to insert her own finger. Joanne was not keen to try this, so the consultant placed her own finger at the vaginal entrance and noted immediately the pelvic muscles contracted much more powerfully than before. She pointed this out to Joanne and explained that there was every likelihood she could overcome this difficulty if she wanted to. She explained that self-examination and use of a finger or a dilator is a very good starting point. They agreed there was no urgency to do a smear.

19.10. Body Image

Physical appearance is more essential to self-esteem, social, and emotional development at adolescence than at any other time. Any part of the body may be perceived as unattractive, however, dissatisfaction with the breasts and genitalia are particularly common in adolescents. At puberty there is wide variation in breast development and dissatisfaction most often centers on size being perceived as too big or too small. Occasionally asymmetry in breast size may occur and cause distress. In boys gynecomastia may cause distress.

The extent of growth and eventual size of the labia minora in pubertal girls also varies widely. Large labia or asymmetric enlargement often causes enormous distress to adolescent girls, which is not helped by explaining range of normality. In the author's experience this distress now results in referral seeking surgical reduction much more than in the past, and possibly this is influenced by a perception that the genitalia are much more visible than in the past with thong and other clothing fashion. There is almost nothing in the literature on management of requests for labial reduction and very little on the outcome of this type of surgery to the labia. Enlargement can be unilateral or bilateral. The girl typically complains of discomfort and difficulties with personal hygiene, especially during menstruation. The most profound symptom, however, is psychological distress. Reassurance that their anatomy is normal and that larger size is entirely physiological is useless in addressing what may amount to profound psychological distress.

These are not simply young women looking for "designer vaginas," although it is not uncommon that they verbalize feeling severely inhibited from entering any sexual relationship owing to the perceived unsightly appearance of their genitalia. The author had one case where the girl's mother burst into tears when she eventually came to surgery, saying that her daughter had verbalized serious suicide intent if she could not get this procedure. While it is clear that reassurance is useless, high satisfaction rates have been reported for surgery (17). If surgery is undertaken then there is very little data to help determine for which cases it is appropriate and at what earliest age or stage of development it should be undertaken. Also to what extent should psychological assessment be undertaken and by whom?

Rouzier et al. define labia as large or hypertrophic when the maximum distance between the base and the edge is at least 4 cm. They advise against surgery when the size is smaller than this. They report a flap technique, while others report a technique that amounts to trimming the edge using a laser (18). A disadvantage of any trimming technique is the potential to create disproportion between the size of the clitoris and the labia. This is avoided by the flap technique. For both procedures very high rates of satisfaction in excess of 90% are reported. The high degree of overall satisfaction supports the use of this procedure, which is often not reflected by gynecologists who may respond very negatively to such requests. This may reflect the fact that gynecologists are unused to patients seeking cosmetic surgery compared with their contemporaries in breast and plastic surgery.

19.11. Vaginal Problems

When young women report difficulty using tampons or establishing vaginal penetration, it is important to exclude anatomical reasons. In the author's experience anatomical variants causing partial obstruction are sufficiently common when this is the presenting complaint that it is never appropriate to consider it a symptom of a psychological difficulty without first performing an examination. The need or otherwise for doing this under anesthesia will depend how confident and comfortable the girl is with her body.

Case Vignette 9

Rachel, age 13, was a competitive swimmer. She was referred because she wished to use tampons but was experiencing difficulty. The GP had examined her but could not see anything wrong. Rachel explained she could get a tampon in but whenever she tried to remove it, it would catch on something causing severe pain. Rachel was relaxed about her body and very confident. She said it would not be a problem if the doctor wanted to look. With gentle down and outward traction on the labia it was possible to see quite a thick fimbriated (ruffled edge) hymen. Only when a swab was passed through the hymen orifice and used to expose the edge of the hymen did it reveal a septum bridging the orifice with a separate opening posteriorly. Rachel was happy for the bridge of skin to be divided with local anesthetic in the clinic, and this resolved her problem.

Rachel was unusual in her confidence and comfort with a procedure many teenage girls would find unacceptable without sedation or anesthesia, perhaps reflecting her successful relationships with peers and in school. She also had a very supportive and understanding relationship with her mother, who helpfully suggested Rachel was mature enough to be seen on her own at the outset. For many young teenagers examination to see the hymen adequately is difficult and examination to exclude a vaginal septum may be impossible. In the circumstance that they have presented with either inability to use tampons or achieve consensual penetration a low threshold for examination under anesthesia is appropriate. This will reveal an anatomical reason, such as a hymen variant causing partial occlusion, in a significant number. Where no abnormality is found, reassurance about the normality of their anatomy is an important aspect of therapy.

Establishing the genital anatomy is particularly a problem for doctors who are asked to examine young people and collect forensic evidence following alleged sexual assault. Where the girl has never previously been sexually active, and especially when she has also not used tampons, obtaining the forensic swabs and adequate visualization of the anatomy is extremely difficult even for the experienced examiner. The Foley catheter technique is generally the best method for visualizing the margins of the estrogenized adolescent hymen for transections or acute bleeding trauma (19,20). Clothing containing secretions is often the most important source of DNA, especially when the girl cannot tolerate the smallest size speculum for taking vaginal swabs. This type of forensic examination in the first 72 h after the event, particularly if before bathing or washing relevant items of clothing, will often prove that there was sexual contact with an alleged assailant. However a medical examination cannot determine consent. Doctors are often pressured to say that injuries indicate lack of consent or that the absence of injury is not compatible with rape but have a duty to clarify the limitations. Rape is a legal concept *not* a medical diagnosis.

19.12. Skin Problems

Adolescence may be characterized to a greater or lesser extent by

- physiologic hyperandrogenism, with a predisposition to acne
- insulin resistance
- acquisition of body fat
- variable anovulation, with a bleeding pattern varying from none to total chaos
- hyperestrogenism
- polycystic ovarian morphology on scan.

For the majority who suffer physical sequelae, the symptoms are transient tending to normalize within 4–6 years of puberty. Those young women who do not resolve spontaneously may be the group for whom a diagnosis of polycystic ovary syndrome is more appropriate. Unfortunately the overlap between diagnostic criteria for PCOS and the common physiologic changes that accompany adolescence leave considerable scope for over diagnosis of a syndrome commonly, but often mistakenly, associated with infertility. This may be an immense source of psychological distress to a teenager.

19.13. Eating Problems

Obesity is the most common chronic disorder in industrialized societies, now considered to have reached epidemic proportions (21), and therefore an issue of public health and political concern (22,23). Apart from the wide range of long-term medical problems associated with obesity, which include cardio-vascular disease, hypertension, dyslipidemia, and insulin resistance leading to type 2 diabetes, there is considerable evidence that obesity increases the risk of social and emotional problems. The psychological consequences are perhaps the most profound to young people themselves and include low self-esteem and social isolation.

The term "Obese" is a rather offensive word which may add to the distress felt by young people struggling with a weight problem. Being overweight is stigmatized, and there is evidence that particularly for teenage girls (more than boys) obesity is related to lowered self-esteem (24). This is not surprising given the pressure on girls to engage with cultural norms of thinness. Adolescents are greatly concerned about appearance norms and large numbers of them attempt to achieve a culturally ideal figure through dieting (25). Thus dieting to lose weight may be a means to gain positive appraisal from others. Yet this attempt to fit norms of appearance can be highly stressful, maybe even more so than having a stigmatized characteristic in the first place. Adolescents with higher BMI are more likely to report poor health (26).

The physical health consequences of being overweight are significant because perceived poor health is correlated strongly with depression (27,28).

Those who feel worse physically are likely feel worse emotionally too. Those at the extreme, with a BMI above the 99.6th percentile, can be referred to a pediatric endocrine clinic. This leaves a considerable number of seriously overweight young people without specialist help, as currently 17% of 15 year olds are obese. Unfortunately experience with specialist obesity clinics for children and adolescents is that it requires huge resources and most of those treated will not lose weight. Most will not stay in treatment (29). The gynecological consequences of obesity are many and include menstrual irregularity, subfertility, and insulin resistance with skin problems due to excess free androgen.

Case Vignette 10

Joanne, age 15, was referred with secondary amenorrhea. Her periods had started when she was 10 and had never been regular. She weighed 125 kg and her blood pressure was 140/90. Joanne came with her mother who was also morbidly obese and stated that it was "a family problem due to polycystic ovaries making them obese."

Joanne was seen alone and confirmed she was not sexually active. Her greatest source of distress was the growth of facial hair and a receding temporal hair line.

Her hormone profile showed normal follicle-stimulating hormone and testosterone levels and an elevated level of luteinizing hormone with low sex hormone binding globulin. The doctor explained this was typical for polycystic ovary syndrome, but also irregular periods were much more common during adolescence than after teenage years. Joanne reluctantly agreed to have a glucose tolerance test which was arranged with the specialist nurse in pediatrics. It was clear that Joanne and her mother would need considerably more time for discussion than was available at a routine clinic appointment. The doctor explained that diet and exercise were key to management of her problem, but at the same time acknowledged this was probably not what she and her mother were hoping to hear. Joanne was prescribed a course of progesterone to induce a bleed and Vaniqua cream to help with her facial hair. It was carefully explained that it would be several months before she would see any improvement in hair growth. She was given an information leaflet about PCOS and diet, and contact information for a support group.

The doctor arranged a double appointment for her follow up. The glucose tolerance test gave a normal result. Joanne had not lost any weight. The doctor acknowledged how difficult it was to change eating patterns but stressed that diet and exercise really were the only solution if Joanne wanted to reduce her longer-term health risks. Joanne was tearful and avoided eye contact with the doctor. Her mother became angry asking why it was doctors blamed overweight people instead of helping with their medical problems. The doctor felt very uncomfortable. She replied that she was not explaining the medical consequences of obesity because she enjoyed doing so, but her discomfort with this did not remove the duty of care to provide clear health information to Joanne. She also explained that helping others is a two-way process that requires effort and motivation from the patient, since no one else could adopt a healthy lifestyle *on her behalf. Most importantly she was attempting to address Joanne's long-term well-being since only lifestyle changes would improve her risks for heart disease, diabetes, and any reproductive consequences of her weight.*

The second appointment left the doctor feeling frustrated and unhappy that Joanne had been rather excluded from the conversation, so she seemed to be addressing the mother's issues instead finding out Joanne's. A few days later she received a letter from the mother stating that they were now seeking laser treatment for Joanne's hair and would not be coming for any further appointments.

19.14.   Conclusion

Young people are disadvantaged in their access to medical care and the services they receive. This is due in part to widespread ignorance of their rights. The spectrum of parental concern spans a range from frank neglect, through appropriate concern about risky behavior, to over concern that stifles the processes by which a child becomes a person in their own right. This is a complex area of health because under-16s do not have absolute rights as determined in statute law for adults. Their rights in common law are dependent on their ability for self-determination. Health professionals generally admit they feel inadequately trained and uncomfortable in their dealings with adolescent patients, particularly about initiating discussion of sexuality and recognizing and managing adolescent distress. A range of psychological and behavioral problems may present challenges. The seriousness of the psychosocial problem may at times be insoluble for the health professional.

Risk taking is an important part of adolescent development. Risky behavior may attract considerable morbidity for sexual and reproductive health. There is scope for opportunistic care. When opportunities arise health-care providers should discuss sexual health with adolescent males and females directly. Remember the overriding need for confidentiality and establish how you can safely contact them with any test result and record this clearly in the notes. The two biggest concerns to young people are confidentiality and body image. Understanding these concerns is crucial if any professional encounter is to engage them successfully. The inclusion of a parent "the three-way consultation" is one of the biggest pitfalls in adolescent medicine. It is imperative that adolescents are seen in confidence for at least part of any consultation, and doctors should have a strategy to facilitate this. Asking questions inappropriately within hearing of an authority figure may significantly compromise a young person.

Unplanned adolescent pregnancies are a particular focus of attention, which rather than being seen as a teenage problem might more accurately be seen as failure of society to accept adolescents as sexual beings and to meet their reproductive rights (30). Adolescent mothers and their children are at risk for many health problems and need readily accessible and nonjudgmental health care.

Reference

1. Martin KA. *Puberty, Sexuality, and the Self: Boys and Girls at Adolescence.* New York: Routledge; 1996.
2. DiClemente RJ, Wingood GM, Crosby R, Cobb BK, Harrington K, Davies SL. Parent-adolescent communication and sexual risk behaviors among African American adolescent females. *J Pediatr.* 2001;139:407–12.
3. Parera N, Suris JC. Having a good relationship with their mother: a protective factor against sexual risk behavior among adolescent females? *J Pediatr Adolesc Gynecol.* 2004;12:267.
4. Whitaker DJ, Miller KS. Parent–adolescent discussions about sex and condoms: impact on peer influences of sexual risk behavior. *J Adolesc Res.* 2000;15:251.
5. DiIorio C, Kelley M, Hockenberry-Eaton M. Communication about sexual issues: mothers, fathers, and friends. *J Adolesc Health.* 1999;24:181.
6. Dittus PJ, Jaccard J. Adolescents' perceptions of maternal disapproval of sex: relationship to sexual outcomes. *J Adolesc Health.* 2000;26:268.
7. Miller BC. Family influences on adolescent sexual and contraceptive behavior. *J Sex Res.* 2002;39:22.
8. Dickson N, Paul C, Herbison P, Silva P. First sexual intercourse: age, coercion and later regrets reported by a birth cohort. *BMJ.* 1998;316: 29–33.
9. Quinn KM. Competence to have an abortion: adolescent issues. *Newslet Am Acad Psychiatry Law.* 1991;16:19.
10. Weithorn LA, Campbell SB. The competency of children and adolescents to make informed treatment decisions. *Child Dev.* 1982;53:1589–1598.
11. United Nations Children's Fund (UNICEF). A league table of teenage births in rich nations. *Innocenti Report Card No. 3*, Florence, Italy; 2001.
12. Tabberer S, Hall C, Prendergast S, Webster A. Teenage Pregnancy and Choice. *Abortion or Motherhood: Influences on the Decision.* York: Joseph Rowntree Foundation, YPS Publishing Services; 2000.
13. Whitehead E. Teenage pregnancy: on the road to social death. *Int J Nursing Studies.* 2001;38:437–446.
14. Crosby RA, DiClemente RJ, Wingood GM, Sionean C, Cobb BK, Harrington K, Davies S, Hook EW 3rd, Oh MK. Correlates of adolescent females' worry about undesired pregnancy. The importance of partner desire for pregnancy. *J Pediatr Adolesc Gynecol.* 2001;14:123–7.
15. Tan LH, Quinlivan JA. Domestic violence, single parenthood, and fathers in the setting of teenage pregnancy. *J Adolesc Health.* 2006;38:201–207.
16. Rickert VI, Weimann CM, Berenson AB. Ethnic differences in depressive symptomatology among young women. *Obstet Gynecol.* 2000;95:55.
17. Rouzier R, Louis-Sylvestre C, Paniel LJ, Haddad B. Hypertrophy of labia minora: experience with 163 reductions. *Am J Obstet Gynecol.* 2000;162:35–40.
18. Pardo J, Sola V, Ricci P, Guilloff E. Laser labioplasty of labia minora. *Int J Gynaecol Obstet.* 2006; 93:38–43.
19. Ferrell J. Foley catheter balloon technique for visualising the hymen in female adolescent sexual abuse victims. *J Emerg Nurs.* 1995;21: 585–586.
20. Jones JS, Dunnuck C, Rossman L, Wynn BN, Genco M. Adolescent Foley catheter technique for visualizing hymenal injuries in adolescent sexual assault. *Acad Emerg Med.* 2003;10:1001–1004.
21. Ebbeling CB, Pawlak DB, Ludwig DS. Childhood obesity: public health crisis, common sense cure. *Lancet.* 2002;360:473–482.

22. National Audit Office. *Tackling Obesity in England*. London: The Stationery Office; 2001.
23. Royal College of Physicians. Storing up problems: the medical case for a slimmer nation. London: Royal College of Physicians; 2004.
24. Strauss R. Childhood obesity and self-esteem. *Pediatrics*. 2000;105(1)15–20.
25. Emmons L. The relationship of dieting to weight in adolescents. *Adolescence*. 1996;31(11):167–178.
26. Vingilis ER, Wade TJ, Seeley JS. Predictors of adolescent self-rated health. Analysis of the National Population Health Survey. *Can J Public Health*. 2002;93:193–197.
27. Ross CE. Overweight and depression. *J Health Soc Behav*. 1994;35(1):63–79.
28. Needham BL, Crosnoe R. Overweight status and depressive symptoms during adolescence. *J Adolesc Health*. 2005;36:48–55.
29. Green S. Obesity in the young. *RCPCH 9th Spring Meeting*. University of York; April 2005.
30. Senanayake P, Faulkner KM. Unplanned teenage pregnancy. *Best Pract ResObstet Gynaecol*. 2003;17:117–129.

20
Unwanted Pregnancy

Audrey H. Brown

20.1. Background

Worldwide, every day, there are over 100 million acts of sexual intercourse, resulting in over 900,000 pregnancies. It is estimated that about 50% of these pregnancies are unplanned and about 25% actually unwanted. As a result, 150,000 pregnancies are terminated by induced abortion every day, that is, over 50 million abortions worldwide every year. The World Health Organization estimates that at least one-third of these abortions are carried out in unsafe conditions.

In the UK (excluding Northern Ireland), induced abortion is carried out under the Abortion Act 1967, whereby two registered medical practitioners (one in the case of an emergency) agree that abortion may be carried out under one of seven clauses (see box below). Annually, over 185,000 abortions are carried out in England and Wales, with a further 12,600 in Scotland (1,2). The vast majority (95%) of these terminations are carried out under Clause 3 of the Abortion Act, where continuation of the pregnancy would involve greater risk to the physical or mental health of the pregnant woman than termination of the pregnancy. A smaller number of terminations (3%) are carried out because of concerns regarding well-being of existing children. Clauses 3 and 4 carry an upper gestational limit of 24 weeks.

The Abortion Act 1967

The Abortion Act 1967 came into effect on 27 April 1968 and permits termination of pregnancy subject to certain conditions. Regulations under the Act mean that abortions must be performed by a registered practitioner in a National Health Service hospital or in a location that has been specially approved by the Department of Health.

An abortion may be approved providing two doctors agree in good faith that one or more of the following criteria apply:

1. the continuance of the pregnancy would involve risk to the life of the pregnant woman greater than if the pregnancy were terminated;

---

2. the termination is necessary to prevent grave permanent injury to the physical or mental health of the pregnant woman;
3. the continuance of the pregnancy would involve risk, greater than if the pregnancy were terminated, of injury to the physical or mental health of the pregnant woman;
4. the continuance of the pregnancy would involve risk, greater than if the pregnancy were terminated, of injury to the physical or mental health of any existing child(ren) of the family of the pregnant woman;
5. there is a substantial risk that if the child were born it would suffer from such physical or mental abnormalities as to be seriously handicapped; or in an emergency, certified by the operating practitioner, as immediately necessary;
6. to save the life of the pregnant woman; or
7. to prevent grave permanent injury to the physical or mental health of the pregnant woman.

In relation to grounds 3 and 4 the doctor may take account of the pregnant woman's *actual or reasonably foreseeable* environment, including her social and economic circumstances.

Women of all reproductive ages undergo termination, with the peak rates in the 18 to 19 and 20 to 24-year-old age groups (31.0 abortions per 1000). The majority are unmarried (77%), although around one-third of these women are with a partner. Almost half of the women have previously had a child (47%), and one-third have had at least one previous termination. Most terminations are carried out in the first trimester of pregnancy, with 87% performed before 13 weeks and 60% before 9 weeks. Abortion forms a large part of the gynecology workload in the UK, and termination of pregnancy is one of the most common gynecological procedures. Although clinicians may have differing degrees of involvement in abortion services, they will all come into contact with women who are currently accessing abortion, have done so in the past, or indeed will do so in the future, and as such require appropriate skills and knowledge to best meet their needs.

20.2. Attitudes to Abortion

20.2.1. Public Opinion

Women seeking abortion often express shame and embarrassment about their situation and feel unable to tell others about their decision, fearing disapproval. However, recent public opinion polls have shown that most people support the right to abortion. A MORI poll carried out in 2001 showed that 65% of those surveyed agreed that if a woman wants an abortion, she should not have to continue with her pregnancy. This survey also confirmed majority approval for right to abortion in a variety of situations, ranging from carrying a pregnancy with severe abnormalities to simply not wishing to have a child (Table 20.1).

More recently, a broadsheet Sunday newspaper commissioned a MORI poll, one item of which asked about gestational time limits for abortion. In this poll, 42% of 1790 adults surveyed thought that abortion time limits should be decreased, 33% thought the current limit is about right, 10% thought abortion is always wrong, 10% did not know, and a smaller number, 4%, thought limits should be increased. This poll did not assess to which time limit people thought abortion should be limited and did not discuss abortion in the context of different situations. For example, some people may support late abortion in a woman who has been raped, but not in someone who changes her mind about pregnancy because she decides to go traveling. The poll was reported under a front-page headline "Women demand tougher laws to curb abortions," when in reality, people answered a question about one aspect of abortion and were not "demanding" anything.

20.2.2. Medical Opinion

Women seeking abortion require the agreement of two doctors before the abortion can proceed, and as most NHS abortion services require external rather than self-referral, women commonly rely on the support of their general practitioner. In a postal survey, 82% of a random sample of British general practitioners described themselves as "broadly prochoice" and 18% as "broadly antiabortion" (3). The British Medical Association guidance "The Law and Ethics of Abortion" advises that "Doctors with a conscientious objection to abortion should make their views known to patients seeking termination of pregnancy and should ensure that the treatment or advice they provide is not affected by their personal views." In this survey, 27% of antiabortion doctors did not agree with this sentiment. Interestingly, of antiabortion doctors, 21% supported women having the right to choose abortion, and around one-third supported the 1967 Abortion Act. General practitioners also showed support for less medical control in the decision-making process, with almost half

TABLE 20.1. Do you approve or disapprove of abortion under the following circumstances?

	Approve (%)	Disapprove (%)	Do not know (%)
Where the woman is under-16	65	20	15
Where there is evidence that the child would be born with serious learning difficulties that used to be known as "mental handicap"	64	21	15
Where there is evidence that the child would be born with serious physical disabilities	70	15	15
Where a woman does not wish to have a child	50	34	16

Source: MORI/bpas

supporting a woman to make her own decision in the first trimester and a further third supporting the woman to make the decision in conjunction with doctor(s). Around a fifth supported continuing the doctor only to have control of the decision. A survey of middle-grade trainee gynecologists carried out in the UK in 1999 showed that around one-third had conscientious objection to abortion, resulting in 28% being unwilling to perform abortion in the first trimester and 38% in the second trimester. Some were willing to be involved in other aspects of care, with four out of five being willing to consent the patient and five out of six willing to clerk the patient. A total of 16% of trainees did not believe abortion should be available on the NHS and 29% did not see abortion to be part of their job. At the British Medical Association annual conference in 2005, 77% of delegates rejected a proposal to reduce the gestational time limit for abortion to below 24 weeks, suggesting that senior medical staff see a need for the small number of women to continue to access late termination.

20.3. Unplanned, Unscheduled, or Unwanted Pregnancy?

For previous generations of women, the situation in which pregnancy occurred dictated society's view of the pregnancy. Pregnancy occurring within marriage was assumed to be accepted and wanted, whereas that occurring in the unmarried woman was unplanned and unacceptable. Today, many unmarried women will have a planned pregnancy, and likewise some married couples will desire no children. With the advent of widely available contraceptive methods, women and couples now have the ability to choose to avoid pregnancy, and the Abortion Act has allowed the opportunity to decide not to proceed with a pregnancy which does occur.

Of course, unplanned and unwanted and planned and wanted may not be synonymous terms. A woman may have an entirely unplanned pregnancy, as a result of contraceptive failure, but be thrilled to find herself pregnant and eagerly embrace motherhood. In contrast, another woman may plan to become pregnant, but shortly after conceiving be offered a fantastic job opportunity overseas and no longer desire a pregnancy. In addition, a woman with a much-wanted pregnancy may feel it necessary to seek abortion, for example, upon breakdown of the relationship or on discovery of fetal abnormality. Work carried out in the 1980s (4) showed that of women who had not intended to become pregnant, 37% were pleased when they found out they were, 47% would rather have become pregnant later, and only 15% were sorry it happened at all. Surprisingly, 14% of couples who had intended to become pregnant had been using some form of contraception around the time of conception. Recent work by Barrett (5) looked at the development and psychometric testing of a contemporary measure of unplanned pregnancy and highlighted six key areas in determining the measure of unplanned pregnancy: expressed intentions, desire for motherhood, contraceptive use, preconceptual preparation, personal circumstances/timing, and partner influences. Applying a blanket term of unwanted pregnancy to women seeking abortion may be too simplistic and can have the effect of "closing the door" or not permitting discussion of aspects of their psyche which wanted or hoped for the pregnancy.

20.3.1.   Psychological Impact of Unintended Pregnancy

Measuring unintended pregnancy is a complex process as outlined above, and assessing the effect on psychological health can be fraught with problems. Psychological well-being, social stability, and partner or family support preconception are all likely to influence the decision to abort or to continue the pregnancy. Recall of pregnancy intendedness may alter by the time delivery takes place, and indeed some women may feel ashamed to acknowledge that the pregnancy was unintended. Those women with unsupportive partners or with partners who reject or deny the pregnancy are more likely to have poor psychological well-being (6). Lack of a positive attitude toward the pregnancy in the partner has been shown to increase maternal perception of pregnancy unwantedness twofold. Depressed mood during pregnancy is a predictor of postnatal depression. A large US study (7) measured intendedness of pregnancy at the time of antenatal booking and assessed psychosocial stressors and depression scores during the pregnancy. Those women with unwanted pregnancies showed higher exposure to stressors, higher depression scores, low partner support, and higher rates of life dissatisfaction (Table 20.2). During antenatal care, it is important that obstetricians and midwives are aware of these factors and can sensitively enquire about intendedness at the time of booking. Women at higher risk of psychosocial sequelae can then be identified and supported through the pregnancy. In addition, children born as a result of an unwanted pregnancy are at higher risk of both physical and psychological problems in the early years, than children who are wanted.

20.3.2.   Psychological Impact of Abortion

Early studies on the impact of abortion compared outcomes with women delivering term pregnancies. As psychological well-being, emotional and social support, and coping mechanisms are likely to have been instrumental in

TABLE 20.2. Intendedness of pregnancy by psychosocial variables

	Intended pregnancy (%)	Unwanted pregnancy (%)
Respondents reporting high exposure to stressors	43.7	56
Respondents with high CES-depression scores	5.4	20.7
Respondents reporting low support from father	42.3	77.2
Respondents not at all satisfied with life	2.4	18.4

Adapted from Orr (7)

informing the woman's decision on how to proceed with the pregnancy, such studies are likely to have major confounding variables. A large study carried out in the UK in the first decade after the Abortion Act compared incidence of major psychiatric sequelae in women undergoing abortion and in women delivering after denial of abortion. The incidence of psychosis was 0.3/1000 in postabortion women and 1.7/1000 in postpartum women (8).

Several groups have looked at pregnancy outcomes in the National Longitudinal Survey of Youth. One analysis compared risk of depression scores for women who had opted to abort their first pregnancy to women who had continued to term an unintended pregnancy. The authors concluded that married women who aborted their pregnancies had higher depression scores than those who continued their pregnancies. No such effect was seen for unmarried women. A subsequent reanalysis of the same data set, with appropriate coding and sampling corrections, failed to find any association between depression and abortion (9). Another study has assessed depression scores before and at time points after abortion and consistently found lower scores postabortion. Several workers have identified preabortion mental health problems as one of the strongest predictors of postabortion problems. Around 17% of women report feeling guilty after abortion, although the majority do not regret their decision. There are a number of reports, particularly from antiabortion pressure groups of "postabortion trauma syndrome". One reputable study employed an evaluated tool, used to assess posttraumatic stress disorder (PTSD) in Vietnam veterans, on postabortion women; 1% of these women showed evidence of PTSD, which is substantially lower than the incidence of PTSD in the general female population. In 1990, the American Psychological Association convened an expert panel to review the published evidence on the psychological impact of abortion. This panel did not find evidence of lasting psychological harm and concluded that abortion is generally "psychologically benign" for most women (10).

A recent Scottish study assessed psychological effects of medical and surgical abortion at 10–13 weeks gestation. Anxiety levels were assessed by visual analog scale before and after termination, and emotional distress was assessed with the hospital anxiety and depression scale. Anxiety levels were higher preabortion in the group randomized to surgical termination but lower in the same group postabortion. There was no difference in the hospital anxiety and depression scale, and the authors concluded that medical abortion does not increase psychological morbidity and should be offered as a choice to all women.

20.4. Identifying Those at Risk of Psychological Sequelae

Although major psychological problems and rates of depression after abortion have not been shown to be higher than the background population risk, there are groups of women who may be at higher risk of coping problems and distress following abortion. The preabortion counseling process can help to identify these women and ensure that appropriate preabortion and postabortion support is offered. As mentioned above, a history of mental health problems is a stronger indicator of risk after abortion. Inevitably, this history may be one of the key factors leading the woman toward the abortion decision. Low self-esteem may also contribute, first by increasing the likelihood of abortion, as the woman will feel less able to cope with the pregnancy and upbringing of a child, but secondly by throwing doubt on her belief about how she will cope with the abortion. Women who are younger, who are unmarried, and who are from a cultural or religious group not believing in abortion are more likely to be isolated and without a significant other in whom to confide. Those undergoing second trimester termination are more likely to experience psychological problems after the termination, as are those who undergo abortion of an initially planned pregnancy. Those women who have had difficulty in making the decision to abort and those who have a negative attitude toward abortion may struggle to cope afterward. Women who have not been free to make their own decision will be vulnerable following the abortion. This control may have been lost due to pressure to abort from family members or a partner or indeed to economic pressures, where a woman has no prospect of being able to support a child. Lastly, women who blame themselves for becoming pregnant and having the abortion may not be able to cope with the decision afterward: identifying what went wrong and agreeing a strategy with the woman to prevent a further unplanned pregnancy can help to give her a structure on which to move forward.

20.5.   Understanding Those Presenting for Repeat Abortion

Around one-third of abortions carried out in the UK are on women who have already had at least one previous abortion. Practitioners can feel frustrated, disappointed, and even angry when a women presents for repeat abortion, especially when they have spent time with the woman at the last visit making a contraceptive plan. Women of course may also feel the same frustrations and disappointment to be in the situation again. Women who undergo repeat abortion are more likely to be older, to already have children, to have relationship issues, and perhaps surprisingly report higher use of contraception than women presenting for a first abortion. Previous studies have not indicated that women who have repeated abortions view it as a method of birth control, contrary to reports in the lay press. A recently reported Canadian study (11) collected information from over 1000 women undergoing abortion and found that women having repeat abortion reported a higher incidence of physical abuse by a male partner and of sexual abuse or sexual violence: those undergoing a third or subsequent abortion were over 2.5 times more likely to report such experience than those undergoing a first abortion. The negative psychological impact of living with such events may affect a woman's ability to prevent a pregnancy and of her likelihood of coping with a pregnancy. Gentle enquiry around such issues may allow a distressed woman to confide her problems and begin working toward a coping mechanism or even an exit strategy.

20.6.   The Unplanned Pregnancy Consultation

Managing a consultation with a woman with an unplanned pregnancy can be a stressful experience for staff. We feel the need to give the woman the time, space, and support to fully consider her options and reach the best decision; but at the same time we have an obligation to convey medical information, explain risks, and describe the procedures. We may also require to scan the patient, book dates for the procedure, obtain consent, and prescribe medication. Combined with a patient who may be upset, defensive, or unable to reach a decision, we may feel somewhat daunted and overwhelmed. We can only begin to imagine how bewildering it must be for the woman.

As clinical staff, we are often used to taking a very structured history, working our way through the responses to a series of closed questions. The unplanned pregnancy consultation will of course require collection of some factual information, such as date of last menstrual period and past obstetric history, but to ensure that the woman's emotions are met and that she feels supported in her decision, some techniques borrowed from basic counseling skills can be applied (Table 20.3).

An RCOG guideline, published in 1994, entitled "The Care of Women Requesting Induced Abortion," recommends that postabortion counseling should be available for the small number of women who develop long-term

TABLE 20.3. Suggested counseling techniques

Ask open-ended rather than closed questions	"How did you feel when you found out about the pregnancy?" rather than "Were you sad about the pregnancy?"
	"What are the circumstances in which you would like to become a parent?"
	"How does that differ from your situation?"
Listen actively to the patient	Ensure that you convey genuine interest in her views
	Show understanding and empathy to the emotions which she expresses
Feedback empathically	This helps to validate the woman's emotions and reassures her that they are normal feelings
	"I understand that you are finding this difficult to talk about"
Encourage patients to ask questions	Try using the open-ended "What would you like to ask me about the options?" rather than "Do you have any questions?"
Be vigilant to circumstances which may indicate vulnerability	Young
	Lack of partner or family support
	Ambivalence
	Member of a religious group
	Initial planned pregnancy

TABLE 20.4. Postabortion assessment: questions to ask women

How did you feel immediately after the abortion? After 1 week? Now? A feelings list may help her to describe how she feels

How have you coped? What has helped you?

Have you told anyone about the abortion? Did that help? Is there someone you wish you could tell?

Has the abortion affected your relationship with anyone else? If you have told your partner, what was his reaction?

If expressing regret, do you feel sad because you got pregnant or because you had the abortion?

Did anyone or anything else influence your decision? Was there loss of control?

Tell me about other losses or deaths you have been through. What did you find helped to get you through that time?

Did religion have any influence on your decision about the abortion? Have you done anything else that your religion would not have approved of? If so, how do you cope with that?

What will help you to move on from here?

Adapted from Harris (12)

postabortion distress. Postabortion counseling can be provided by a range of practitioners including trained counselors, nurses, or midwives trained in the technique and doctors with counseling training or experience and can allow the client permission to grieve for the loss of the pregnancy and to achieve self-forgiveness. Harris (12) suggests a selection of questions and discussion points to guide the woman in achieving resolution (Table 20.4).

20.7. Summary

Unplanned and unwanted pregnancies are common and lead to around 200,000 abortions annually in the UK. Initial distress and guilt around the time of termination procedure are common, but significant long-term psychological sequelae are unusual. Certain personal and circumstantial factors predispose to psychological morbidity, and practitioners should be sensitive to these issues, ensuring appropriate preabortion and postabortion support for women. The nongovernmental organization Ipas (13) reminds us that respecting the rights of the client is essential to the quality and continuity of abortion care and that every woman has the right to:

1. *Information*: To learn about her reproductive health, contraception, and abortion options
2. *Access*: To obtain services regardless of religion, ethnicity, age, and marital or economic status
3. *Choice*: To decide freely whether to use contraception and, if so, which method
4. *Safety*: To have a safe abortion and to practice safe, effective contraception
5. *Privacy*: To have a private environment during counseling and services
6. *Confidentiality*: To be assured that any personal information will remain confidential
7. *Dignity*: To be treated with courtesy, consideration, and attentiveness
8. *Comfort*: To feel comfortable when receiving services

9. *Continuity*: To receive follow-up care and contraceptive services and supplies for as long as needed
10. *Opinion*: To express views on the services offered

References

1. Government Statistical Service for the Department of Health. Abortion Statistics, England and Wales: 2004. Available at: http://www.dh.gov.uk/ PublicationsAndStatistics.
2. Scottish Health Statistics, 2005. Available at: http://www.isdscotland.org/isd/info.
3. Francome C, Freeman E. British general practitioners' attitudes toward abortion. *Fam Plan Perspect*. 2000;32(4):198–191.
4. Cartwright A. Unintended pregnancies that lead to babies. *Soc Sci Med*. 1988;27(3):249–254.
5. Barrett G, Smith SC, Wellings K. Conceptualisation, development and evaluation of a measure of unplanned pregnancy. *J Epidemiol Community Health*. 2004;58:426–433.
6. Collins N, Dunkel-Shetter C, Lobel M, Scrimshaw S. Social support in pregnancy: psychological correlates of birth outcomes and postpartum depression. *J Pers Soc Psychol*. 1993;65:1243–1258.
7. Orr S, Arden Miller C. Unintended pregnancy and the psychosocial well-being of pregnant women. *Womens Health Issues*. 1997;7(1):28–46.
8. Brewer C. Incidence of post-abortion psychosis: a prospective study. *BMJ*. 1977;1:476–477.
9. Schmiege S, Russo N. Depression and unwanted first pregnancy: longitudinal cohort study. *BMJ*. 2005;331:1303–1306.
10. Adler N, David H, Major B, Roth S, Russo N, Wyatt G. Psychological responses after abortion. *Science*. 1990;248(4951):41–44.
11. Fisher W, Singh S, Shuper P, et al. Characteristics of women undergoing repeat induced abortion. *CMAJ*. 2005;172(5):637–641.
12. Harris A. Supportive counselling before and after elective pregnancy termination. *J Midwifery Womens Health*. 2004;49(2):105–112.
13. Talluri-Rao S, Baird T. *Information and Training Guide for Medical-Abortion Counseling*. Chapel Hill, NC: Ipas; 2003.

21
Early Pregnancy Loss

Ian Ainsworth-Smith

A high proportion of all pregnancies will end spontaneously early in the pregnancy, possibly even before the woman is aware that she is pregnant. At the time that she miscarries, staff may see her medical management as "routine." Almost certainly, as far as she and her partner are concerned, it is anything but routine. The memories and experience may be lifelong.

Loss in early pregnancy can involve any of the following:

- A departure from the normal
- The loss of expected outcome
- The loss of quality of life in the short term and possibly in the longer term
- The loss of a loved one
- The loss of a hoped-for family unit

21.1. Reacting to Loss

There are as many ways to react to loss early in pregnancy as there are people. Some parents may mourn deeply and obviously; others may be unsure of their emotions. There is no "right" or "wrong" way to grieve and no set time for how long grief should take. Some parents may mourn a little just after the loss and then the feelings of grief may return months or years later. A lot of things happening in the woman's life, or indeed a rapid subsequent pregnancy, may delay mourning. If her history is not carefully taken and if she is not listened to with attention, her natural delayed mourning reaction under these circumstances may become labeled, usually unhelpfully as a postnatal depression Typically, physical recovery and feelings of loss and grief do not necessarily run together. Physical reactions may include exhaustion and fatigue, changes in appetite, restlessness, and weight loss or gain. Emotional reactions may involve denial, guilt, a sense of failure, decreased self-esteem, anger, irritability, and sadness.

Couples may experience many and varied emotions following the loss of a baby through miscarriage or ectopic pregnancy. A woman's feelings may be very different to those of her partner who may feel that he needs to be "the strong one." This may make it hard for them to share their grief even with each other. It is very common for the grief to be relived in the following months, especially significant times may be the date the baby was due and the anniversary of the miscarriage. It is sometimes hard on first meeting to distinguish between appropriate sadness (being full of feelings) and depression (which involves much more the lack of any feelings). Like all losses, miscarriage may produce physical, emotional, social, and spiritual reactions. Most of what is required of staff who encounter women who have gone through an early pregnancy loss is informed and imaginative common sense.

The increasing use of antenatal scans means that many parents would have seen their baby's image and indeed have heard a heartbeat. For some people it will be helpful to have had a real experience to look back on and indeed something more tangible to say goodbye to. Others might quite understandably regret ever having formed an attachment to their unborn baby. Some women may be admitted to hospital after a miscarriage for an evacuation (ERPC) and be more distraught that there was nothing to mourn. I well remember a lady who had been admitted following a 9-week miscarriage simply saying "I have nothing to remember or mourn—it went down the toilet without my knowing. . ."

Research and practical experience do not support the assumption that the earlier the pregnancy at the time of miscarriage the less the potential grief. This may well not be the case. Lost potential may be as poignant as a loss that happens later in a pregnancy. It is not sufficient to assume that a woman who is distraught at a 9- or 10-week miscarriage is overreacting. The baby may well represent a very powerful hope for the woman. Another assumption may be that, at the time of miscarriage, a baby who was unexpected may also have been unwanted. Again, this may not always be so. It can also be difficult for women with an unwanted pregnancy. Miscarriage does not bring relief that nature has taken its course, but often intense guilt that the feelings of rejection caused the miscarriage. Staff, all the time, should avoid making assumptions but be prepared to look beyond what seemed obvious.

Staff may find the move from being a "healer" to being a supporter and comforter a challenging one. A good rule of thumb may be that the more helpless one feels, the more use one is likely to be. There is overwhelming evidence that women and their partners who experience early pregnancy loss will find staff who can be "human" the most reassuring and healing.

21.2. Language and Vocabulary

In most situations a good starting point when approaching the patient will be to think and talk "baby" unless the woman makes it absolutely clear that she does not find it helpful to think in that way. An important distinction should be made between loss early in pregnancy (miscarriage or ectopic pregnancy or even early termination) and stillbirth and neonatal death. In the latter event there is likely to be the presence of a baby and/or pictures or images. Where a baby is lost early in the pregnancy its existence may go unrecognized and often unacknowledged because of the lack of a recognizable body to visualize. Furthermore, early loss may not draw in social supports and rituals which may accompany the death of any loved person. The lack of a supported experience of loss may well have consequences during a subsequent pregnancy, especially at a time in the pregnancy when the previous loss occurred, or at or near term. (A number of studies seem to suggest that parents who have lost a baby earlier may report a greater dissatisfaction with their care.) The differences involved between surgery and medical evacuation of retained products may be significant. The emotional load of carrying on for a long time with a number of scans which may give an equivocal answer may be heavy. However difficult it is, it is very helpful when staff can say supportively and thoughtfully that they do not know exactly what is happening.

Most women do not talk or think about "carrying a fetus," but "expecting a baby." Terminology is important at the outset. The medical term for a miscarriage is "spontaneous abortion," a term that is capable of very mixed interpretation. I remember being called to see a distraught lady who had been asked repeatedly by a junior doctor "When did you have your abortion?" (referring to an earlier miscarriage) at the time when she was losing a much-wanted baby. It is also important not to insert one's own preconceptions as to how the woman and her partner may or should be feeling and what could be helpful for them. For example, some women may choose to deal with the experience by appearing to ignore it. Others, for religious and cultural reasons, may find the idea of referring to the loss or developing their feelings about it quite unacceptable. Although there are some useful guidelines there is no set or normal way of coping with a miscarriage. Practitioners need to be sensitive to feelings of loss without that loss necessarily being made into a tragedy. There can be very good reasons why people do not "grieve" openly at the time of an early pregnancy loss. Denial can sometimes be a valuable psychological mechanism!

Euphemisms frequently have a way of protecting carers from their own feelings of loss and helplessness. Alternatively staff may try to protect themselves by an over use of jargon. Terms like "incomplete abortion" or "missed abortion" may need careful explaining and defining. Careless use of medical terms can get in the way of good communication. Expressions like "vanishing twin," "incompetent cervix," and even "We cannot see the baby's spine" during ultrasound examination can all be misunderstood and misinterpreted.

There is no simple way of breaking bad news. It should be remembered that women may receive the news of the pregnancy loss in ways as diverse as hemorrhage or equivocal ultrasound examination. A few suggestions may be helpful.

a. Choose the time, place, and situation with care. The middle of a formal ward round is not normally the best situation. Think about who may be available to offer support, both to the woman and to those close to her.

b. Avoid euphemisms (e.g., "We think you may have lost the baby") and be as direct as possible.

c. Make it quite clear that you are available for further discussion and will offer information as it becomes available.

d. Gently open up the possibilities and be prepared to answer the question "What happens next?"

Do remember that the time you spend when breaking the bad news is critical, and what you say and do not say will be remembered long afterward. Equally, it is important to avoid offering false reassurance, such as "This pregnancy was only very early and you can always have another one." Even if you feel that you may have said the wrong thing, this may not make the situation irrecoverable. It may be quite possible to go back and restate something or to acknowledge that you have not expressed the situation as clearly as you might.

21.3. When a Miscarriage is not Complete or Further Intervention is Needed

Some women may find the experience of "incomplete" miscarriage even more distressing because of the prospect of surgical intervention. Approximately, 1 in every 80 pregnancies is now thought to be ectopic. In addition to the loss of a baby, frequently when news of the pregnancy comes as a complete surprise, the woman may also be in considerable pain, and pain control needs to be addressed as rapidly and competently as possible. Another particularly difficult circumstance for the patient is that she may be told "You have lost your pregnancy, but we need to continue doing scans and blood tests to check your tube." The other factor which distinguishes ectopic pregnancy is that the condition can be life threatening. The woman may also face loss or damage of part of her reproductive anatomy and face the possibility of surgery or medication, even with the possibility of sterility as the outcome. The future may seem particularly daunting under these circumstances. Close encounter with new life and the possibility of the mother's life being threatened can be devastating news.

21.4. Miscarriage and the Family

It is clear from talking and listening to many women that their miscarriage can become part of a family secret. Family secrets typically are what nobody ever talks about but everyone knows about them and someone will behave as if they are true. It is not unknown for colleagues working with the elderly to find women talking about their miscarried babies, sometimes in very vivid terms, from many years previously. Babies also have a place in the family context. A miscarriage may have implications for a husband or partner too and potential grandparents. Their needs to acknowledge the loss may also need recognizing.

Other children in the family may well become aware that something is happening to their mother but not be told about what is going on. Because of the age of the women concerned, it is quite likely that they will have other young children. It is easy to imagine, incorrectly, that just because children have not been told what is going on they do not experience the loss. Parents may feel, understandably, somewhat at a loss to know how to explain a miscarriage to a young child. Most children would not be interested in the gynecological details but can deal with a simple explanation which would explain that the baby that their mother was expecting had died. Parents should never be forced into telling such things but may well value carefully timed support from health care professionals. Children may well find it helpful to draw or paint a picture expressing how they feel. Some women may not wish to "mark" the end of the pregnancy but others may find it very helpful to be offered a ritual for saying goodbye. The value of a ritual is that it may put the "unsayable" into action. This may be inside a formal religious context, but then it need not be. Some will know exactly how they wish to mark the event, others may appreciate contact with a hospital chaplain or spiritual adviser.

21.5.   Loss Due to Antenatal Testing

In many planned and happily anticipated pregnancies parents may, as a result of antenatal testing and examination, be placed in the unenviable position of being given painful information about the development of the baby and the possibility of having to make difficult choices about the future. A woman and her partner in this situation might reasonably expect:

- To be treated with dignity
- To be given simple explanations
- To be spared innocuous small talk
- To feel able to express whatever feelings come naturally
- To be guided through unfamiliar issues and painful decision-making
- To know that their privacy will be respected, but support and comfort rather than isolation are available to them

21.6.   The Formal/Legal Framework for Miscarriage

The loss of a baby before birth does not need formal registration before 24-week gestation. (It is important to remember that a baby delivered before this time showing any signs of life should normally be registered as a neonatal death.) However, it is increasingly seen as good practice to offer a funeral for a baby delivered before this. Normally, an individual funeral is possible for a baby delivered any time from 16-week gestation onward. The attending doctor or midwife should sign a formal "To Whom It May Concern" letter stating the woman's name, the date of delivery, and her wish for a funeral to take place. This should provide sufficient documentation for a burial or cremation to take place, which may be either arranged by the parents themselves or by the hospital. A rather basic point which can be distressing to raise but should be made gently is that cremated tiny babies do not create any ashes. Occasionally, difficulty is experienced subsequently if this point is not sensitively made at the time. Some parents may choose to attend such a funeral; others may not but may equally be relieved to know that a funeral is taking place. Such a funeral would take place according to the parents' wishes and may or may not be formally "religious." A member of the hospital chaplaincy team, the hospital bereavement officer, and local funeral directors are usually well equipped to offer advice and support as to the options that are available. Even if a funeral does not take place, some women may appreciate the opportunity to light a candle, possibly have some prayers said, or generally have some time for quiet reflection away from a busy hospital ward. There is considerable scope here for imaginative practice. If there is a recognizable entity, the mother should be offered a chance if she wishes to see the miscarried baby. This may be more distressing for staff who may wish to protect their own feelings. However, there is no place for forcing parents to view when they do not wish to and when it may also be culturally unacceptable and quite possibly shocking and may cause trauma. Little recognition is given to the time, effort, and sensitivity required from staff in looking after these women and the emotional load that these staff may find themselves bearing. Too often the opposite is true, this work is belittled as "touchy feely" or dismissed as a luxury. This betrays the feelings and defenses of those who do not recognize the work.

It is now considered good practice for proper procedures to be in place for the care of the previable fetus. Many women will not ask at the time what will happen to their baby, but it is important to have procedures that can be discussed quite openly and honestly. Common practice is for previable fetuses to be buried or cremated at regular intervals and frequently an appropriate memorial is put in place. (The normal custom is for parents to be informed that the funeral will take place at some point in the future. Parents would not normally be invited on this occasion, so it is particularly important that any parent who wishes to arrange an individual funeral should have the opportunity of doing this as soon as possible.) The burial or cremation takes place without a religious service but is witnessed by a member of the hospital staff.

21.7. Abnormal Grief

"Abnormal" grief is always difficult to identify after early pregnancy loss. Confusion may frequently arise between appropriate and overwhelming sadness, being "full" of feelings and clinical depression, which may present itself as "emptiness" of feelings. The woman's social history and any pre-existing psychiatric history may be relevant. However, it is important not to rush to conclusions. Hospital liaison psychiatrists, psychologists, obstetric and gynecological counselors, and chaplains are frequently in a good position to help the woman clarify what is going on for her. If long term the woman deals with the loss by withdrawing from other activities in her life, for example, family commitments; this would be a good indicator of the need to seek further help.

21.8.   Recurrent Loss

The experience of recurrent loss can have profound implications for the woman's view of herself and her body. Some women describe quite simply feeling "punch drunk" after each miscarriage. It may well be that the recurrent miscarriages may only be acknowledged much later, possibly long after a "successful" pregnancy.

21.9.   Having Another Pregnancy

Some women will wish to cope with the miscarriage by immediately wanting to think about another pregnancy. Equally, others may find the possibility beyond their reach or imagination. Each view should be respected. One woman, after an early miscarriage, commented to me that the prospect of another pregnancy felt similar to the possibility of making a new relationship having been jilted in a previous one. With one's head one might know that it would happen; with one's feelings it is impossible to contemplate.

In a subsequent pregnancy, staff may need to be aware of how her early experience may mean that the woman's relationship with staff, her partner, and/or family and the unborn baby may be different.

21.10.   Summary

It is important to think as widely as possible about the implications of early pregnancy loss when faced with a woman who is going through this experience. The sequelae of pregnancy loss are not just encountered in obstetrics and gynecology.

At the time of loss:

- Competent physical care
- Psychological support
- The offering of spiritual (not identical with religious!) support
- Practical support (funerals and identification of the possible needs of the wider family)

Follow-up:

- "Open door" to professionals (medical, nursing, and midwifery, psychological, and spiritual)
- Ceremonies and memorial events
- Support for changed or changing family
- Help when ready with thinking about/planning the next pregnancy
- Possibility of genetic or other counseling

Bibliography

1. Royal College of Obstetricians and Gynaecologists. *The Management of Early Pregnancy Loss.* October 2000.
2. Kohner N. *A Dignified Ending.* Stillbirth and Neonatal Death Society; 1992.
3. Henley A. *When a Baby Dies.* Routledge; 2001.
4. Ainsworth-Smith I, Speck P. *Letting Go: Care of the Dying and Bereaved.* SPCK; 1999.
5. Raphael-Leff J. *Psychological Processes of Childbearing.* Chapman and Hall; 1991.
6. Woods JR, Esposito Woods JL, eds. *Loss During Pregnancy or in the Newborn Period.* Jannetti Publications; 1997.

22
A Biopsychosocial Approach to Premenstrual Problems

Myra S. Hunter

22.1. Prevalence, Definitions, and Diagnosis of Premenstrual Problems

It is estimated that approximately 95% of women in western cultures report some changes in their physical and emotional well-being in the days before some or all of their menstrual periods. The range of possible premenstrual symptoms is wide, but the most common *physical* symptoms include bloating, weight gain, mastalgia (breast pain), abdominal discomfort and pain, lack of energy, headache, and exacerbation of chronic illnesses such as asthma, allergies, epilepsy, or migraine. The most commonly reported *emotional* and *behavioral* changes are depressed mood, irritability, anxiety, tension, aggression, and feelings of being unable to cope and having a sense of loss of control. It is these emotional symptoms, which often prompt women to seek medical intervention (1). Moderate premenstrual changes are reported to be between 40 and 75% of women (2), and between 2 and 10% of women experience severe premenstrual symptoms that interfere with life and meet the diagnostic criteria of Premenstrual Dysphoric Disorder (PMDD) (Table 22.1) (3). Clearly the way that premenstrual problems are defined will determine the prevalence rates.

Since Frank first coined the term premenstrual tension or PMT in 1931, numerous terms have been proposed including Premenstrual Syndrome (PMS), Late Luteal Phase Dysphoric Disorder (LLPDD), and Premenstrual Dysphoric Disorder (PMDD) (see Table 22.1)—which is the current term used in the clinical and research literature.

However, the lay terms used by women and many health professionals still tend to be PMT and PMS. In this chapter PMS will be used as shorthand to refer to a broad group of premenstrual symptoms, and PMDD will be used when the diagnostic definition is strictly applied. Clear definitions aid communication and diagnosis but labels, such as PMDD, are controversial because the relevant symptoms do not have the empirical integrity to be described as a syndrome, and it is also debatable whether they should be categorized within a psychiatric classification.

TABLE 22.1. Diagnostic criteria of PMDD

A. In most menstrual cycles during the past year, 5 (or more) of the following symptoms were present for most of the time during the last week of the luteal phase, began to remit within a few days after the onset of the follicular phase, and were absent in the week postmenses, with at least 1 of symptoms being either 1, 2, 3, or 4:

    1. markedly depressed mood, feelings of hopelessness, or self-deprecating thoughts
    2. marked anxiety, tension, feelings of being "keyed up" or "on edge"
    3. marked affective lability (e.g., feeling suddenly sad or tearful, irritable or increased sensitivity to rejection)
    4. persistent and marked anger or irritability or increased interpersonal conflicts
    5. decreased interest in the usual activities (e.g., work, friends, hobbies)
    6. subjective sense of difficulty concentrating
    7. lethargy, easy fatigability or marked lack of energy
    8. marked change in appetite, overeating, or specific food cravings
    9. hypersomnia or insomnia
    10. subjective sense of being overwhelmed or out of control
    11. other physical symptoms such as breast tenderness or swelling, headaches, joint or muscle pain, a sensation of "bloating," weight gain.

B. The disturbance markedly interferes with work or school or with usual social activities and relationships with others (e.g., avoidance of social activities, decreased productivity and efficiency at work or school).

C. The disturbance is not merely an exacerbation of the symptoms for another disorder- such as major depression disorder, panic disorder, dysthymia disorder or a personality disorder (although it may be superimposed on any of these disorders).

D. Criteria A, B, and C must be confirmed by prospective daily self-ratings during at least two consecutive symptomatic cycles. (The diagnosis may be made provisionally prior to this confirmation).

As shown in Table 22.1, the PMDD definition includes the nature of the symptoms, their severity (interference with daily functioning), and the timing of the symptoms. When assessing women with PMS, 2 months of prospective daily diary ratings of symptoms are recommended in order to confirm the diagnosis. Assessment measures, such as the Menstrual Distress Questionnaire (MDQ), the Premenstrual Assessment Form (PAF), and the Calendar of Premenstrual Experiences (COPE), are described in detail in Haywood et al. (4). Diaries can provide invaluable evidence for the woman and the clinician about the relationships between symptoms and the phases of the menstrual cycle. For example, studies of PMS have found that less than half of the women presenting with the complaint of PMS often actually have the disorder. For example, the symptoms may fail to improve following menstruation or the problem may be continuous, occurring across the monthly cycle. A symptom-free period during the follicular phase of the menstrual cycle is considered essential in differentiating PMDD from pre-existing anxiety and mood disorders. However, in clinical practice it is often the difference between the follicular and the luteal phases that is more important. Differential diagnoses include clinical depression, anxiety disorders, alcohol and substance misuse, and personality problems. For example, a woman with features of borderline personality disorder might present with extremes of mood (not necessarily linked to the menstrual cycle), difficulties in interpersonal relationships, and a history of abuse or neglect. Again the monthly diary can help to show the extent to which the problems are premenstrual or more general. The option of referral to another health professional can then be discussed.

22.2. Theories and Treatments

Medical, psychological, and sociological theories have all been developed to explain PMS resulting in quite diverse and often polarized approaches. Is a woman with PMS "mad" or is she imagining her symptoms or is it her hormones (5)? It is only recently that these disciplinary divides are diminishing and theories emerging that acknowledge a multifactorial biopsychosocial perspective of PMS.

22.2.1. Medical Theories and Therapies

The precise etiology of PMS remains unclear. While hormonal explanations were dominant in the past, no hormonal substrate of PMS has been identified. Early treatments such as progesterone have not been found to be effective, and other medical treatments such as estradiol patches and GnRH agonists serve to disrupt the menstrual cycle and are not popular amongst younger women. Nevertheless, moderate to severe PMS or PMDD is associated with the cyclic pattern of ovarian hormones, and there is evidence of a decrease in serotonin uptake in the premenstrual phase of the cycle in women reporting PMDD. There is a growing consensus that it is differential sensitivity to circulating progesterone metabolites rather than abnormal hormone concentrations, which can cause PMS, and there is increasing evidence that serotonin (5-hydroxytryptamine) could be related to the differential sensitivity and is important in the pathogenesis of PMS. There is now a body of evidence demonstrating that serotonin reuptake inhibitors (SSRIs) are effective in the treatment of PMS (daily or for the second half of the cycle only) and are recommended as the treatment of choice for women who present with PMDD (6). For specific symptom relief, diuretics can alleviate water retention during the luteal phase, and dopamine agonists may relieve mastalgia.

Herbal remedies, vitamins, and complementary therapies are widely used, but there is inconclusive evidence of their efficacy [see Domoney et al. (7)]. For example, there is inconsistent evidence for the effectiveness of oil of evening primrose and evidence that vitamin B6 is not more effective than placebo. However, Agnus castus fruit extract has been found to be more effective than placebo in reducing premenstrual symptoms and warrants further research (8).

22.2.2. Psychological Theories and Treatments

Psychosocial factors have been implicated in the etiology of PMS. PMS occurs more often in women between their late 20s and early 40s, those with at least one child, those with a family history of a major depression, or women with a past medical history of either postpartum depression or an affective mood disorder. There is evidence that psychological and social factors are associated with premenstrual symptom reports; these include stress, life events, marital dissatisfaction, attribution of negative moods to the menstrual cycle, as well as individual differences in beliefs and coping strategies. It has been suggested that stress and personality factors might combine to make some women more sensitive to premenstrual changes. Psychological treatments based on cognitive behavior therapy (CBT) have been developed as treatments for premenstrual problems. For example, coping skills training, relaxation therapy, and cognitive therapy have been found to be more effective than control conditions. In a recent study (9) we found that CBT was as effective as fluoxetine (an SSRI) in the treatment of women with moderate to severe premenstrual problems (defined by PMDD criteria). Furthermore, at 1 year following cessation of treatment, significantly more of those having had CBT maintained improvement compared to those having had fluoxetine.

Figure 22.1 represents the components of a cognitive behavioral model of premenstrual problems, which has at its centre a woman's view of her symptoms and self during the premenstrual phase. This model is in fact a biopsychosocial model as it acknowledges the influences of biological, psychological (thoughts, emotions, and behavior), and social and cultural factors upon the perception of premenstrual symptoms. It is suggested that women with premenstrual problems may be appraising cyclic physiological changes (for example, bloating, breast changes, increased autonomic nervous system

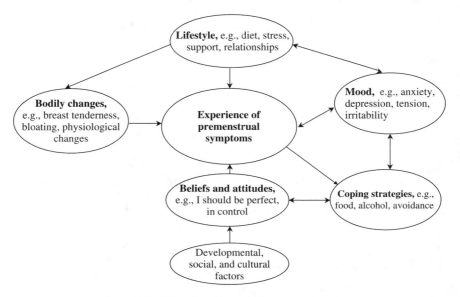

Figure 22.1. A biopsychosocial model of premenstrual problems.

arousal, and decreased serotoninergic activity) in the premenstrual phase in ways that exacerbate emotional reactions to them. For example, thoughts such as "I can't cope", "If I'm not in control people won't like me", can lead to increased anxiety. Such beliefs may be learned through various life experiences and influenced by social and cultural values. For example, if a woman thinks that she should be "perfect", should always "put other people's needs first", or "shouldn't be angry", then this makes it more difficult to tolerate cyclic changes in mood and might lead to further depression, anger, and anxiety. In addition, lifestyle factors are important such as exercise, diet, and relaxation. Relationships can be an important source of social support but also can be a source of stress particularly if there is a lack of understanding or different ways of understanding PMS between the women and her partner, friends, or family. It seems that general levels of stress and social problems influence the extent to which PMS is manageable. Problems, which appear to be surmountable during the follicular phase of the cycle, can be overwhelming during the premenstrual phase. Finally, the coping strategies used to deal with emotional reactions during the premenstrual phase can feed into a vicious circle. For example, women may avoid activities and other people, or use alcohol, or binge eating. These behaviors can feed into a downward spiral of negative thinking and low mood.

In contrast women often see themselves as being fine during the follicular phase of the cycle. They often feel that they are two people or have a "split personality" and question, "who is the real me?" because they see themselves as being polar opposites across the monthly cycle. Generally, it is the nonpremenstrual state that is seen as the "real me", but women are often confused and anxious about their ability to cope and the impact of PMS upon their family, friends, and work colleagues.

22.3.   A Biopsychosocial Approach to Assessment and Treatment of Premenstrual Symptoms

The goals of assessment are outlined in Box 1. The success of helping women with PMS rests on the development of a shared understanding of PMS and a holistic or biopsychosocial approach. Asking her to describe her experience of PMS, her history of seeking help, and her views about the factors causing or affecting her PMS can set the scene for introducing the biopsychosocial model which acknowledges a range of influences. If she has seen a range of different health professionals and been offered quite different opinions, it is important to acknowledge that this can be confusing and irritating. Some women might well be angry and frustrated by the time they see you, and this needs to be addressed first by listening and empathizing with their situation. You can acknowledge that there are different views about PMS, and that the research evidence supports the view that a range of factors can influence PMS. Exploring the individual factors affecting her PMS can help

---

Box 1 Goals of assessment

- To help the woman to feel understood—by listening first to *her understanding* of her symptoms, that is, what she experiences and what she thinks are the factors causing them or making them worse.
- To assess the extent and severity of premenstrual symptoms—using the PMDD criteria can make women feel that their problem is being taken seriously.
- To exclude other problems—take a detailed history including the development of the symptoms and presence of physical or psychiatric disorder.
- To confirm the diagnosis—by asking the woman to complete 2 months of daily diary ratings of key symptoms and key events and activities.
- To share a simple biopsychosocial model of PMS—this is best carried out at the second visit when woman and doctor can look at the diary to understand the relationships between symptoms, the menstrual cycle, and other events.
- To give her choices and to agree on a treatment plan.

---

the woman to feel understood and that she is being taken seriously. It is worth spending a bit more time during an assessment which will take two clinic visits—the first to take a history and to explore her symptoms and to present the biopsychosocial model, the second to review this in the light of 2 months of daily diary records. When completing the diaries she can be encouraged to note events or factors, for example, particular stresses, activities, holidays, and so on, that make her symptoms better or worse during the whole month. Women frequently report feeling relief in response to their problems being taken seriously and find it useful to understand and normalize their reactions in the context of their lifestyles.

The treatment plan is informed by the particular factors identified in the model. These are presented in common goals of treatment and include a wish to be in control, to have more moderate reactions, and to be less angry or depressed. Keeping a diary of daily symptom and noting daily activities and stressful events can be useful to examine the relationships between moods and situations across the menstrual cycle. The patient can be encouraged to make lifestyle changes to see how effective they are during the following 2 months. This can increase her sense of being in control as can being offered the choice of treatments. Some women feel so desperate that they wish to have a medical treatment such as an SSRI straight away, others might prefer a more gradual approach, making lifestyle changes and then if needed being offered cognitive behavior therapy. Relaxation therapy and stress management are helpful for many women to reduce tension and anxiety and to try out alternative strategies to deal with psychosocial problems, such as managing children's demands, tackling problems at work. It is often

---

Box 2 Treatment approaches for PMS

- Information and advice about PMS.
- Lifestyle changes: health diet, regular meals rich in complex carbohydrates and low in salt, fat, and caffeine, regular exercise, limit alcohol, regular sleep.
- Complementary therapies: there is some evidence that agnus castus is helpful, approaches such as massage, aromatherapy, and yoga can increase relaxation and help deal with stress.
- Stress management and problem-solving across the whole cycle: relaxation, identifying problems causing stress and seeking solutions, support groups.
- SSRI (can be used during luteal phase only): Fluoxetine 20 mg per day, Citalopram 10—30 mg per day, Paroxetine 1030 mg per day, Sertraline 50—150 mg per day.
- Cognitive behavior therapy: refer to clinical or counseling psychologist.
- Hormone therapies: Danazol (100 mg twice a day), GnRH agonist for 2–3 cycles disrupts the menstrual cycle but have side effects. Estrogen patches can be used which also disrupt the cycle.
- Surgery: In extreme circumstances some women opt for hysterectomy and oophorectomy but this requires careful consideration and informed consent when all other options have been explored.

---

easier to begin to tackle such problems during the follicular phase. Educating friends and family, and being able to communicate to others what is helpful, and becoming more assertive across the cycle, can increase social support. In a study of what changes during CBT for premenstrual problems (10), we found that learning to use active behavioral coping strategies, such as relaxation, talking about problems, and active problem-solving, was associated with good outcome and maintenance of improvement at 1 year post-treatment. If an SSRI is the treatment choice, regular follow-up appointments should be offered with daily diary symptom records in order to monitor effectiveness as well as any side effects. Having regular monitoring enables the patient and doctor to work together on finding the best combination of treatment strategies.

22.4. Summary

Helping women to manage premenstrual problems can be rewarding detective work. Spending time during the assessment phase can benefit the patient and the doctor, because the patient is likely feel understood, to feel in control and involved in her treatment, and the doctor shares the responsibility of the decisions and can be creative in exploring a range of factors that can affect

PMS. However, it is also important to be clear about one's own expertise, for example, offering information and advice about PMS and dealing with emotional problems (see Web sites) is very helpful, but psychological therapy and psychiatric assessment require specific expertise. Ideally, multidisciplinary teams (comprising a gynecologist, psychologist, and nurse) could provide PMS assessments and a choice of treatments. But until these are widely available the informed gynecologist can provide a valuable service to this group of women who in the past have been misunderstood and negatively stereotyped. I hope that readers will take up this challenge.

References

1. Hunter MS, Swann C, Ussher JM. Self report and help-seeking behaviour of women attending a premenstrual syndrome clinic. *Sexual & Marital Therapy* 1995;10:253–262.
2. Steiner M, Born L. Diagnosis and treatment of premenstrual dysphoric disorder: an update. *International Clinical Psychopharmacology.* 2000;15:5–17.
3. Wittchen H-U, Becker E, Lieb, R, Krause P. Prevalence, incidence and stability of premenstrual dysphoric disorder in the community. *Psychological Medicine.* 2002;32:119–132.
4. Hayward A, Slade P, King H. Assessing the assessment measures for menstrual cycle symptoms: a guide for researchers and clinicians. *Journal of Psychosomatic Research.* 2002;52:223–237.
5. Ussher J, Hunter MS, Browne S. Good, bad or dangerous to know: representations of femininity in narrative accounts of premenstrual syndrome (PMS). In: Squire C, ed. *Culture and Psychology.* London: Routledge; 2000:87–99.
6. Wyatt KM, Dimmock PW, O'Brien PMS. Selective serotonin reuptake inhibitors for premenstrual syndrome, [Review]. *Cochrane Database of Systematic Reviews.* 2002;4:CD00139.
7. Domoney CL, Vashisht A, Studd JW. Use of complementary therapies by women attending a specialist premenstrual syndrome clinic. *Gynecological Endocrinology.* 2003;17:13–18.
8. Schellenberg R for the study group. Treatment for the premenstrual syndrome with agnus castus fruit extract: prospective, randomised, placebo controlled study. *British Medical Journal.* 2001;322:134–137.
9. Hunter MS, Ussher J, Browne S, Cariss M, Jelley R, Katz M. A randomised comparison of psychological (CBT), medical (fluoxetine) and combined (CBT and fluoxetine) treatment for women with Premenstrual Dysphoric Disorder. *Journal of Psychosomatic Obstetrics & Gynaecology.* 2002;23:193–199.
10. Hunter MS. Ussher J, Browne S, Cariss M, Jelley R, Katz M. Medical (fluoxetine) and psychological (cognitive behaviour therapy) treatments for Premenstrual Dysphoric Disorder (PMDD): a study of treatment processes. *Journal of Psychosomatic Research.* 2002;53:811–818.

23
Infertility: A Psychosocial Viewpoint

Michael E. Pawson

When a young woman has anorexia she stops ovulating; her psyche recognizes that she is not fit either for pregnancy or to support a child and therefore prevents it. Likewise a woman mourning the death of her family in some disaster may also suppress ovulation for some considerable time. She is not yet ready to replace her lost children. The demand of science for a hypothesis then subjected to proof or disproof is very hard to satisfy with respect to psychogenic subfertility. However, I believe that it is reasonable to suggest that emotional trauma less obvious than the above examples may also inhibit conception.

23.1. The Effect of the Psyche on Fertility (Box 1)

Box 1 Effect of psyche on infertility

Female

- Superficial

  Anorexia
  Bereavement

- Deeper level

  Guilt
  Shame
  Fear
  Unresolved relationships

- Profound level

  Generativity

Male

- Direct impotence
- Indirect? spermatogenesis

Female factors: the psyche affects fertility at three different levels:

1. At a superficial level: there is a direct organic effect as in the example above, anovulation following a life disaster.
2. At a deeper level: unconscious factors.

   a. Suppressed guilt or shame related to previous events such as a concealed abortion.
   b. Family history distortions: a relative who died in childbirth (especially mother)
   c. Horror stories about labor and birth through friends or the media.
   d. There may be both guilt and regret about deferring pregnancy for a career or material success.
   e. Unsatisfactory and unresolved relationships with the mother. My own experience, supported by Dinora Pines, is that more women than I would have expected, give a history of an unsatisfactory relationship with their mother. Dinora Pines suggested that these women often put their creative energy into being high achievers and have a complex emotional world around fertility and motherhood, unconsciously despising their mother whilst envying their fertility.

3. At a profound level: psychological development.
   In his epigenetic theory Erik Erikson describes the seventh stage of development as adulthood where the individual is ready to establish and guide the next generation. This he called "generativity." If the individual has not yet reached the stage of generativity, this may be a psychogenic cause of not conceiving; such a person is not emotionally ready to be a parent.

All of the above backgrounds require a lot of time to tease out in the history.

Male factors: there are two psychogenic routes affecting fertility in the male.

a. *Direct*. The demand for sex at the time of ovulation may cause temporary impotence whilst potency is normal at other times in the cycle. The effect of the psyche on sexual performance is well documented.
b. *Indirect*. The effect of the psyche on semen quality is poorly understood and needs more research, but azoospermia has been reported in men awaiting execution and, less dramatically, the quality of semen when produced at egg collection for IVF can be poorer than previously observed.

No doctor should now allow themselves to consider a disorder of function without considering also the emotional, social and cultural environment.

23.2. The Motivation for Having a Child

In order to understand the psychological aspects of infertility better, it is necessary to explore the motives that drive us in wanting children. The society in which we live still expects us to have children. To be regarded as successful in this world, however trivial and superficial it may be, we need to be rich, beautiful and have children. We are also conforming to the expectations of our parents. There is a lifelong expectation of a woman that the ultimate fulfillment of her femininity will only be achieved by a child. Onerous expectations can be pinned on a child, the mother seeing it as a chance to fulfill her own frustrated ambitions and wasted opportunities. In the case of the young girl, leaving home prematurely as a teenager, there is often the desire to do better than her mother did. She has not been in a loving environment; she does not feel nurtured or well mothered. She sets out to remedy this by having her own child. She will then have something that loves her and needs her. It is, of course, a recipe for trouble because there is a failure to differentiate between the romantic idea of proving fertility by conceiving and the reality of pregnancy and bringing up a child (Box 2).

Box 2 Motivation to conceive

- To conform to expectations
- To do better than one's mother
- To ensure "genetic immortality"
- But there is always some ambivalence

There are also complex existential issues that underlie the motivation to have a child. Post-Darwin there is a decreasing belief in the soul and in an afterlife in "Christian" society. The only chance most of us have of being remembered after death is by passing on half our genes. For many there is an awful finality when denied this. Our life is rationed, we have only so much life, there is a powerful drive to be creative, better still, procreative. Nature overcomes death not by giving us immortality, but by enabling us to procreate. Birth and new life is welcomed and celebrated across all cultures worldwide, and generation of new life is the consummation of marriage or a union between a woman and a man.

There are existential "givens" in life which include

1. We are alone in this life.
2. There is no clear purpose to our existence.
3. We are mortal; death is inevitable.

Those with deeply held religious faith might dispute this, but for many in the west the above statements are true. A child may alleviate the pain of these stark facts to some extent by adding purpose to life and by ensuring genetic immortality for at least another generation. Failure to conceive requires a direct confrontation with these existential problems. These are issues difficult to reflect upon when you do have a child, but even more so without that solace.

Whilst motivation is high at many levels, it is important to recognize that this is tempered by a natural ambivalence. In seeking help for infertility the woman has not only to expose her body but also her marriage and her intimate self to strangers. She will have to ask her partner to produce a semen sample. She enters a clinical world with which she is not familiar. She suppresses the ambivalence and the negatives initially because she will do anything that the doctor says. With increasing intrusions, procedures, drugs these negatives return and the positive optimism of the early days fades.

Nor is everything wonderful about having a baby. A baby can take up time, money and interrupt a promising and fulfilling career. Pregnancy and labor for some can be uncomfortable, painful, undignified and frankly distasteful. Brazelton and Als studied the psychological health of a group of primiparous women through pregnancy, they were alarmed to find multiple anxieties and expected a lot of problems in the early childhood years. However, those women who had recognized their anxieties and expressed them did well in the long term, those who suppressed their feelings did less well. Recognizing the negative side of ambivalence has a better outcome than denial. The couple themselves may deny their natural ambivalence for fear that the doctor may misinterpret their feelings for a lack of commitment and motivation. It is not only a failure in the patient to recognize ambivalence that may lead to problems in the future but also a failure in the doctor.

23.3. The Effect of Subfertility on the Psyche (Box 3)

Box 3 Effect of infertility on psyche

- Mourning/grief
- Depression
- Personal identity changes
- Loss of sexual fulfillment
- Loss of "control"
- Stress, guilt, shame.
- Living a lie
- Relationship problems
- Irrational pursuit of treatment

---

a. *Mourning of the baby/child.* Many women have an image of the baby that they will one day have. If that baby is not to be then there is a mourning process to go through. In some ways this may be worse than the mourning that we experience for those whom we have known and loved. This is because there are no memories of happy occasions, of shared intimacies, there is nothing realized to mourn. All that the woman can do is to grieve for what might have been. This grief can be very prolonged, is renewed at the menopause, and resurfaces when her friends are becoming grandparents.

b. *Depression.* The cycle has been monitored carefully and social life and sex timed to fit in with ovulation. There is often a severe reactive depression when it is clear that a period is coming. There is also a more general depression of the infertile.

c. *Changes in construct of personal identity.* In one sense the woman feels that she is different because she is "not like everybody else" because she has no child. In another sense, however, she is the same as everyone else because science, or her God if she believes in one, is failing her in not treating her as special. She has to face the fact that we all have to face at some time, and she is not different in that there is no fairy godmother waving a magic wand for her.

d. *Loss of sexual fulfillment.* What used to be "making love" now becomes "having sex." Sex becomes an obligation and only reminds the couple of the problem rather than creating comfort and closeness. There is a third person in the bed telling you when and when not to make love. The doctor and the staff in the clinic are all present in your private life trying to help you make a baby. It is not surprising that relationships may falter under such conditions and may not survive.

e. *Loss of control.* Increasingly the modern woman delays pregnancy in order to pursue a career. She is used to being in control and expects to conceive when she makes the decision. Society encourages this by publicizing pregnancy in the older celebrity while failing to present the other side of the picture. However, she does not have control over her psyche. Her failure to control reproduction becomes a great personal disaster. Her expectation of having a child as her own mother did is vital to her feminine development and concept of her own worth.

23.4. More General Effects

1. *Stress of everyday life.* Although the choice of not having a child has become much more acceptable, there is still a stigma attached to childlessness. Friends and family can be very thoughtless and unaware of the pain that their comments can cause. Assumptions are made that the couple do not want children, that they have opted for a selfish, materialistic lifestyle when, in fact, nothing could be further from the truth. The unguarded comment may be less painful than the obvious avoidance of talking of children at all.

2. *Guilt.* Guilt may be felt at "not conforming" but more so at not producing grandchildren and continuing the generations.

3. *Irrational pursuit of treatment.* As the woman's desire for a baby becomes increasingly frustrated, so she may idealize it and pursue conception at the expense of all other aspects of her life. If she is used to being in control of her life, she wants to regain that control. If she does succeed she will find that a child is an "out-of-control" experience. Furthermore, if she has not come to terms with out-of-control events there may be problems with bonding, parenting and post natal depression.

4. *Shame.* There may be shame associated with not conceiving naturally.

5. *Self-esteem.* The woman feels empty, sterile and of no worth. This affects both her relationship and her work.

6. *Relationship problems.* The whole process through which the couple has gone has the potential to be very destructive. The partnership is incomplete without a child. Conflict may be engendered because one partner may have wanted a child more than the other.

"I went through all this only for you."

7. *Unacknowledged grief.* The woman in particular finds herself leading a double life and to some extent a lie. She tries to lead a "normal" life whilst underneath is great sadness. This grief, shame, jealousy, frustration; this anger that science has helped others but not her may all be internalized. It is then reflected at her partner, friends, children, and colleagues at work.

Joan Rafael Leff sums up many of these feelings when she writes of "the violation of the expectation of generativity as a fundamental, normal human property."

23.5.   The Management of Investigation and Treatment (Box 4)

There should be at least three investigators, patient, partner and doctor

---

Box 4 Treatment

- Listen
- Avoid Cartesian dualism
- Empathy. Empathy. Empathy.
- Outline plan and end points
- Counselor available
- Confront failure
- Guide acceptance of failure.

23.5.1. The Couple

The woman attending a fertility clinic for the first time is going to be nervous, embarrassed and frightened of bad news, indeed very vulnerable. If she is accompanied by her husband or companion she will be less so. My preference has always been to see the woman alone in the consulting room on the first visit, because she may talk about things that she might not want her husband or others to hear. I then talk to the couple together and see them together for the second visit to discuss the results and the plan of treatment. The partner is also given the opportunity for a consultation on his own.

The management and reception of the woman at the first visit is of paramount importance to her and to the future relationship she will have with you. When she enters the consulting room she is crossing a threshold, she is leaving her own world and entering yours, she is becoming something different—a patient. (The word "patient" seems to have become a word to avoid, but it is not disparaging, it means one who is suffering and those with a fertility problem are certainly suffering.) The doctor should welcome her into his world by standing up, greeting her by name, introducing himself and shaking her hand. This latter is important. Intimate and deep issues will be discussed and this physical contact increases trust. At least 20 minutes and preferably 30 should be allowed for this initial consultation.

The history taken at this visit is the lynch pin of the whole diagnostic and management procedure. This is when confidence and rapport will be established. Let the patient talk and listen to her story. The most important diagnostic tools in medicine are still the spoken word and the listening ear. Time spent on the history at the first visit is a far better investment than 10-minutes reeling off a series of tests on the computer followed by instructions to return in 6 weeks. Ask the woman how she actually *feels*. Be gentle but firm in asking about the sexual side of the marriage. I always talk of "making love" rather than "having sex" or "intercourse." You do need to know how often they make love, and it can be difficult to know how to approach this. Rather than ask a direct blunt question you may be able to introduce the subject with a statement such as "You both seem to lead very busy lives, perhaps that makes it difficult to make love as often as is ideal when you are trying to conceive" This reverses the questioning and allows her to ask how often is ideal and the discussion continues from there.

Again, you can say something like "Often there is a strain when you are trying to time making love to conceive. I have had couples when the husband/partner has found it difficult to maintain an erection when he knows it is so important. I wonder whether you have had any problems like that?" This sort of observation provides an opening to discuss possible sexual problems. However, do treat the answers that you get with some circumspection. I was once assured by a woman at her first visit that there were no sexual problems in her marriage of 4 years, only to discover on examining the husband that he was a female with congenital adrenal hyperplasia.

23.5.2.   *The Doctor*

The doctor is often perceived as being a godlike, life saving baby maker. The doctor is trained in the scientific method to observe physical signs, to correlate them, and then to treat. She/he is not trained to observe, recognize, and help with the psychology and the social and cultural environment, with the personality, character and emotions, despite the evidence so far that this is intrinsically bound up in the fertility process. The purpose of this book is to *help* the young doctor recognize how vital such observations are and to give advice as to how these aspects of care are best approached.

Doctors and staff in a fertility clinic can become very totalitarian, a rigid and inflexible regime is less complicated for us. We often overwhelm the patient with tests and treatments without stopping to think and consider. The natural hierarchy and pecking order within the clinic can make the godlike baby maker arrogant and insensitive. Some women even refer to "your baby, doctor" and this paternalism is enhanced when doctors sit in an office surrounded by photographs of the clinic's successes. This reinforces the patient's failure; it is as though the doctor is saying "I have made all these babies, so it is your fault you are not getting pregnant not mine"

Most dangerous of all is when infertility is unexplained and the doctor does not really know what to do for the best. This is when desperate remedies may be applied, when a psychological problem may be authenticated by physical treatment such as IVF.

Finally the doctor may have to confront failure with the patient. None of us like failure, and there is a great temptation to discard our failures into a medical wastepaper basket. I will return to this issue later.

The doctor needs to be aware of the incidence of transference, which occurs frequently in a fertility clinic. (This means the unconscious instilling of their feelings into you, e.g., you are wonderful/a god because you are going to solve this very deep and important problem of our immortality.) Do not be flattered by this and be aware of both the benefits and risks of transference. In the very emotional environment of the fertility clinic it can be difficult for the doctor to remain humble. A degree of arrogance is an accusation often made against doctors "playing God." But remember that, while only Mozart could have composed his sublime music, someone else would have described gravity if Newton had not done so. In the same way, any doctor with the training can do what you are doing in the clinic from a technical point of view. Not all doctors have the empathy and understanding to make the distressed and unique patient sitting opposite them feel cared for and understood, releasing her anxiety and maximizing her chances for the best resolution to her problem, with or without a pregnancy.

Avoid the Cartesian dualism with which Medicine is so encumbered. This separated the mind, soul, and emotions from the body and the physical world. As Medicine advanced it has become increasingly a science and not an art, so the emotional and spiritual being has been overlooked. In reproductive medicine technology is moving very fast; this must be balanced by caring for the nonphysical in the patient. Avoid also the attitude on which my generation was brought up, namely that you are the patient and I am the doctor and there is rightly a barrier between us. Remember that the patient may well be sharing feelings and fears with you that she has never confided to anyone before.

The treatment of the couple with fertility problems has necessarily become multidisciplinary. No single doctor can be an expert in all the aspects of investigation and treatment. Input may be required from an endocrinologist, gynecological surgeon, the assisted reproduction team, and urologist or specialist in the problems of the male. Some may even work in different hospitals. It is essential that there is a doctor in overall charge to whom the couple can always refer if they want. Ideally that doctor should be the one who sees them on their first visit. Other professionals should not be threatened by this relationship, which can be very supportive for a couple. The plan for investigation and treatment should be discussed with the patient at her first visit. She and her partner should have a schedule with clear end points and the options after each step should be explained. The couple should be sympathetically warned of the indignities they may have to face. These are much better handled if anticipated.

The benefit of leaflets in the clinic is limited. There is a danger that the staff may use these rather than explaining the complexities of a condition such as endometriosis verbally. Leaflets should complement discussion, being referred to during the explanation. They should not replace explanation and dialogue, and certainly should not be given with a casual "go home and read this."

Patient groups, both within the clinic and externally, can be extremely beneficial in alleviating the stress and anxiety that couples inevitably experience. Such groups are not useful for all couples but they do provide a forum where experiences are shared. "Oh, you felt that too/experienced that problem too did you? So we are not the only ones" Such an exchange of feelings is reassuring. These groups also act as a focus for giving information in a less formal atmosphere. For this reason a member of the fertility clinic team should be present at the meetings within the clinic. It is ideal if the team rotate so that the embryologist is present at one meeting, the urologist at the next, and so on.

Counseling from someone trained in the area of infertility must be available. In this respect the help that can be given, even by experienced staff, is limited. The doctor's ear is invaluable in listening; in valuing the couple and helping them not to feel a failure; in validating their feelings and reassuring them that such feelings are not abnormal; and in helping them work out a solution that is consistent with their own life and values. But there must also be a trained "neutral" counselor, someone who can understand the depth of the psychic problems they are facing, who can help them understand this and why they feel how they do. Patients may also hold back some feelings for fear of upsetting one of the staff, whereas they will be less inhibited with a counselor.

The Royal College of Obstetricians and Gynaecologists has recognized the value of counseling and has stated the following:

1. All clinics providing IVF and donor treatment must provide the opportunity for counseling.
2. Fertility treatment can cause significant stress. Counseling reduces that stress and may alter the outcome.
3. Counseling should be available throughout the treatment and after treatment has ended, either through pregnancy or through acceptance of failure.

The second and third of these statements are applicable to all couples having fertility treatment not exclusively those having IVF or donor treatment.

The outstanding and widely publicized achievements of assisted reproductive technology have led to very high expectations. Stories of "miracle babies" give the impression that nothing is impossible. These expectations need to be balanced by a more realistic and broader perspective. This is best provided by the doctor in overall charge and the counselor.

23.6. Intractable Infertility in One Partner

If the problem is totally one sided, as in azoospermia or the premature menopause, then the option of gamete donation needs particularly experienced counseling and discussion. It is especially difficult for the partner who appears to be the sole cause of the infertility. There can be no blame to whichever partner it is, but it is a hard blow to overcome.

At this stage the options are going to be

- Ovum, embryo or sperm donation
- Adoption
- Surrogacy
- Acceptance

The first three need comprehensive explanation in both a legal and a counseling context. There are guidelines and clear written information provided by the HFEA on gamete and embryo donation and on surrogacy and similar guidelines in respect of adoption. All of these should be available in the clinic.

23.7. Intractable Infertility in the Couple

Both patient and doctor have to confront failure, there will be many that do not succeed in conceiving. Patients will opt out of treatment at different stages. Some will not proceed to IVF seeing it as a step too far, creating a baby rather than procreating. No doctor is happy facing up to failure, and there is a great temptation to discard the patient as soon as it is agreed that treatment should end. The couple are dropped into the medical waste paper basket and forgotten. Those who come back to visit with babies are welcome, the "failures" who may return seeking solace or comfort are less so. To discard a couple once infertility is recognized as intractable is as bad medicine as to perform skilful surgery but then to neglect to close the wound. The couple facing the intractable nature of their problem are deeply wounded and the doctor bears some of the responsibility to help the healing process.

23.7.1. Acceptance

Guiding the couple toward accepting the fact, or the likelihood, that they will remain childless is very difficult and has to be handled with extreme sensitivity. Some couples will be content to leave and to make their own way through the grief they feel. There are, however, two other avenues that the doctor might consider discussing with the couple.

The first of these is that mourning the image of the child that is not to be might be helpful. The understanding and management of stillbirth has been revolutionized in the last 25 years. Before that the stillborn baby was hidden from the mother because it was believed that it was too distressing for the mother to see her dead child. The hospital would arrange the funeral and the body usually placed in the coffin of a recently deceased adult. The baby remained unacknowledged. The much more open approach now adopted makes the tragedy of stillbirth easier to bear. Likewise the grief associated with miscarriage has benefited from a more enlightened approach.

The fetus in a late miscarriage can now have a funeral. Nondenominational services are held in many hospitals annually for parents who have lost a pregnancy at whatever stage. If such approaches are truly beneficial, then the childless couple might be helped by a mourning process for the child they have imagined. Many women do have a mental picture of "their child," the gender, physical attributes, and behavior. Describing this and sharing it acknowledges this important fantasy life and facilitates the grief process. It is wise to warn the couple of the normal grief reaction of anger, disbelief, despair, and resolution. The fact that this dream exists and is important is borne out by the fact that the image a woman may have of her idealized baby is discussed in preadoption counseling, in this case to demonstrate that the adopted child is unlikely to live up to the fantasy. But the fantasy can be mourned. A childless patient of mine, confronted with the imperative of a hysterectomy, was helped very much by writing a letter to her fantasy child explaining to him why he was never to be.

The second approach is group or couple psychotherapy. As described by Christie and Morgans this has therapeutic benefit, in as much as there is a significant pregnancy rate, even in failed IVF, and if there is no conception it helps the couple accept childlessness. It is important as it may well be the first time that ambivalence and innermost feelings about pregnancy are discussed.

Both of these approaches deserve and need more research. Managing our failures is as important as achieving our successes.

23.8.   Lessons to Learn from This Chapter:

- There are psychogenic causes of infertility.
- Infertility may be very distressing. It may be destructive to both partners.
- The history is as important as the investigations.
- One doctor must be in overall charge.
- A trained infertility counselor must be available.
- If treatment fails or infertility is intractable the couple must have other options discussed.
- Couples must be helped and guided in accepting childlessness. The doctor's responsibility does not end with failure of treatment.
- Creation and procreation are not the same.

Bibliography

1. Brazelton TB, Als H. Four early stages in the development of mother–infant interaction. The psychoanalytic study of the child. 1979. 34, 39.
2. Christie GL, Morgan A. *Australas J Psychother.* 2006;25(1).
3. Christie GL, Pawson ME. The psychological and social management of the infertile couple. In: Pepperell RJ, Hudson B, Wood C, eds. *The Infertile Couple.* Edinburgh: Churchill Livingstone 1987:313–319.
4. Erikson, E. Childhood and society (2nd edition). Paladin 1984;222–247.
5. Pawson ME. In: Haynes J and Miller J, eds. *Inconceivable Conceptions.* Hove and New York: Brunner Routledge; 2003:60–72.
6. Pines D. Emotional aspects of infertility and its remedies. *Int J Psycho-anal.* 1990;71:561–568.
7. Rafael LJ. The baby makers: an in depth single case study of conscious and unconscious psychological reactions to infertility and "baby making" technology. *Br J Psychother.* 1992;8(3):278–294.
8. Stanton AL, Dunkel-Scheffer C. *Infertility Perspectives from Stress and Coping Research.* New York: Plenum Press; 1991.

Suggested Further Reading

1. Haynes J, Miller J, eds. *Inconceivable Conceptions.* London: Brunner Routledge; 2003.
2. Snowden R, Snowden CM. *The Gift of a Child.* Exter: Exeter University Press; 1993.

Useful Addresses

Intercountry Adoption Society, 64-66 High St, Barnet, Herts Tel: 0870 516 8743, www.icacentre.org.uk

Overseas Adoption Support and Information Service, Tel: 0870 241 7069, www.adoptionoverseas.org

Surrogacy UK, Tel: 01531 821889, www.surrogacyuk.org.

Human Fertilisation and Embryology Authority, 21 Bloomsbury St, WC1B 3HF, Tel: 0207 291 8200, www.hfea.gov.uk

24
Sexual Violence

Catherine White

24.1.   What is Rape, Incest?

Sexual Offences Act 2003

2003 Chapter 42

PART 1

Sexual offences

Rape

1. Rape

(1) A person (A) commits an offence if

(a) He intentionally penetrates the vagina, anus, or mouth of another person (B) with his penis

(b) B does not consent to the penetration, and

(c) A does not reasonably believe that B consents.

(2) Whether a belief is reasonable is to be determined having regard to all the circumstances, including any steps A has taken to ascertain whether B consents.

(3) Sections 75 and 76 apply to an offence under this section.

(4) A person guilty of an offence under this section is liable, on conviction on indictment, to imprisonment for life.

Assault

2. Assault by penetration

(1) A person (A) commits an offence if

(a) He intentionally penetrates the vagina or anus of another person (B) with a part of his body or anything else

(b) The penetration is sexual

(c) B does not consent to the penetration, and

(d) A does not reasonably believe that B consents.

(2) Whether a belief is reasonable is to be determined having regard to all the circumstances, including any steps A has taken to ascertain whether B consents.

(3) Sections 75 and 76 apply to an offence under this section.

(4) A person guilty of an offence under this section is liable, on conviction on indictment, to imprisonment for life.

24.2.   Rates of Sexual Assault

The 2001 British Crime Study (BCS) Interpersonal Violence Module (IVM) found that 7% of the women sampled had suffered rape or serious sexual assault at least once in their lifetime. In the year 2004/2005, 60,946 sexual offences were recorded by the police in England and Wales, of which 14,002 were offences of rape (1). Sexual violence is massively underreported by both female and male victims. The 2001 BCS IVM found that only about 15% of rapes came to the attention of the police. Forty percent of those who had suffered rape in the 2001 study had told no one about it.

24.3.   How Might a Rape or Sexual Assault Victim Present?

Rape can affect any age and crosses all social strata. At the St Mary's Centre, the youngest client to date was 7 months old, the eldest a 93-year-old man. A victim may present in various ways.

Acute, direct	Acute, nondirect
Via complaint to police	Request for emergency contraception
A&E	A&E complaining of vaginal bleeding
GP	A&E with other injuries
Self-referral to a Sexual Assault	Police complaining of another crime, e.g.,
Referral Centre (SARC)	burglary
Historical, direct	Historical, nondirect
SARC	Chronic pelvic pain
GP	Pregnancy
Counseling services	TOP request
Voluntary services	Dyspareunia
	Sexually transmitted infection
	Infertility
	Psychiatric problems
	Depression, anxiety, self-harm,
	posttraumatic stress disorder (PTSD), etc.

24.3.1.   Response of the Clinician to Direct Disclosure

The initial response that a person receives when they first disclose that they have been assaulted will have a massive impact on that person's subsequent actions. Therefore, it is vital that a doctor who is confided in reacts appropriately. This will include being seen to be interested, to believe, and to listen. The doctor should not react in a judgmental manner. Rape and sexual assault are about loss of power and control by the victim. It is important to empower the victim and start the recovery process by restoring choice and control. The doctor can do this by helping her to be aware of her choices and options and allowing her to decide what will be best for her in her personal circumstances. It is not up to the doctor to decide what he/she thinks is the correct line of action for the victim. A paternalistic attitude by health-care staff can enhance the feeling of helplessness. The options available to a victim will be dependent on local services and time between assault and disclosure.

Any disclosure made by a patient should be recorded verbatim. The doctor should not take on an investigative role as it is the police who have these skills. However, any questions asked by the doctor in establishing basic facts should be kept as "open" as possible and recorded, along with any answers, also verbatim. The doctor should make a note of who gave the information, when, where, and who else was present. How much information the doctor needs to seek will depend on what other services are available. For example, if there is the ability to refer to a SARC, then the original doctor's involvement may be minimal.

In discussing with any victim what their needs might be, the doctor will have to consider both forensic and therapeutic issues.

Forensic	Therapeutic
Liaison with law enforcement	Treatment of injuries
Identification and documentation of injuries	Emergency contraception
Forensic samples	Unwanted pregnancy
Retrieval	Postexposure prophylaxis (PEP)
Storage	HIV
Documentation	Hepatitis B
Chain of evidence	STIs
	Screening for sexually transmitted infections
	Psychological needs
	Crisis intervention
	Counseling
	Practical support
	Needs of significant others

Of course, where the victim is a child, or it is thought that there are ongoing risks to children, the doctor will have to abide by local child protection procedures and the victim's confidentiality may not be guaranteed. This should be discussed with the victim prior to the passing on of information.

24.3.2. Nondisclosure but Abuse Is a Possibility

As has already been discussed, the majority of sexual assault victims do not disclose the abuse. This could be for a whole host of reasons including the following:

- Fear of not being believed by

  o Police
  o Family
  o Friends, work colleagues

- Stigma of being an assault victim
- Fear of retribution by the assailant
- Shame, guilt, self-blame.

A high index of suspicion around the possibility of assault will enable the doctor to recognize these patients. But what action should the doctor take if they do suspect?

The doctor's response will be dependent on the needs and circumstances of each individual patient. However, there are some general guidelines. If the doctor is able to preplan the discussion, then ensuring the setting is conducive to discussion is of benefit, that is, a quiet room, minimal interruptions, adequate time set aside. The doctor needs to have adequate knowledge of local resources to be able to deal with the information that may be given by the patient. These include follow-on services for counseling, phone numbers for legal advice, housing, local SARC, and the police. Some patients may appreciate direct questions. Many may appreciate a less direct approach. It may be helpful to talk in a rhetorical manner. For example, Doctor:

> 'Some of our patients who have these types of symptoms (chronic pelvic pain, dyspareunia), have in fact been abused in the past. This can sometimes be at the root of their problems' pause.... 'Sometimes they are frightened of talking about it as they think they will get into trouble or that we will call the police and they don't want us to'.... Pause 'What we can do is help them look at their choices, it might be that they would want counselling, or legal advice. Sometimes they just want to talk to someone about it and nothing else and that is fine. We will only do what they want us to do, we would never force them to do anything that they didn't want to.'

This approach, talking about the problem in the third person, allows the patient to explore the pros and cons of disclosing in a safe nonthreatening manner. It is important to give people space to think and to allow them to come back to you at a later point if they feel able to speak out. This can be particularly useful for adolescents. A note of caution, however, is never to make a promise that you are unable to keep. For example, absolute confidentiality when there are child protection issues or that the perpetrator will be caught and punished or even that things will get better.

24.4.   Therapeutic Needs of Rape Victim

- Injuries
- PEP
- Contraception
- Termination
- Crisis support
- Counseling.

It is assumed that the reader will understand the management of injuries, PEP, contraception, and termination. Crisis support and counseling can be provided by referral to the nearest SARC or through Rape Crisis Network Europe.

24.5.   Forensic Aspects of Rape Examination

The purpose of the forensic examination of the sexual assault complainant is for the doctor to be an *independent observer* on behalf of the court and

1. Document any injuries
2. Record any significant negative findings
3. Collect forensic samples.

A forensic examination should be carried out only by examiners who have received thorough training and have a sound understanding of general forensic principles. There is much at stake for both the complainant and the defendant. The doctor must be aware that their notes may be scrutinized many years later, by many professionals, indeed in the highest court in the land. The forensic examination should only take place once fully informed consent has been gained. During the discussion process regarding consent for examination, the complainant should be aware of who may see the documentation, what confidentiality there is, and what else the records may be used for, for example, research, teaching, peer review. The examination should be undertaken after an appropriate history has been taken. This would include the nature of the alleged assault, the actions of the complainant since that time (e.g., changed clothes, washed), and a relevant medical history in order to put any findings into context. This is a detailed process. All note-keeping should be contemporaneous, clear, and legible. It is often useful to use a proforma as an aide memoir.

24.5.1.   Injuries

It is not in the scope of this book to give a detailed account of injuries. Excellent texts already exist on this to which the reader can refer. However, any doctor working with clients who may be assault victims should have a working knowledge of injury types. A misconception held by many is that victims of rape or sexual assault will always have injuries, especially genital injuries, and that they will be extensive. This is not the case. The doctor needs to be aware of this as it is not unusual for a complainant to be concerned that her lack of injuries will discredit her story. The doctor also needs to reassure any accompanying relatives and police that lack of injuries does not dispute the allegations.

Data from studies done at St Mary's, looking at adult females, examined within 48 h of alleged rape, found that less than 25% had any genital injuries.

Indeed, even looking at adolescents who stated that they had not been sexually active prior to the sexual assault, approximately half had no genital injury (2).

24.5.1.1. Injury Types

1. *Bruises*: A bruise is caused by force onto tissue resulting in damage to the blood vessels. Blood then leaks out into the surrounding tissue. When a large collection of blood occurs, this is then a *hematoma*. Bruises may take some time to appear after an injury, particularly if the damaged tissue is deep to the surface of the skin. The blood may then track down tissue planes and appear at the surface, some distance from the site of initial impact. Determining the age of a bruise is fraught with difficulty. Bruises may go through a range of color changes but do so at different rates. Two bruises acquired at the same time can change color differently. Much research has been done on this. So far, the only scientific certainty is that a bruise with yellow coloration is at least 18 h old. The converse is not true; a bruise without yellow coloration may also be 18 h or more old (3). Petecheal hemorrhages are bruises that are 1–2 mm in diameter. These are caused by increased venous pressure. They may be seen in suction injuries "love bites" or strangulation attempts.

2. *Abrasions*: This is an injury which only involves the outer layers of the skin, in lay terms often referred to as a graze or scratch. They are due to the skin moving over a rough surface or vice versa. When the skin is damaged, serum is exuded. This will go on to become a scab. Due to the corrugated nature of the epidermis, they can sometimes involve small blood vessels and therefore bleed. Very superficial abrasions may barely damage the skin and are called *brush* or *scuff* abrasions. When documenting an abrasion, it is important to look for any piling up of the skin at one end of the injury or the other. This may assist in determining the direction of travel of the skin against the rough surface.

3. *Lacerations*: These are caused by a blunt force splitting the full thickness of the skin. They are often confused with incisions. However, there are features of lacerations that should help differentiate, for example, a laceration often has bruised crushed edges that are ragged as the skin has torn. There may be bridges of tissue across them.

4. *Incisions*: These are caused by sharp cutting weapons, such as a knife or glass. There are different types of incision. A stab injury is deeper than it is wide whilst a slash injury is wider than it is deep.

24.5.1.2. Documentation of Injuries

This should be done contemporaneously. Any injury should have the following noted:

Body charts are a useful means of recording injuries. Photo-documentation can also be very useful. Consideration must be given to the secure storage and

Type of injury	Shape
Size	Tenderness
Swelling	Color
Distance from fixed bony point	Signs of healing

confidentiality of any highly sensitive images. It is useful to record any normal findings and important negative findings. For example, if persons say they have been punched several times in the face only a few hours previously, yet they have no facial injuries, then that would be an important negative finding.

The use of a colposcope as a bright, magnified light source is often used during the external genital examination of children.

Bite marks are also fairly common in sexual assaults. If possible these should be photographed by someone trained in bite mark photography. They should be swabbed for saliva. The advice of a Forensic Odontologist should be sought.

24.5.2. Forensic Sampling

This is done on the principle of the French surgeon Edmond Locard, "Every contact leaves a trace" (Figure 24.1).

Depending on the nature of the allegation, time delay between assault and examination, and the consent of the victim, swabs should be taken to try to link the victim to either the crime scene or the alleged assailant, for example, skin swabs where she has been kissed or licked, genital swabs for semen/DNA, mouth swabs if fellatio has occurred. If alcohol or drugs are associated or suspected to be involved in the assault, then toxicology samples are vital, for example, blood, urine, hair samples. Sample collection is a time-consuming specialized process and should only be done after appropriate training to ensure that the chain of evidence is intact and that any such samples can be relied upon in court.

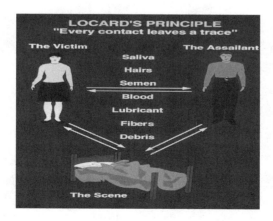

FIGURE 24.1. Locard's principle.

24.5.3.   Court Attendance

Most doctors will feel apprehensive on having to attend court as a witness. There are a few tips that will make the experience more tolerable. The doctor should not be partisan or dogmatic. Read over your contemporaneous records and also any statement made from them prior to attendance. Take to court any original documents, not photocopies.

The following maxim is good advice: Read up, dress up, stand up, speak up then shut up.

For those doctors who are required to attend court on a regular basis, attending a court room skills course is advisable.

24.6.   Psychological Consequences

Individuals will respond to the trauma of rape in various ways. Often victims of acquaintance rape, rather than stranger rape, find it harder to re-establish intimate relationships after the assault. On reflection this is logical. If a person whom the victim had trusted violates that trust, then it throws into question their judgment of other aspects of their life. A betrayal by a trusted friend is far worse than that of a stranger. Another aspect is where the assault occurred. A person who has been raped outside by a stranger may avoid that situation in the future to minimize the risk of another attack. But what options are open to the victim raped by someone known to them in their own home? Where do they now feel safe?

Various other factors will also influence a person's response.

Pre-existing individual variables	Prior psychiatric history
	Previous exposure to trauma, including sexual abuse
Stressor variables	Unpredictability
	Suddenness
	Threat to life (real or perceived)
	Receiving intentional harm
	Relationship to perpetrator
Responses of external world	Lack of support
	Institutional avoidance
	Victim blaming
Specific experiences of the individual	A sense of hopelessness and resignation
	Attributions
	Cultural beliefs

24.6.1.   Rape Trauma Syndrome

This was first described by Burgess and Holmstrom in 1974(5). It is a form of PTSD. PTSD (see Appendix) is a *normal* human reaction to an *abnormal* event. Rape trauma syndrome is recognized to have four stages, each may involve physical, psychological, and behavioral symptoms. The length of each phase will vary and people may move back and forth between stages.

1. Acute phase
2. Intermediate phase
3. Reorganization phase
4. Integration/resolution phase.

1. *Acute phase*: This is characterized by a disorganization of lifestyle and can last from 1 to 6 weeks. There are a range of symptoms which may effect the way in which a victim responds. This may account for the "unexpected" response a doctor may note in a rape victim. In this immediate phase the victim may respond in one of three ways:

   a. Controlled—subdued feelings, masked, or hidden
   b. Expressed—restless, tense, crying
   c. Mixed—a combination of the above two, so 1 minute laughing, the next crying or sobbing. This may be confusing for both the victims and their carers.

Their responses can be categorized into three groups.

Psychological	Physical	Behavioral
Loss of control/powerlessness	Sleeping difficulties and nightmares	Unable to go out alone and/or with others
Fear	Eating disorders	Change in personal hygiene routine
Shame	Symptoms specific to assault	Carrying on as "normal"
Guilt "I should have done something"	Possible physical injury	
Denial	May present at GP, accident, and emergency, family planning, etc., with a range of symptoms and not disclose rape or sexual assault	
Anger		
Frustration		
Numbness		

2. *Intermediate phase*: This can last from 6 weeks to 6 months or more, possibly a lifetime. There is some readjustment to normal life but also continued changes to lifestyle. There may be persistent symptoms such as nausea and headaches and gynecological symptoms. Phobias may start to develop or obsessional compulsive disorders. There may be spontaneous flashbacks, fear of sex, fear of men, or global fears. There may be re-experiencing of the assault triggered by sights, sounds, or smells.

3. *Reorganization phase*: Here the victim may be experiencing any of the symptoms mentioned in phase 1 or 2 and some patterns may now be well established. The victim may be appear "normal" until an event triggers off some reaction, for example, a TV program or the anniversary of the event. They may be depressed, hypervigilant to danger, and have diminished capacity to enjoy life. Factors which will influence the reorganization process will be the nature of the assault, the developmental stage of the victim, the social and cultural background of the victim, and so on.
4. *Integration/resolution phase*: Here the rape becomes another bad event in the victim's life. They may resolve the rape and the effect it has had on their life.

In Burgess and Holmstrom's study, they recontacted victims 4–6 years after the rape. Thirty-seven percent felt that their recovery had taken "months," 37% felt it had taken "years," and 26% felt that they had not recovered from the assault.

Psychological consequences of childhood sexual abuse. Depression and anxiety are common short-term effects of childhood sexual abuse. Other sequelae include behavioral problems such as sexualized behavior, social withdrawal, sleep disturbance, acting-out, and anger. Deliberate self-harm may also be a sign of sexual abuse. Long-term effects of CSA have shown that the adult survivors are more prone to mental health problems, including depression, anxiety disorder, substance abuse, sexual dysfunction, and interpersonal difficulties (4).

When the sexual abuse is repeated over a period of time, especially in the context of what should be a trusting relationship, for example, father–daughter, the psychological sequelae can be greatest.

24.7.   Contact Details, Useful Web sites, and so on

- The Journal of Clinical Forensic Medicine
  http://www.harcourt-international.com/journals/jcfm
- Faculty of Forensic and Legal Medicine. This is new, no web site at present, should be one soon
- Diploma in Medical Jurisprudence

  The Worshipful Society of Apothecaries
  registrar@apothecaries.org
  http://www.apothecaries.org.uk
  0207 236 1180

- Masters or Diploma in Clinical Forensic Medicine and Bioethics

  University of Central Lancashire
  tfarrell@uclan.ac.uk
  01772 892792

- Royal Society of Medicine

  http://www.rsm.ac.uk
  christine.davenport:rsm.ac.uk
  0207 290 3935

- Association of Forensic Physicians

  aps@glasconf.demon.co.uk
  http://www.apsweb.org.uk
  01355 244101

- British Association of Forensic Odontologists

  http://www.bafo.org.uk

- British Association for Sexual Health and HIV
- http://www.bashh.org
- http://www.nice.org.uk/pdf/CG026NICEguideline.pdf.
- Rape Crisis Network Europe

  rcni@eircom.net
  http://www.rcne.com

References

1. Crime in England and Wales 2004/5. Home Office Statistical Bulletin; July 2005. http://www.homeoffice.gov.uk/rds.
2. White C, McLean I. Adolescent complainants of sexual assault; injury patterns in virgin and non-virgin groups. *J Clin Forensic Med.* 2006;13:172–180.
3. Langlois NEI, Gresham GA. The ageing of bruises: a review and study of the colour changes with time. *Forensic Sci Int.* 1991;50:227–238.
4. Browne A, Finkelhor D. Impact of child sexual abuse: a review of the research. *Psychol Bull.* 1986;99:66–77.
5. Burgess AW, Holmstrom L. Rape trauma syndrome. *Am J Psychiatry.* 1974;131(9):981–985.

Appendix: Diagnostic Criteria from Diagnostic and Statistical Manual for Mental Disorders DSM-IV

Posttraumatic Stress Disorder

A. The person has been exposed to a traumatic event in which both of the following were present:

1. The person experienced, witnessed, or was confronted with an event or events that involved actual or threatened death or serious injury or a threat to the physical integrity of self or others.

2. The person's response involved intense fear, helplessness, or horror.

   Note: In children, this may be expressed instead by disorganized or agitated behavior.

B. The traumatic event is persistently re-experienced in one (or more) of the following ways:

1. Recurrent and intrusive distressing recollections of the event, including images, thoughts, and/or perceptions

   Note: In young children, repetitive play may occur in which these or other aspects of the trauma are expressed.

2. Recurrent distressing dreams of the event

   Note: In young children, there may be frightening dreams without recognizable content.

3. Acting or feeling as if the traumatic event was recurring (includes a sense of reliving the experience, illusions, hallucinations, and/or dissociative flashback episodes, including those that occur on awakening or when intoxicated)

   Note: In young children, trauma-specific re-enactment may occur.

4. Intense psychological distress at exposure to internal or external cues that symbolize or resemble an aspect of the traumatic event
5. Physiological reactivity on exposure to internal or external cues that symbolize or resemble an aspect of the traumatic event.

C. Persistent avoidance of stimuli associated with the trauma and numbing of general responsiveness (not present before the trauma), as indicated by at least three of the following:

1. Efforts to avoid thoughts, feelings, and/or conversations associated with the trauma
2. Efforts to avoid activities, places, and/or people that arouse recollections of the trauma
3. Inability to recall an important aspect of the trauma
4. Markedly diminished interest or participation in significant activities
5. Feeling of detachment or estrangement from others
6. Restricted range of affect (e.g., inability to have loving feelings)
7. Sense of a foreshortened future (e.g., does not expect to have a career, marriage, children, or a normal life span).

D. Persistent symptoms of increased arousal (not present before the trauma), as indicated by at least two of the following:

1. Difficulty falling or staying asleep
2. Irritability or outbursts of anger
3. Difficulty concentrating
4. Hypervigilance
5. Exaggerated startle response.

E. Duration of the disturbance (symptoms in criteria B, C, and D) is more than 1 month.
F. The disturbance causes clinically significant distress and/or impairment in social, occupational, and/or other important areas of functioning.

> *Acute*: Duration of symptoms is less than 3 months
> *Chronic*: Duration of symptoms is more than 3 months
> *Delayed onset*: Onset of symptoms is at least 6 months after the incident.

25
Chronic Pelvic Pain

R. William Stones

25.1. How Has This Patient Ended Up in My Clinic?

Chronic pelvic pain (CPP) is common in the general population, as shown by surveys principally in the USA and the UK, but only a subpopulation come to medical attention by consulting their general practitioner, and a further subgroup will be referred on for hospital assessment. Working backward and taking a "'chronic pelvic pain" threshold of 6 months' symptom duration in order to exclude more acute or isolated problems such as dysmenorrhea or dyspareunia, we estimated that around 5% of new referrals to general gynecology clinics were for CPP in Southampton. At the level of primary medical care, the best data are those from the Oxford research group. Consulting patterns were studied using the UK national data from 284,162 women aged 12–70 who had a general practice contact in 1991 (1). Contacts over the subsequent 5 years were analyzed and showed a monthly prevalence rate of 21.5/1000 and a monthly incidence rate of 1.58/1000. The prevalence rate for general practice consultations is comparable to other "common" conditions such as migraine, back pain, and asthma. The gynecological stereotype is that CPP is a problem of the mid reproductive years, but in these primary care based data older women were more prominent: for example, the rate was 18.2/1000 in the 15–20 age group and 27.6/1000 in women over 60 years of age. This association was thought be due to persistence of symptoms in older women, the median duration of symptoms being 13.7 months in 13 to 20-year olds and 20.2 months in women over the age of 60 (2). It is clear that future population-based studies need to include older women.

Going one step further back to population surveys, in the USA 17,927 households were contacted by telephone, yielding 5325 women aged 18–50 who agreed to participate, and of these 925 reported pelvic pain of at least 6 months' duration, including pain within the past 3 months (3). Having excluded those pregnant or postmenopausal and those with only cycle-related pain, 773/5263 (14.7%) were identified as suffering from CPP. From the UK, a postal survey approached 2016 women randomly selected from the Oxfordshire Health Authority register of 141,400 women aged 18–49 (4). CPP was defined as recurrent pain of at least 6 months' duration, unrelated to periods, intercourse, or pregnancy. For the survey, a "case" was defined as a woman with CPP in the previous 3 months, and on this basis the prevalence was 483/2016 (24.0%). It is probably inappropriate to exclude women with "isolated" dysmenorrhea or dyspareunia from data collection, as while it is confusing and inappropriate to classify their problem simply as CPP, analysis of the Oxfordshire survey showed strong statistical associations between CPP and both dysmenorrhea and dyspareunia.

As indicated above, many women do not seek care despite having symptoms: among 483 women with CPP participating in the Oxfordshire population study discussed above, 195 (40.4%) had not sought a medical consultation, 127 (26.3%) reported a past consultation, and 139 (28.8%) reported a recent consultation for pain (5). The US population-based study discussed above also drew attention to the large number of women who have troublesome symptoms but do not seek medical attention: 75% of this sample had not seen a health-care provider in the previous 3 months. It might be thought that not seeking care would be an indicator of milder symptoms, and indeed in the US study those who did seek medical attention had higher pain and lower general health scores than those who did not. We noted a gradient of deteriorating scores for the mental and physical components of the SF-36 health-related quality of life considering those from the Oxfordshire study who had not sought care through to those who had, through to those seen in general hospital gynecology clinics (6).

Our understanding of the individual factors that lead women to seek care for CPP is very limited. One can hypothesize that pain intensity might be important or the extent of quality of life impact, but without the benefit of detailed community-based qualitative research these remain speculative. There is a range of other social and psychological drivers to care seeking that need to be taken into account, as well as biological or disease factors.

25.2.   A Conceptual Framework

It is useful to illustrate a biopsychosocial approach in CPP by considering a condition which can be a normal part of reproductive experience, but which can become a medical problem and shade into the spectrum of CPP. Dysmenorrhea is an extremely common experience for menstruating women, of whom perhaps half self-medicate with over-the-counter analgesics at least intermittently, and around 15% are thought to seek medical advice for severe or troublesome symptoms. A smaller subgroup finds that "dysmenorrhea" starts to mean pain lasting for half or more of the menstrual cycle and is associated with substantial disruption of normal function, so that one can then consider it as CPP. Figure 25.1 illustrates some of the factors that might contribute to "dysmenorrhea." Current pathology might be relevant: adenomyosis may cause heavy painful periods but only be confirmed by the pathologist following hysterectomy; currently, only a tiny minority of cases are positively confirmed using MRI owing to very limited access to this form of imaging in routine clinical practice. Endometriosis is much more amenable to positive diagnosis via laparoscopy, and other possible causes include cervical stenosis (now much less common since knife cone biopsy has been superseded by diathermy loop excision) and interstitial cystitis, which may be associated with a wide range of pelvic pain symptoms (7).

There may be no currently active disease, but past problems may have left residual pain and tenderness giving rise to clinically significant "dysmenorrhea." Examples include previously treated endometriosis, chlamydial infection, recurrent urinary tract infection, and obstetric injury (while noting that primary "dysmenorrhea" tends to improve following childbirth). Our understanding of the neurophysiology of visceral sensation is much less developed than that of somatic nociception, but there is clear animal experimental evidence for processes such as central sensitization of afferents following noxious stimulation in both bladder and vagina (8). Normal physiology also plays a part: strong uterine contractions are associated with menstrual cramps, and spasm of pelvic floor musculature can maintain the duration of pain symptoms.

Sociocultural context plays a part in the understanding and interpretation of bodily pain: there is a literature to support positive constructs of "pain mastery" in labor pain and there may be a similarly positive dimension for some in "dysmenorrhea," representing a reassuring manifestation of normal reproductive function. Consulting behavior is heavily influenced by messages from family members about the significance of symptoms, and previous adverse experiences such as abuse may play a part. Finally, these various influences are mediated through psychological processes including vigilance, motivation, and catastrophizing, all of which are amenable to formal psychometric study.

The conceptual framework presented in Figure 25.1 has a gray boundary around what might be regarded as constitutional or background factors that

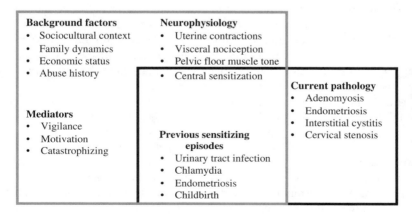

Figure 25.1. Conceptual framework for dysmenorrhoea

might predispose to care seeking, while the black boundary might include the conventional medical notion of "pathology." These boundaries are presented to allow mapping of the present discussion to conventional disease concepts and also to illustrate how arbitrary such distinctions really are. In practical terms, the traditional distinction between "primary" and "secondary" dysmenorrhea is clearly seen to be a gross oversimplification, and indeed this is an element of medical tradition that is no longer useful.

25.3.   Assessment in the Clinic

The following are steps that can be followed to maximize concordance between the patient and gynecologist. Firstly, the history needs to focus on the impact of symptoms as well as their presence: as medical students learn, an uncritical systems review can generate a long list of symptoms that are immediately filtered by the experienced history taker. But in a surgically oriented specialty there is a particular imperative in determining with the patient whether a particular symptom is a real problem, especially before embarking on invasive tests or treatment. It is good practice to ask directly about the patient's objectives for the consultation: is she primarily in search of symptom control, or of diagnosis, advice, and explanation? It is sometimes surprising to hear an individual with apparently disabling symptoms explain why she is reluctant to take painkillers, for fear that these will mask some hitherto undetected disease.

Secondly, the history needs to be broad enough to include the range of potentially relevant issues as raised in the conceptual framework. Questionnaires and rating scales can be particularly useful for formal assessment of pain intensity and symptom impact, as well as mood disturbance. A "pack" sent to patients before the consultation can be efficient, and also provides the opportunity to give the patient some information about pelvic pain, and what might happen during the consultation. Recent RCOG guidelines for the initial management of CPP are now available for download (see http://www.rcog.org.uk) and a corresponding information sheet for patients will shortly be available. Other often neglected points for history taking include full details of gastrointestinal and urinary systems, where there is huge scope for misdiagnosis leading to inappropriate investigation.

Thirdly, physical examination should be used as a tool to confirm or refute likely diagnoses suggested from the history. It is not uncommon for the initial impression to be changed considerably by the findings on physical examination. For example, a patient presenting with pain in the right iliac fossa associated with a 4 cm "cyst" seen on ultrasound might turn out to have an abdominal wall "trigger point" arising from an ilioinguinal nerve entrapment, and an entirely non-tender pelvic examination, strongly suggesting that the "cyst" is functional and of no relevance. By contrast, a patient minimizing the impact of her dysmenorrhea and tolerating painful intercourse with stoicism might turn out to have nodularity in the pouch of Douglas and restricted mobility of the uterus, suggesting gross endometriosis. In patients presenting with CPP, especially with an acute exacerbation, a cautious one-finger digital examination may be all that can be tolerated, and the speculum examination for endocervical swabs although important might need to be deferred. A two-finger digital examination is almost always inappropriate.

25.4.   Does the Patient Have a Problem Or Is It the Doctor?

CPP seems to be a problematic condition for both general practitioners and gynecologists. Some specific medical attitudinal issues were identified in qualitative research (9) and it would seem to be the individual doctor's consulting style that is associated with favorable or unfavorable outcomes in CPP rather than obvious variables such as grade or gender of the doctor (10). Women well remember their initial hospital consultations, and while the value of information materials has been emphasized above, it was the doctor's affect and the extent to which expectations were met that led to positive recollections of consultations at follow-up, rather than the amount of information provided (11). From these findings it is appropriate to reiterate the importance of establishing the patient's own goals for the consultation at the outset so that her expectations can more effectively be met; at the same time, less experienced or more junior practitioners can be reassured that there is no magic formula and encouraged to have the confidence to draw on their consulting skills, perhaps acquired in other medical settings, and use these to bring about a good outcome.

25.5.   Commonly Encountered Challenges

25.5.1.   Does This Patient Need a Laparoscopy?

There is conflicting research evidence as to whether a negative diagnostic laparoscopy is useful in providing symptom relief through reassurance. This can be counterproductive, as many women are very distressed when told at the postoperative ward round that there is no "pathology" to be seen and will interpret such statements as dismissive. Preprocedure information to set the likely outcomes in context can be useful so that expectations are not inappropriately raised. Showing pictures of the procedure may add to rather than relieve the anxiety (12). More fundamentally, it is important to ensure that laparoscopy is offered as part of a diagnostic plan based on the clinical picture. It is often preferable practice to defer this investigation to see how the pattern of symptoms evolves.

25.5.2. How Can I Encourage This Patient to Seek Psychological Help?

Across the UK health services, access to clinical psychology is extremely limited. For example, services are sometimes provided for very closely defined patient groups such as those with alcohol dependence or a history of sexual abuse. The research evidence in support of cognitive approaches to pain management is very good, but access to psychology in UK pain clinics is nevertheless very patchy (13). Even where a local service is available, many women with CPP respond negatively to the suggestion of referral, receiving an unintended message of dismissal. Perhaps the only practical way forward is to include the psychologist in a multidisciplinary assessment set-up, where patients are reassured that they are not being dismissed, and they can receive a greater depth of information provision and its consistent repetition by different members of the team. Concepts in chronic pain such as the Gate Theory can provide a useful structure for patients as well as doctors to understand the interactions between psychological state and pain perception. A small subgroup of patients will need liaison psychiatry referral for indications such as potential self-harm, psychiatric adverse effects of medication, or underlying psychiatric conditions such as somatization disorder. Again, there are practical problems in overcoming the stigma associated with such referral.

25.5.3. What Are the Principles of Chronic Pain Management, and Will My Patient Accept Them?

Women with CPP that has not resolved after initial investigation and treatment often find it difficult to reorientate their expectations toward chronic pain management, and away from a further quest for diagnosis and cure. This reorientation is critical to the success of a pain management program, as the active participation of the patient is essential. Also, positive outcomes in pain management are often considered to lie less in symptom relief than improvement in functional capacity and coping skills. When a patient is ready to accept this approach, she can be supported by regular "time contingent" rather than "pain contingent" follow-up. Continuity of care is very important, as it is unsatisfactory for the patient to have to reiterate the whole story for a new doctor. Sometimes this can more readily be delivered by a nurse rather than medical follow-up. The approach just described is wholly at variance with the structure of most gynecological clinics, where the emphasis is on rapid progression to a surgical procedure followed by discharge, so the pain clinic may be a better setting. There is, however, a need to recognize that some women will require ongoing gynecological as well as pain clinic support, for example, in severe endometriosis or when decisions about preserving fertility change. In these circumstances, joint consulting and decision-making is very valuable.

25.5.4.   What About Sex?

Should dyspareunia be considered a psychosomatic or even psychiatric diagnosis? The historical answer is in the affirmative, codified in DSM-IV: "Dyspareunia (Not Due to a General Medical Condition) 302.76." Seen from both a chronic pain and disease-oriented gynecological perspective there are many questions around this way of thinking. Most especially, when do we know that dyspareunia is not "due to a general medical condition"? As discussed above, there is an association at the population level between dyspareunia, dysmenorrhea, and CPP. In a large-scale population survey from India there was symptom overlap between dyspareunia, urinary leaking, and urinary sensory symptoms, but each had a distinct pattern of social and demographic associations (14). There is no reason to think that the full range of elements of the conceptual framework described for dysmenorrhea would not also apply here. For example, chlamydial infection might have left a patient with a "tender uterus" owing to central sensitization of visceral afferents, and her tendency to vigilance and catastrophizing has ensured that this sensitivity is all too evident as dyspareunia. But will hysterectomy relieve the problem, or should the emphasis be on psychosexual counseling or cognitive approaches? Here, there are more questions than answers.

25.6.   Conclusion

In this chapter the author has tried to convey an approach rather than a manual of treatment: for the latter the reader is directed to the current RCOG guideline, the main gynecology texts, and the Cochrane review (15). An emphasis on careful clinical method is critical, including a full history with details of symptoms from all relevant organs, a physical examination that aims to localize tenderness, and cautious use of relevant investigations. Meeting the expectations of patients in a supportive manner, even where the diagnosis remains elusive, will set the best conditions for a positive outcome.

References

1. Zondervan KT, Yudkin PL, Vessey MP, Dawes MG, Barlow DH, Kennedy SH. Prevalence and incidence of chronic pelvic pain in primary care: evidence from a national general practice database. Br J Obstet Gynaecol. 1999;106:1149–1155.
2. Zondervan KT, Yudkin PL, Vessey MP, Dawes MG, Barlow DH. Kennedy SH., Patterns of diagnosis and referral in women consulting for chronic pelvic pain in UK primary care. Br J Obstet Gynaecol. 1999;106:1156–1161.
3. Mathias SD, Kuppermann M, Liberman RF, Lipschutz RC, Steege JF. Chronic pelvic pain: prevalence, health-related quality of life, and economic correlates, Obstet Gynecol. 1996;87:321–327.

4. Zondervan KT, Yudkin PL, Vessey MP, et al. Chronic pelvic pain in the community—symptoms, investigations, and diagnoses. *Am J Obstet Gynecol.* 2001;184(6):1149–1155.

5. Zondervan KT, Yudkin PL, Vessey MP, et al. The community prevalence of chronic pelvic pain in women and associated illness behaviour. *Br J Gen Pract.* 2001;51(468):541–547.

6. Stones RW. Chronic pelvic pain (Chapter 60). In: Shaw RW, Soutter WP, Stanton SL, eds. *Gynaecology.* 3rd ed. Edinburgh: Churchill Livingstone; 2003.

7. Parsons CL, Dell J, Stanford EJ, Bullen M, Kahn BS, Willems JJ. The prevalence of interstitial cystitis in gynecologic patients with pelvic pain, as detected by intravesical potassium sensitivity. *Am J Obstet Gynecol.* 2002;187:1395–1400

8. Stones RW. Female genital pain (Chapter 17). In: Fillingim RB, ed. *Sex Gender and Pain. Progress in Pain Research and Management,* vol. 17. Seattle: IASP Press, 2000.

9. Selfe SA, van Vugt M, Stones RW. Chronic gynaecological pain: an exploration of medical attitudes. *Pain.* 1998;77:215–225.

10. Selfe SA, Matthews Z, Stones RW. Factors influencing outcome in consultations for chronic pelvic pain. *J Womens Health.* 1998;7:1041–1048.

11. Stones RW, Lawrence WT, Selfe SA. Lasting impressions: influence of the initial hospital consultation for chronic pelvic pain on dimensions of patient satisfaction at follow-up. *J Psychosom Res.* 2006;60:163–167.

12. Onwude L, Thornton J, Morley S, Lilleyman J, Currie I, Lilford R. A randomised trial of photographic reinforcement during postoperative counselling after diagnostic laparoscopy for pelvic pain. *Eur J Obstet Gynecol Reprod Biol.* 2004;112:89–94.

13. Stones RW, Price C. Health services for women with chronic pelvic pain. *J R Soc Med.* 2002;95:531–535.

14. Padmadas SS, Stones RW. Matthews Z. Dyspareunia and urinary sensory symptoms in India: population based study. *J Sex Med.* 2006;3:114–120.

15. Stones W, Cheong Y, Howard FM. Interventions for treating chronic pelvic pain in women. *The Cochrane Database of Systematic Reviews 2005,* Issue 3. Art. No.: CD000387. DOI: 10.1002/14651858.CD000387.

26
Communicating with Cancer Patients

Dimitrios Doumplis and J. Richard Smith

The diagnosis of cancer is a devastating event for the individual with many different consequences both physical and psychological. Emotions such as anger, anxiety, and guilt affect the relationship of the patient with both her family and social environment. Whatever the professional or educational level of the woman, she will always feel isolated and helpless with numerous questions and need for support. The degree of distress depends on the specific meaning of cancer to the individual, her previous exposure to the diagnosis, her coping mechanisms, and the support from those around her.

There are certain characteristics of gynecological cancer which should be considered in order to have some understanding of how the patient feels about herself as a woman and with respect to childbearing, before planning specific therapy. The uterus, vagina, and ovaries are directly connected with femininity, motherhood, and sexuality; so cancer of the genital organs often results in feelings of guilt relating to sexual or reproductive activities such as venereal diseases, abortions, or extramarital activities. Understanding of these issues must be part of counseling for both the patient and her partner in order to prevent sexual dysfunction and encourage resumption of sexual activity. Concerns about whether genital cancer is contagious or sexual intercourse might prevent healing or result in recurrence should be clarified and reassurance given.

Having had a previous positive or negative experience with similar situations, either in herself or her environment, could be of vital importance in trying to assess the emotional status of a cancer patient. This emphasizes the importance of taking an accurate medical and family history, as it indicates the direction for psychotherapeutic intervention.

The type of the patient's personality must be considered very carefully by the oncologist who is trying to establish a relationship with the cancer patient. The levels of her dependence, her suspicion, her isolation, or self-punishment are crucial in the way her coping mechanisms adapt. The sense of loss that cancer itself represents is enormous with several aspects such as loss of autonomy, good health, self-esteem, relationships, employment, and social status. Some people tend to respond to all these with anger while others tend to deny the reality, resulting in delays in terms of diagnosis or treatment.

Good patient–doctor communication is vital because it enhances a patient's experience of and satisfaction with care, and increases informed consent and cooperation. There are three different aims: creating a healthy interpersonal relationship, exchanging information, and the treatment itself—all related decisions. Doctors in gynecological oncology must build a relationship with the patient based on the human qualities of trust and mutual respect, friendliness, genuine interest, and acceptance. They must aim to transmit information to the patient in a way that the patient determines the nature and the depth of the conversation, and they must support the patient and her family throughout her ordeal. The doctor must give time to allow the patient to describe her symptoms, concerns, and preferences and effectively present the scientific details regarding the disease and treatment options in a comprehensive way.

Making treatment-related decisions presupposes exchange of information which should be tailored to the patient's needs or values, taking into account the individual's variability in terms of personality, health status, and sociocultural background. Doctors must be able to make a rapid assessment of personality types and then utilize such information therapeutically. The treatment options should be clarified; benefits, dangers, possible side effects, and so on should be thoroughly discussed before reaching a consensus regarding the preferred option. Most patients feel that actively participating in the treatment decision-making results in them having control over the disease itself.

Support is extremely important for the cancer patient. Sometimes the relatives' view of what is best for the patient is at variance with what the doctor thinks appropriate, and it needs extensive discussion with them in order to agree on the best management. Cultural differences can make things particularly difficult.

The first task is to break the news of the diagnosis to the patient. The setting should be planned carefully involving an appropriate place with privacy, the presence of right people, and the right way of presenting the bad news. The patient and the preferred supporter should be present, and preferably a specialist nurse. It is always difficult to break bad news because distress makes us all feel uncomfortable. This may result in "cushioning" the bad news by avoiding discussion of such difficult topics as prognosis or falsely reassuring the patient that the situation will improve. Doctors have to walk a narrow path between the truth and not destroying hope or being too blunt. They have to be realistic but also positive so as not to give false hope but at the same time to preserve an optimistic feeling. Time must be given to the patient to take in the situation and it is probably best to avoid giving statistics when asked about prognosis and chances.

After breaking the bad news and coping with the first reactions, the oncologist must proceed to the second difficult task which is to discuss the treatment plan and prognosis. We have found a model called the four-cusp approach very helpful in this respect (see Table 26.1).

TABLE 26.1. The four-cusp (cusps A to D) approach to doctor–patient communication in cancer care

	Cusp A ⟷	Cusp B ——⊬→	Cusp C ——→	Cusp D
Status	Potentially curable	Living with cancer	Preterminal	Terminal
Duration	Weeks to years	Months to years	Weeks to months	Days
Treatment	Radical surgery	Adjuvant or palliative	Supportive care	Terminal care
	Adjuvant therapy	Chemotherapy or radiotherapy		
Aims	Cure	Prolong survival	Improve quality of life	Improve quality of dying
	Prolong survival	Improve quality of life		End-of-life issues

Golden Rules

1. Never say never—if you believe and act as if the situation is hopeless, it is!

    You never know how the patient will respond to treatment unless you treat them!

2. Never tell lies.
3. Always tell the truth.
4. Always tell everybody the same thing, that is, the truth.
5. Take the team with you—everybody—the patient, her family, the nurses, and junior doctors must all be onside.
6. Ask the patient what is troubling her, do not presume to read the patient's mind.

26.1. The "Four-Cusp" Approach

26.1.1. Cusp A: Potentially Curable/Cured

The first cusp applies to most patients from the first clinic visit when the surgeon imparts the probable diagnosis and discusses with the patient the plan of action to achieve staging and hopefully removal of the tumor. An honest appraisal of the possibilities is required, coupled with a plan of action. This should include date of surgery, length of time in hospital, and when final and definitive histological and cytological reports will become available. The aim is to achieve these results within 2 weeks of the first visit. The concept of cancer staging should be explained and that the stage and type of tumor will influence the necessity for further treatment with radiotherapy or chemotherapy. If treatment by surgery alone is achieved there is usually the presumption of cure, which can only be confirmed by the passage of time. A high level of positivity and an optimistic approach are recommended both before and after surgery for those with complete resection of tumor, although the need for careful follow-up and the possibility of relapse should be discussed.

Case 1

A woman is referred to the gynecological oncology clinic with post-coital bleeding and a suspected cervical cancer. On examination a small cervical tumor is found which is approximately 2–3 cm in diameter. The uterus and cervix are mobile and there are no other detectable abnormalities. A colposcopy and biopsy are performed.

Following the examination, the consultation should continue, usually by asking the patient if she has any idea what the diagnosis might be.

This is generally a good juncture to sensitively discuss the possibility of a diagnosis of cancer and that the biopsy will confirm or exclude this within the next few days. It is then possible to say that the initial examination suggests that this is eminently curable cancer and to outline the plan of action. Explain that there are four stages of cervical cancer, that stage 1 is the best and stage 4 the worst. Explain that you believe the tumor to be stage 1 and therefore highly curable, probably by surgery alone, but possibly requiring further treatment with chemoradiotherapy. Ask the patient to have her next of kin present at the post-staging ward round if they are not there at the clinic. The patient should be invited to ask any questions and encouraged to write down any questions she thinks of when she is at home and to ask them when she is admitted. A good practice is to copy the letter written to the referring doctor to the patients themselves. Involvement of the clinical nurse specialist affords the patient a point of contact and invaluable support.

The patient will have the usual prestaging investigations such as radiographic scans and will then be admitted for a staging examination under anesthesia. These findings along with the histology are communicated to the patient that day. The date for radical hysterectomy is then set and an explanation of this given, including the prognostic significance of nodal status and its impact on likely adjuvant therapy. To complement the discussion the patient may be provided with information leaflets. It should be explained that, although a good idea of where the patient stands immediately following surgery is known, definitive answers require histological confirmation and that usually takes 7 days. The operation is then performed and the findings explained to the patient either the same day or the following day. A few days later the full histological picture is given.

Scenario 1: the histology report shows complete resection of a 2 cm well-differentiated squamous carcinoma with adequate resection margins and negative nodes (Cusp A).

This patient can be told that you believe a cure has been achieved and while long-term follow-up is warranted you expect to see her in the clinic for the next 5–10 years following which time she may be discharged from care once "fit and well."

Scenario 2: the histology report shows complete resection of a moderately differentiated squamous cervical carcinoma with 3 positive metastatic nodes out of 40 removed.

This information is imparted and the patient told that although there is complete removal of the tumor, further treatment is required with combination chemoradiotherapy. Such patients can be told that you believe a cure is likely but that there is no denying they do have a higher chance of relapse than if their nodes had been negative. The concept of adjuvant therapy following radical surgery may be explained as an insurance policy to mop up any tumor cells that might have escaped the surgery (see table above).

Case 2

A general practitioner refers a 55-year-old woman with abdominal swelling, which she has noticed in the last few weeks. She has no other symptoms. Abdominal examination suggests the presence of ascites. Vaginal examination reveals a mass arising from the right adnexa, probably ovarian in origin, and nodules are felt in the pouch of Douglas.

The patient is informed that there are findings suggestive of an ovarian mass and that it requires urgent investigation. The patient should be told that you suspect cancer and that the investigations you are about to request will aid in making the diagnosis.

Investigations include hematological and biochemical tests, tumor markers, an ultrasound scan with color flow Doppler, and a CT scan of the abdomen and pelvis to detect any lymphadenopathy. The patient is reviewed shortly thereafter and the risk of malignancy index calculated. The findings are highly suggestive of a stage 1c ovarian cancer.

Staging of ovarian cancer is explained to the patient, together with the three possible outcomes of the operation that is required:

1. Complete macroscopic resection of tumor
2. Resection of tumor down to nodules less than 1–2 cm in diameter
3. Inadequate debulking

The latter two possibilities seem unlikely bearing in mind the optimistic findings of the investigations. Full staging will be complete a few days after surgery when all the cytological and histological results become available. Patient consent is obtained for a total abdominal hysterectomy, bilateral salpingo-oophorectomy, omentectomy, and debulking as required.

Scenario 1: at surgery a smooth-walled cyst is found with some free fluid in the pelvis. There is no evidence of any tumor elsewhere in the abdomen on macroscopic examination.

Postoperatively the patient can be told that she falls into the first category (fully macroscopically resected tumor) and a few days later the histological report confirms a well-differentiated ovarian epithelial carcinoma, with negative peritoneal cytology. The patient is informed that she has a stage 1a tumor and should have no further problems. She remains at *Cusp A* (see table on p. 299).

Scenario 2: At surgery on opening the abdomen 500 ml of straw-colored fluid is noted and some fluid is sent for cytology. Abdominal exploration reveals small tumor deposits on the diaphragm and a small omental deposit. A total hysterectomy, bilateral salpingo-oophorectomy, and omentectomy are performed with minimal residual tumor left at the end of the operation.

The patient is informed postoperatively that she falls into the second category with tumor debulked to less than 1 cm, and that she probably has a stage 3 tumor depending on results and almost certainly will require further treatment. A few days later the histological and cytological reports confirm that the clinical impression was correct. The patient is informed and chemotherapy is arranged. She should be informed that she has now entered the *Cusp B*, "living with cancer," and that she may regain *Cusp A* following chemotherapy and the elapse of 5 years in complete remission, but only time will tell (see table on p. 299).

26.1.2.   Cusp B: Living with Cancer

The second cusp is for treated patients who are in remission but who may not be cured, that is, "living with cancer," but not terminal. A positive approach is appropriate, but the long-term goals are less optimistic. The patient should be informed that it is impossible to determine how long she will remain in remission; however, many patients are alive several years after chemotherapy and some have returned to Cusp A, that is, presumed cured. Sadly some patients may not survive so long. The longer the patient is in complete remission the better the outlook. Unfortunately neither the patient nor the doctor knows which category she is in until time elapses, but the importance of following through with treatment must be appreciated.

The role of psychology, religion, and spirituality in the care of the cancer patient is the provision of an additional coping mechanism. They have no impact on the disease prognosis but patients utilizing any of the above appear to cope better with their cancer.

The patient described in *Case 2, scenario 2* above then undergoes chemotherapy.

Scenario I: the patient goes into complete remission for 5 years.

This patient is one of the lucky ones and is presumed cured (*Cusp A*)(see table on p. 299).

Scenario 2: the patient goes into complete remission which lasts for 3 years and then at the follow-up in the oncology clinic she is found to have an elevated Ca125 and a palpable nodule in the pouch of Douglas. Staging investigations reveal radiological evidence of a solitary nodule. She therefore has a second laparotomy with complete excision of the tumor, followed by a further course of chemotherapy. Again the patient enters complete remission.

She can be told that she appears to have a relatively non-aggressive tumor and can expect to remain in the Cusp B for a good time longer (see table on p. 299).

Scenario 3: following the first-line chemotherapy the patient achieves a partial remission, which lasts for 5 months when she is seen at follow-up in the oncology clinic with abdominal swelling and an elevated Ca125 level. Radiological investigation suggests that there are widespread metastatic peritoneal nodules.

This patient may be given the choice of whether to be observed until she develops symptoms or to have second-line chemotherapy. The role of chemotherapy is to palliate symptoms and improve the quality of life rather than prolong survival in this context and the balance between the possible benefits and toxicities of the chemotherapy should be explored with the patient. The patient declines further chemotherapy and then deteriorates over the next few weeks. She needs to be informed that she has moved to *Cusp C* (see table on p. 299).

26.1.3.   *Cusp C: Preterminal Phase*

The third cusp applies to patients with virtually no chance of cure, who have entered the "preterminal phase." It is important that the patient is made aware that she has a limited time left to live and that she is given the opportunity to "put her house in order"–see relatives and friends, make a will, and so on. No patient should ever be told that there is nothing more that can be done. She should be informed that while she has virtually no chance of cure, there are various measures available to ameliorate symptoms of pain, nausea, or bowel dysfunction. The therapies that are appropriate at this phase are supportive measures to improve the quality of life without causing toxicity. The role of the palliative care specialists and their various strategies is highly beneficial to patients at this stage.

Scenario: a patient with a stage 3 carcinoma of the cervix presents 3 years after radical radiotherapy with urine passing permanently per vaginam. On investigation and examination under anesthesia she is found to have extensive recurrence of tumor both in the para-aortic region and on the pelvic sidewall. She also has a large unrepairable vesicovaginal fistula and deteriorating renal function.

The patient is informed that she has recurrent cancer and there are no curative treatments available. She says she had guessed that anyway and is clearly very upset. She is then asked the vital question for *Cusp C*: what in addition to the fact that she is dying is bothering her most? She replies that she accepts death as inevitable but this does not make her most upset, what makes her most upset is her permanent incontinence which is preventing her from going out and seeing family and friends. She is referred to the interventional radiologist and has bilateral nephrostomy tubes inserted, which render her dry. The patient goes home and returns 4 weeks later, in a terminal condition.

She has now entered *Cusp D*. She reports having had a great 4 weeks, which included daily visits to the pub and meeting up with all her friends. She dies 24 h later.

26.1.4.   Cusp D: Terminal Phase

The terminal phase of life lasts from hours to days and all interventions are only designed to "ease the passing." Patients in general are very conscious of this; however, the relatives may sometimes need help accepting it. Care is focused on emotional support rather than medical intervention, and frequently most of the patient's medication can be stopped apart from analgesia and sedatives. Involvement of a palliative care specialist is most helpful. Assessment of religious and spiritual needs is essential. The patient's choice of place of death should be given full consideration. The death of a patient whose physical symptoms are well controlled and who is spiritually calm is an achievable goal to which we should all strive.

Bibliography

1. Fallowfield LJ. Giving sad and bad news. *Lancet.* 1993;341:476–478.
2. Maguire P, Faulkner A. Communication with cancer patients: handling bad news and difficult questions. *Br Med J.* 1988;297:907–909.
3. Maguire P, Faulkner A. Communication with cancer patients: 2. Handling uncertainty, collusion and denial. *Br Med J.* 1988;297:972–973.
4. Nordin A, ed. *Gynaecological Cancer. Patient Pictures.* Oxford: Health Press; 1999.
5. Slevin ML. Talking about cancer. How much is too much? *Br J Hosp Med.* 1987;July:56–59.
6. Smith JR, Del Priore G. *Women's Cancer: Pathways to Healing.* London: Springer; 2006 (in press).
7. Smith JR, Del Priore G, Curtin JP, Monaghan JM. *An Atlas of Gynecologic Oncology, Investigation and Surgery.* London: Taylor and Francis; 2006.

Some of this text was previously reproduced in Smith JR, Del Priore G, Curtin JP, Monaghan JM. *An Atlas of Gynecologic Oncology, Investigation and Surgery.* London: Taylor and Francis; 2006.

27
Psychosocial Aspects of the Menopause

Michael Dooley and Bronwyn B. Bell

'I am now 50 years old and feel not quite so well as before. I love dreaming and brooding, however, if I have come to a certain point I begin to become sad, because my reflections are black and, if the reality shows only the gloomy side, my soul must lose the fight.'

This is what George Sand, lover of Frederic Chopin and of the poet Alfred de Musset, writes in her history of *My Life*. Sadly Virginia Woolf, at the age of 59, ended her life in one of her deep depressions. She had panic attacks and felt a great emptiness in her life—it is hoped that this chapter will not portray such gloom.

The aim of this chapter is to give a general background about the menopause, to address its cultural issues, and then to cover two particular areas in more detail. These are sexual problems and depression and mood changes. It is hoped that the reader will realize that a true integrated approach to the management of the menopause is required and just resorting to the prescription pad and providing a course of hormone replacement therapy (HRT) is not the answer. Spending time with the patient, a listening ear, and realizing that this is a multifactorial problem is essential. Notman (1) argues that psychological distress experienced during the menopause may be more closely linked to psychosocial changes than to biological changes. This has been supported by other workers and Cooke (2) demonstrated that the gynecological phenomenon of the menopause and climacteric are elusively tied to psychosocial phenomenon. Consideration of the physical and psychosocial features of these experiences will enhance our understanding of them.

27.1. What is the Menopause?

Menopause comes from the Greek "menos" meaning "monthly" and "pausis" meaning "ending." The menopause is defined as "the permanent cessation of menstruation resulting from loss of ovarian follicular activity." A natural menopause is recognized to have occurred after 12 consecutive months of amenorrhea, for which there is no other obvious pathological or physiological cause. The menopause is the final menstrual period and is known in certainty only in retrospect a year or more after the event. The climacteric is the phase in aging of women marking the transition from the reproductive to the nonreproductive state.

Early references to the menopause do exist. Aristotle referred to the age of the menopause as being 40 years. Medical interest in the condition increased considerably in the mid-nineteenth century and in the 1930s people started referring to it as a deficiency disease. Consequently various replenishing therapies emerged, including testicular juices and crushed animal ovaries. In 1938 synthetic estrogen was developed, and in the 1970s the menopause was recognized by the medical profession with the establishment of the International Menopause Society (3).

The median age at which the menopause occurs is 52 years. It has been shown that the age of the menopause can be determined in utero. Growth restriction in late gestation, low weight gain in infancy, and starvation in early childhood may be associated with an earlier menopause. The menopause also occurs early in women with Down's syndrome and in smokers. Japanese race and ethnicity may be associated with a later age of natural menopause. With female life expectancy being approximately 82 years, and it is increasing with an estimated age of 85 years by 2031, British women can expect more than 30 years of postmenopausal life.

The human menopause has been considered to be an evolutionary adaptation and Shaw (4) has indicated that there is a benefit not particularly to a menopause, but to a rapidly declining reproductive capacity to enable care of women's own second generation. Also the menopause follows from the extreme dependence of human babies, coupled with the difficulty in giving birth due to the large neonatal brain size and the growing risk of childbearing at older ages. There may be little advantage for an older mother in running the increased risk of a further pregnancy when existing offspring depend critically on her survival. An alternative theory is that with kin groups the menopause enhances fitness by producing postreproductive grandmothers who can assist their older daughters.

27.1.1.   Biochemical Changes

The menopause is caused by ovarian failure. The ovary has a definitive endowment of germ cells with a maximum number of 7 million ovarian follicles at 20 weeks of fetal life. From mid-gestation onwards there is a logarithmic reduction in germ cells until the oocyte store becomes depleted, on average at the age of 51 years. A resulting fall in production of estradiol and inhibin occurs and gonadotrophin levels increase. The ovary gradually becomes less responsive to gonadotrophins several years before the last menstruation. These changes in circulating hormone levels frequently occur in the face of ovulatory menstrual cycles. Complete failure of follicular development eventually occurs and estradiol production is no longer sufficient to stimulate the endometrium leading to amenorrhea, and FSH and LH levels become persistently elevated. FSH levels >30 iu/l are generally considered to be in the postmenopausal range.

27.1.2. Physical Changes

Common physical and psychological changes can be seen in Tables 27.1 and 27.2.

27.1.3. Cultural Differences in Menopausal Experiences

Although the body of all women works in the same way, women's experience of menopause varies dramatically. Research comparing different cultures shows that symptoms from hot flushes and insomnia to low mood and loss of

TABLE 27.1. Physical changes during the menopause

Period changes
Hot flushes/night sweats (50–75% of women)
Insomnia
Difficulties with short-term memory and concentration
Less energy/fatigue
Aches and pains
Weight changes
Bowel changes
Skin/hair changes
Decreased libido
Vaginal dryness (dyspareunia, vaginitis)
Pain with intercourse
Bladder problems (frequency, urgency, dysuria, cystitis and incontinence)
Possible long-term health problems: osteoporosis, heart disease, general health problems

TABLE 27.2. Psychological changes during the menopause

Depression and anxiety
Mood swings
Relationship shifts
Loneliness
Children moving on/empty nest syndrome
Realization of an end to fertility
Self-image changes, both physically and emotionally
'Peter Pan' worries: difficulty accepting the aging process
Sexual changes
Family problems with sick/old parents and/or friends
Work/career changes/problems
Financial problems
Facing retirement

libido vary between countries and ethnic groups. The cross-cultural experiences of the menopause are relevant because they give clear signposts about what natural approaches can help women to cope well with the menopause. Two of the biggest factors regarding experience of the menopause are that: (1) what women believe about the menopause has a direct bearing on how they experience it and (2) there is a clear link between lifestyle—including diet, physical activity, and well-being—and the frequency and severity of symptoms, both physical and psychological.

Social scientists believe that a woman's attitude towards the menopause can directly influence the sort of experience she has—troublesome and negative or liberating and positive. Low mood and depression around the menopause may well be due as much to her expectation of suffering—seeing it as a disease with physical symptoms that need treating, the end of femininity, a downhill to old age—as to fast declining estrogen and/or tough life events.

Western doctors, in tandem with the pharmaceutical industry, tend to medicalize the change of life. The menopause is considered an "estrogen deficiency disease" and the array of symptoms—physical, mental, and emotional—is put down simply to that lack. It is unsurprising that Western women see the menopause as the start of old age and degeneration. In contrast traditional cultures see the menopause as a natural life transition that often brings benefits, including worry-free sex, less work, and more respect. Typically women in such cultures are far less likely to have distressing symptoms and, if they do, will take them in their stride rather than look for medical help. Symptomatology of the menopause differs in different areas of the world. For example, hot flushes in the West, shoulder pain in Japan, and low vision in India are the hallmarks of the menopause.

Among the Hmong hill tribes of Laos, women become "clean like a man" when they have stopped menstruating and they can relax more. Mayan women in an ancient farming culture in south-eastern Yucatan, Mexico, generally said they looked forward to the menopause, comparing it to being young and free again. None reported hot flushes and they reported better sexual relations with their husbands because they were not worried about getting pregnant. In a recent American study, black women of African descent, who reached the menopause significantly earlier than white Americans, said their mothers told them how to cope with menopausal symptoms. They felt they could generally cope on their own and were unwilling to follow their doctors' advice and take HRT. In Pakistan few women see the menopause as a medical condition requiring treatment, whereas the majority consider it a natural transition in a woman's reproductive life. In Puebla, New Mexico, there is a high value placed on both external appearances and familial responsibility among menopausal women, and negative characterizations of the menopause reflect these values. In a Danish study the strongest predictors of the way in which women experienced the menopause, including sexuality, were their general health earlier in life, their social circumstances, and their expectations of menopausal changes. The menopause was seen as a symbol of aging; a minority suffered serious problems, typically originating earlier in life. A

Swedish study's results support the view of the menopause as a developmental phase associated with an increased self-awareness and a stronger personal identity. More than half the women held a positive view of the menopause, whereas the remaining women had either a negative or a neutral attitude.

Only a small percentage of Arabic women know about the menopause and HRT use, probably because of the relatively low rate of counseling and information provided and their lack of knowledge. Loss of regular bleeding is beneficial for some Muslim women and Orthodox Jewish women, as they are no longer seen as "impure" during menstruation and can enter the temple, handle and prepare food, or continue to have sexual relations throughout the month.

The menopause for most African women marks the end of reproductive potential. For the grand multiparous women deprived of modern contraceptive technologies it is also a relief from pregnancies. But to the childless women it may be the beginning of a depression. In some cultures menopausal women are finally awarded equal status with men. Since menstrual flow is commonly viewed as a cleansing process that keeps a woman healthy, the cessation of menses may be associated with ill health. In some cultures postmenopausal bleeding is viewed as a sign of witchcraft, leading many women who in fact have endometrial or ovarian cancers to delay seeking medical care.

As the East/West divide becomes progressively blurred, Western culture erodes traditional beliefs. In Thailand the menopause has historically been accepted as a normal life stage. However, in a recent study, Thai women in Bangkok reported hot flushes, headache, joint pain, and backache. In Beirut, Lebanon, 45% reported hot flushes, 39% sought medical help, and 15% used HRT.

There is wide variation as to how older women are treated around the world, ranging from extreme reverence and respect to abandonment and deprivation. When 70 perimenopausal Australian women were compared over 3 years with the same number of Filipinos, some interesting differences emerged. The Australian women had fewer children and tended to live alone or with a partner, whereas the Filipinos lived with an average of four others. While Filipinos were almost all practising Catholics, the Australians were much less committed. In terms of symptoms, although the physical experiences were reported as very similar, emotionally they contrasted. Almost all the Filipinos were positive in outlook and said they felt only minor, if any, psychological irritations, whereas one in four of the Australians was symptomatic. They found it difficult to come to terms with the aging process, saying they experienced depression, irritability, fear of aging, loneliness, mood swings, and unhappiness as well as loss of self-esteem, respect, and admiration.

Chinese women report far fewer difficulties during the menopause than Western women. The Japanese too have a much lower incidence of hot flushes and depression. One study suggests that 85% of Japanese women have no symptoms at all. Diet maybe a potent factor. In much of Asia, food is low in fat, low in sugar, and rich in phyto (plant) estrogen, including soya and wholegrains such as brown rice and legumes. Several studies have shown a decrease in the frequency of hot flushes in women consuming soya, either in food or supplements.

Research studies suggest that women who had fewer menopausal symptoms were leading more active lives. In primitive cultures, physical activity is a necessary part of daily survival, not an add-in as it tends to be in the West.

There are also many negative myths regarding sexuality and the menopause. These have evolved from different political, religious, cultural, and moral values and need to be discussed with the woman. Post-Victorian society and religious households have indicated that sex is for procreation only and sexual activity, apart from intercourse, is unnatural, with masturbation being a sin.

27.2.   Depression and the Menopause

'Then she realised that she must weep in deep, helpless depression'. This was written by Doris Lessing in her book 'Golden Notebook' depicting climacteric depression. The French writer Marguerite Duras in 'A Quiet Life' talks about her severe depressive mood and a body that disgusted her.

Depression and the menopause can be a difficult area for research as the definition of depression can vary. Depressed mood is a feeling of sadness familiar to everyone. Depressive disorder is a syndrome that is less common but far more serious (5). High rates of depression do occur in those women attending menopause clinics (6) and among middle-aged women attending gynecology clinics (7). However, other studies which have included interview surveys in different countries, have found that there is no excess of depressive disorder at the menopause (8,9). However, the data are not consistent with some studies suggesting that milder mood changes expressed as decreased well-being are more common after the menopause than before (10–15).

Psychologically the menopause may induce depression if the woman regrets the loss of her fertility or thinks she is losing her femininity. Research has demonstrated that such reactions are uncommon in women undergoing an artificial menopause due to a hysterectomy with or without bilateral oophorectomy (16). However, data from the Massachusetts menopause study suggests that there may be a significant increase in symptoms of depression after surgical menopause (17).

It is important to remember that depression can occur and must not be missed. The menopause is often called "the change." This is due to the fact that around this time in a woman's life several events occur including a change of job, retirement, and her parents may be ill or dying. Children may leave home, there may be a decrease in sexual activity, and there is the so-called "redundancy syndrome" or the "empty nest" syndrome. Other problems can occur including demanding workload, economic problems, and coming to terms with aging in a culture that values youth and fertility. There may also be educational or marital difficulties of young adult offspring.

This demoralization resulting from the belief that there is no longer anything useful to do can be a particular problem. That is why it is important to spend time discussing this at the consultation. Research has demonstrated that depressed mood and depressive disorder in middle-aged women are related less to the menopause than the vicissitudes of life (18,19).

Lack of estrogen may lead to depression due to the physical effects of hot flushes, night sweats, dry vagina, and poor sleep. Biochemically this may cause a reduced tryptophan concentration or effect on the monoamine brain receptors. Estrogen promotes cell growth and replication in neurons. A neurological effect can occur by blocking calcium channels in cell membrane receptors where it also alters chloride, potassium, and sodium channels (20–22). Ovarian hormones also affect brain blood flow (23). Other studies have demonstrated the effect of estrogen on the peripheral nervous system. When age-matched women with adequate ovarian function were compared with postmenopausal women there was a significant decrease in vibration sense which was restored with estrogen replacement therapy.

27.2.1. Treatment of Depression

27.2.1.1. Estrogen

Can estrogen therapy improve a depressed mood even if it does occur? Overall there is evidence that estrogen may alleviate depressed mood and induce a sense of well-being. The opposite to this, however, needs to be remembered. For some women the menopause can mean a new lease of life, bringing freedom from menstruation and childbearing. Cultural effects are important with some societies giving postmenopausal women an enhanced status as indicated above (24,25).

However, the benefits may be a domino effect on improvement of the vasomotor symptoms. Contribution of estrogen to psychological health is controversial (26). A meta-analysis on HRT and depression did demonstrate an improvement in mood with estrogen therapy, the greatest effect being on perimenopausal women rather than on postmenopausal women. The benefit was greatest in those with a natural rather than a surgical menopause. However, Yonkers et al. (27) in a quantitative review demonstrated that the benefits of estrogen were more consistent in the surgical menopause.

In a randomized controlled study (28) the conclusion was that estrogen improved depression equally in women with or without vasomotor symptoms. Morris and Rymer (29) reviewed the published literature on the effect of estrogen on psychological symptoms. There were no randomized control studies on estrogen treatment in women with clinically proven pure depression. Other studies were statistically too weak to draw any firm conclusions. There are four randomized control studies that did demonstrate a significant improvement in quality of life among women treated with estrogen compared with baseline or placebo (30–33).

27.2.1.2. Other Medical Treatments

For depression, SSRIs such as fluoxetine may be of benefit, and Venlafaxine (a serotonin and noradrenalin receptor uptake inhibitor) will also improve depression and may help hot flushes.

27.2.2. Complementary and Alternative Therapies

Counseling, stress management, and psychotherapy may be of benefit.

27.2.2.1. Exercise

The aging process is associated with decreased serotonin synthesis and an increased serotonin metabolism (34). Reduced serotonin levels have been shown to be associated with depression (35). Exercise leads to higher brain concentrations of both noradrenalin and serotonin in rats, and studies in humans have demonstrated an increase in peripheral concentrations of catecholamines and beta-endorphins (36–39) which are believed to contribute to the mood-elevating effects of exercise. Exercise should be encouraged strongly for postmenopausal women because not only may it have an effect on depression but it will also have a positive effect on the cardiovascular system, bone health, and general well-being and there is evidence that it may reduce the incidence of hot flushes.

27.2.2.2. Phytoestrogens

Phytoestrogens are plant substances that have an effect similar to those of estrogens. There has been recent interest in phytoestrogens as people from populations that consume a diet high in phytoestrogens, such as the Japanese, have a lower rate of menopausal vasomotor symptoms, cardiovascular disease, osteoporosis, breast, ovarian, and endometrial cancers. Different "over the counter" products such as Menoherbs 2 by Victoria Health (http://www.victoriahealth.com) have a mixture of 10 phytoestrogens and may be beneficial in patients who want to consider alternative and complementary therapies.

27.2.2.3. Herbal Remedies

Herbal remedies do need to be used with caution in women with a contraindication to estrogen as some herbs, for example, ginseng, have estrogenic properties. *Ginkgo biloba* may be beneficial but it needs to be used carefully with patients who are on warfarin or aspirin or other high blood pressure tablets.

Ginseng (panax) can be beneficial but it reduces the blood concentrations of alcohol and warfarin. *Hypericum perforatum* (St John's wort) can be beneficial but again one needs to be careful in patients taking warfarin or digoxin and in those on the oral contraceptive pill who have planned pregnancies.

Black cohosh (*Actaea racemosa*) can alleviate menopausal symptoms and some studies are demonstrating this to be beneficial.

27.2.2.4. Acupuncture

Acupuncture is a stimulation of special points in the body, usually by the insertion of fine needles, and originates in the Far East about 2000 years ago. Although studies have not been convincing there may be some general improvement in well-being.

27.2.2.5. Reflexology

Reflexology aims to relieve stress or treat health conditions with an application of pressure to specific points in the feet. This has been used for thousands of years and can help pain, anxiety, and premenstrual syndrome although convincing studies have yet to be done.

27.2.2.6. Yoga

Yoga may have a beneficial effect on depression and general well-being.

27.2.3. Sexual Problems

Sex and the older woman used to be a taboo subject but attitudes are changing in a positive way. This is manifested by the increasing number of books on the high street that discuss the subject (40). A woman's sex life does not end with the menopause and we need to be aware of this and address her needs. It has been demonstrated that many postmenopausal women have an increased sexual responsiveness. The exact reason is not clear but it may include reduced fear of pregnancy, no longer needing contraception, and the end of menstrual distress. The National Council on Ageing and American Association for Retired Persons concluded that 60% of men and women over the age of 50 were satisfied with their sex lives (41); 60% reported that sex was good or better than when they were young and 70% had sex at least once a week. Many older people indicated that they enjoyed greater sexual experimentation in their relationship. New relationships can also cause concern with anxiety of "adequate performance" and the risk of sexually transmitted diseases.

But many women do experience sexual dysfunction both before and after the menopause (42). The exact incidence of female sexual dysfunction, defined as distress and impairment resulting from a disturbance in sexual desire and the emotional and psychological changes of the sexual response cycle, is unknown. In a US probability sample study of sexual behavior in a cohort of almost 2000 women between the ages of 18 and 59 the prevalence of female sexual dysfunction was estimated at 43%. Low sexual desire was identified as the most common disorder for women with a prevalence of 22%. Sexual problems associated with the menopause include loss of libido, decreased sexual response, painful intercourse, decreased sexual activity, and reactive sexual dysfunction of a woman's partner (43). The psychological significance of loss of sexual function can be deeply meaningful and can contribute to postmenopausal depression and anxiety. Dyspareunia is the most common sexual complaint of older women who seek gynecological advice. Changing body shape of their partner may play a role and reduced passion in everyday life is possible. Libido is a multifactorial loss of sexual desire and sexual attractiveness to men and may cause other psychological symptoms.

27.2.4.   The Holiday Sex Syndrome

A particular interest of one of the authors (MD) is the relationship between holidays and sexual problems in the postmenopausal woman. The scenario goes: the holiday is booked, partner on holiday demands more sex, the female partner develops increased anxiety preholiday, pelvic and vaginal pathology appear, and they need to see a doctor. This leads to cancellation of the holiday because of their sexual fears.

Sexual problems increase with age and these include

- *Problems with desire and arousal*: This can lead to anguish if there is a discrepancy between partners. Often it is also a physical problem such as poor vaginal lubrication.
- *Problems with orgasm*: Reduction in the intensity of orgasm is common with the menopause and about 10% do not experience any orgasm at all.
- *Painful sex*: This can occur with poor lubrication or infection. Vulvodynia can occur with extreme pain on touch. Drug treatment or psychotherapy can help.
- *Vaginismus*: Vaginismus due to painful involuntary spasm of the pubococcygeus muscles renders penetration painful or impossible. It responds well to physical and psychological intervention.

Etiologies may include psychological problems such as depression or anxiety disorders, conflict within the relationship, issues relating to prior physical or sexual abuse, stress, fatigue, lack of privacy, medical illness, medications, substance abuse, a partner's sexual dysfunction or physical problems that make sexual activity uncomfortable, for example, atrophic vaginitis.

27.2.5.   Androgens and Effects on Sex

Androgen levels do not decline with the menopause specifically, but they do decrease with ageing. Older women have a lower level compared with younger women (44) with some indicating it can be less than 50% of the level produced in the early twenties (45).

No population study has clearly demonstrated a relationship between androgen levels and satisfactory sexual function (46). Comparing women who have had a hysterectomy, with or without a bilateral oophorectomy, provides useful data although ovarian function may be compromised even with conservation of the ovaries. Women who have had a bilateral salpingo-oophorectomy have an approximately 50% reduction in testosterone concentrations (47). In another study, women who have had a bilateral salpingo-oophorectomy reported significantly decreased libido and sexual satisfaction despite estrogen treatment, when compared with those whose ovaries were conserved (48). A number of studies have evaluated the effects of androgens and the treatment of psychological symptoms associated with the menopause (49).

27.2.5.1. Androgen Treatment

Controlled studies are limited but several studies have demonstrated a role of testosterone and dehydroepiandrosterone (DHEA) in disorders of sexual desire, arousal, and response (50–55). In one single-blind study testosterone implants were given for 2 years in postmenopausal women with estradiol implants. The testosterone group reported significantly greater scores for sexual activity, satisfaction, pleasure, and orgasm compared with women receiving estradiol alone (56). At present, only testosterone implants are licensed for use although the careful use of testosterone gel with blood monitoring and appropriate counseling with regard to licensing may be acceptable. Oral DHEA has been shown to increase circulating androgen levels to the physiological range in women with adrenal dysfunction (57). It is not licensed in the UK but can be obtained via the Internet or over the counter. Regulation is poor and packages have been shown to contain no DHEA at all to 50% of the labeled claim (58). Phase 3 trials of transdermal patches of testosterone for menopausal women with hypoactive sexual desire are currently under way.

27.2.6.   Drugs that Can Help Sexual Satisfaction

Tibolone is a steroid agent that produces specific androgenic, estrogenic, and progesterogenic effects. It can be beneficial and a number of studies have found that it can enhance sexual function as well as significantly increase vaginal blood flow in response to erotic fantasy.

Other treatments include the use of vaginal estrogens to help vaginal lubrication. Sildenafil is first selective inhibitor of phosphodiesterase 5 and is mainly used in erectile dysfunction. Evidence is conflicting but it may help women with female sexual disorders. Bupropion is an antidepressant and may have a role in sexual dysfunction.

27.2.7.   Psychosexual Therapy

Sex therapists can assess and treat the whole gamut of sexual dysfunctions regardless of whether the main cause is physical, psychological, or relational. There is evidence base for its success.

27.2.7.1. Self-Help

Self-help includes education. A number of excellent books are available, and videos and DVDs addressing both personal sexual growth and couple issues.

27.2.7.2. Enhancing Arousal

A vast range of products are available that can help arousal. These include vibrators, clitoral stimulators, lubricants, games, and fantasy lingerie.

27.3. Conclusion

The treatment of the menopause requires an integrated approach and a "magic pill" of HRT is definitely not a "fix all." A careful history must be taken in order to tease out the particular problems and the use of counselors should be encouraged.

An examination is essential to ensure there are no other physical problems. Treatment requires a patient-focused integrated approach.

References

1. Notman M. Midlife concerns of women. Implications of the menopause. *Am J Psychiatry*. 1979;136:1270–1274.
2. Cooke DJ. A psychosocial study of the climacteric. In: Broome A, Wallace J, eds. *Psychology and Gynaecological Problems*. London : Tavistock Publications; 1984:243–265.
3. Rees M, Purdie DW, eds. *The Management of the Menopause. The Handbook.* 4th ed. British Menopause Society Publication. The Royal Society of Medicine Press Ltd; 2006.
4. Shaw LMA. Menopause as an evolutionary adaptation. *Hum Reprod.* 2006;21(Suppl. 1):i33.
5. Gath D, Iles S. Depression and the menopause. *Br Med J*. 1990;300:1287–1288.
6. Jones MJ, Marshall DH, Nordin BEC. Quantitation of menopausal symptomatology and response to ethinyl oestradiol and piperazine oestrone sulphate. *Curr Med Res Opin*. 1977;4(Suppl. 3):12–20.
7. Byrne P. Psychiatric morbidity and the menopause: survey of a gynaecological outpatient clinic. *Br J Psychiatry*. 1985;144:28–34.
8. Kaufert PA, Gilbert P, Tate R. The Manitoba project; a re-examination between the link between menopause and depression. *Maturitas*. 1992;14:143–155.
9. Avis NE, Brambilla D, McKinlay SM, Vas, K. A longitudinal analysis of the association between menopause and depression. Results from the Massachusetts Women's Health Study. *Ann Epidemiol.* 1944;4:214–220.
10. Hunter M. The South-east England longitudinal study of the climacteric and postmenopause. *Maturitas*. 1992;14:117–126.
11. Holte A. Influences of natural menopause on health complaints; a prospective study of health Norwegian women. *Maturitas*. 1992;14:127–141.

12. Ballinger CB. Psychiatric aspects of the menopause. *Br J Psychiatry.* 1990;156:773–787.
13. Dennerstein L, Smith AM, Morse C et al. Menopausal symptoms in Australian women. *Med J Aust.* 1993;159:232–236.
14. McKinlay SM, Brambilla DJ, Posner JG. The normal menopause transition. *Maturitas.* 1992;14:103–115.
15. Collins A, Landgren BM. Reproductive health, use of estrogen and experience of symptoms in perimenopausal women: a population-based study. *Maturitas.* 1994;20:101–111.
16. Gath D, Cooper P, Bond A, Edmonds G. Hysterectomy and psychiatric disorder II. Demographic and physical factors in relation to psychiatric outcome. *Br J Psychiatry.* 1982;140:343–350.
17. Avis NE, Brambilla D, McKinlay SM, Vass K. A longitudinal analysis of the association between menopause and depression: results from the Massachusetts Women's Health Study. *Ann Epidemiol.* 1994;4:15–21.
18. McKinlay JB, McKinlay SM, Brambilia D. The relative contributions of endocrine changes and social circumstances to depression in middle aged women. *J Health Soc Behav.* 1987;28:345–363.
19. Green JS, Cooke DJ. Life stress and symptoms of the climacterium. *Br J Psychiatry.* 1980;136:486–491.
20. McEwen BS, Colrini H, Schumacher M. Steroid effects on neuronal activity; when is the genome involved? *Ciba Found Symp.* 1990;153:3–12.
21. McEwen BS, Colrini H, Westlind-Danielsson A et al. Steroid hormones as mediators of neural plasticity. *J Steroid Biochem Mol Biol.* 1991;39:223–232.
22. Naftolin F, MacKlusky NJ, Learanth CZ et al. The cellular effects of estrogens on neuroendocrine tissues. *J Steroid Biochem.* 1988;29:215–228.
23. Sarrel PM, Lufkin EG, Oursler MJ, Keefe D. Estrogen actions on arteries, bone, and brain. *Sci Am Sci Med.* 1994;1:44–53.
24. George T. Menopause: some interpretation of the results of a study among non-western groups. *Maturitas* 1988;10:109–116.
25. Beyene Y. Cultural significance and psychological manifestation of menopause. A biocultural analysis. *Cult Med Psychiatry.* 1986;10:47–71.
26. Zweifel JE, O'Brien WH. A meta-analysis of the effect of HRT upon depressed mood. *Psychoneuroendocrinology.* 1997;22:189–212.
27. Yonkers KA, Bradshaw KD, Halbreich U. Oestrogens, progestins and mood. In: Steiner M, Yonkers K, Eriksson E, eds. *Mood Disorders in Women.* London: Martin Dunitz; 2000:207–232.
28. Westlund TL, Parry BL. Does estrogen enhance the antidepressant effects of fluoxetine? *J Affect Disord.* 2003;77:87–92.
29. Morris E, Rymer J. Menopausal symptoms. *Clin Evid.* 2003;9:2074–2086.
30. Karlberg J, Mattsson L, Wiklund I. A quality of life perspective on who benefits from estradiol replacement therapy. *Acta Obstet Gynecol Scand.* 1995;74:367–372.
31. Derman RJ, Dawood MY, Stone S. Quality of life during sequential hormone replacement therapy: a placebo-controlled study. *Int J Fertil Menopausal Stud.* 1995;40:73–78.
32. Hilditch JR, Lewis J, Ross AH et al. A comparison of the effects of oral conjugated equine estrogen and transdermal estradiol – 17 beta combined with an oral progestin on quality of life in postmenopausal women. *Maturitas.* 1996;24:177–184.

33. Wiklund I, Karlberg J, Mattsson L. Quality of life on postmenopausal women on a regimen of transdermal estradiol therapy: a double-blind placebo-controlled study. *Am J Obstet Gynecol.* 1993;168:824–830.

34. Robinson DS, Nies A, Davis JN et al. Aging, monoamines and monoamine oxidase levels. *Lancet.* 1972;i:290–291.

35. von Praag HM. Korf J. Monoamine metabolism in depression: clinical application of the probenecid test. In: Barchas J, Usdin E, eds. *Serotonin and Behaviour.* New York: Academic Press; 1973.

36. Dimsdale JE, Moss J. Plasma catecholamines in stress and exercise. *J Am Med Assoc.* 1980;243:340–342.

37. Kindermann W, Schnabel A, Schmitt WM, Biro G, Casens J, Weber F. Catecholamines, growth hormone, cortisol, insulin and sex hormones in anaerobic and aerobic exercise. *Eur J Appl Physiol.* 982;49:389–399.

38. Carr DB, Bullen BA, Skrinar GS et al. Physical conditioning facilitates the exercise-induced secretion of beta-endorphin and beta-lipotropin in women. *N Engl J Med.* 1981;305:560–563.

39. Farrell Pa, Gates WK, Maksud MG, Morgan WP. Increases in plasma β-endorphin/β-lipoprotin immunoreactivity after treadmill running in humans. *J Appl Physiol.* 1982;52:1245–1249.

40. Tomlinson JM, ed. *Sexual Health and the Menopause.* London: RSM Publishers; 2005.

41. American Association for Retired Persons. *Healthy Sexuality and Vital Aging.* Washington, DC: American Association for Retired Persons; 1999.

42. Shifren JL. The role of androgens in female sexual dysfunction. *Mayo Clin Proc.* 2004;79(Suppl.):S19–S24.

43. Sarrel PM. Psychosexual effects of menopause: role of androgens. *Am J Obstet Gynecol.* 1990;180:319–323.

44. Zumoff B, Strain GW, Miller LK, Rosner W. Twenty-four-hour mean plasma testosterone concentration declines with age in normal premenopausal women. *J Clin Endocrinol Metab.* 1995;80:1429–1430.

45. Ismail KMK, Crome I, O'Brien PMS. *Psychological Disorders in Obstetrics and Gynaecology.* Higham J, ed. London: RCOG Press; 2006.

46. Shifren JL. The role of androgens in female sexual dysfunction. *Mayo Clin Proc.* 2004;79(Suppl.):S19–S24.

47. Judd HL, Lucas WE, Yen SS. Effect of oophorectomy on circulating testosterone and androstenedione levels in patients with endometrial cancer. *Am J Obstet Gynecol.* 1974;118:793–798.

48. Nathorst-Boos J, von Schoultz B, Carlstrom K. Elective ovarian removal and estrogen replacement therapy – effects on sexual life, psychological well-being and androgen status. *J Psychosom Obstet Gynaecol.* 1993;14:283–293.

49. Sherwin BB, Gelfand MM. The role of androgen in the maintenance of sexual functioning in oophorectomized women. *Psychosom Med.* 1987;49:397–409.

50. Sherwin BB, Gelfand MM, Brender W. Androgen enhances sexual motivation in females: a prospective, crossover study of sex steroid administration in the surgical menopause. *Psychosom Med.* 1985;47:339–351.

51. Davis SR, McCloud P, Strauss BJ, Burger H. Testosterone enhances estradiol's effects on postmenopausal bone density and sexuality. *Maturitas.* 1995;21:227–236.

52. Lobo RA, Rosen RC, Yang HM, Block B, Van Der Hoop RG. Comparative effects of oral esterified estrogens with and without methyltestosterone on endocrine profile

and dimensions of sexual function in postmenopausal women with hypoactive sexual desire. *Fertil Steril.* 2003;79:1341–1352.

53. Arlt W, Justl HG, Callies F et al. Oral dehydroepiandrosterone for adrenal androgen replacement: pharmacokinetics and peripheral conversion to androgens andestrogens in young healthy females after dexamethasone suppression. *J Clin Endocrinol Metab.* 1998;83:1928–1934.

54. Lovas K, Gebre-Medhin G, Trovik TS et al. Replacement of dehydroepiandrosterone in adrenal failure: no benefit for subjective health status and sexuality in a 9-month, randomized, parallel group clinical trial. *J Clin Endocrinol Metab.* 2003;88:1112–1118.

55. Hunt PJ, Gurnell EM, Huppert FA et al. Improvement in mood and fatigue after dehydroepiandrosterone replacement in Addison's disease in a randomized double blind trial. *J Clin Endocrinol Metab.* 2000;85:4650–4656.

56. Davis SR, McCloud P, Strauss BJ, Burger H. Testosterone enhances estradiol's effects on postmenopausal bone density and sexuality. *Maturitas.* 1995;21:227–236.

57. Arlt W, Callies F, van Vlijem JC et al. Dehydroepiandrosterone replacement in women with adrenal unsufficiency. *N Engl J Med.* 1999;341:1013–1020.

58. Parasrampuria J, Schwartz K, Petesch R. Quality control of dehydroepiandrosterone dietary supplement products [letter]. *J Am Med Assoc.* 1998;280:1565.

About the Editors

Jayne Cockburn, FRCO5, has been a Consultant in Obstetrics and Gynaecology for 12 years. Whilst a senior registrar, she became one of a few obstetricians and gynaecologists to receive training in psychotherapy and has been researching and presenting since 1990. She is on the national committee of the British Society for Psychosomatic Obstetrics and Gynaecology. She has also been a principle organiser for 10 years for the Nixon Club, which is a forum for training obstetricians and gynaecologists in psychosomatic O&G. Having spent much effort over the last 10 years trying to get recognition and improvements in training for psychological problems in O&G, this book was conceived and written to be useful in the improvement of training.

Michael E. Pawson, FRCOG, now retired from the Chelsea and Westminster Hospital, London, has a long-standing interest in the subject. He is particularly active teaching and writing in his specialist area, psychological aspects of infertility and reproductive technology. He is a past president the British Society for Psychosomatic Obstetrics and Gynaecology and an organising member of the International Congress of Psychosomatic Obstetrics and Gynaecology, 2004.

Index

Printed in the United States of America.